Semiotic Foundations of Drug Therapy

Approaches to Semiotics
112

Mouton de Gruyter
Berlin · New York

Semiotic Foundations of Drug Therapy

The Placebo Problem in a New Perspective

by

Klaus Schonauer

Mouton de Gruyter
Berlin · New York 1994

Mouton de Gruyter (formerly Mouton, The Hague)
is a Division of Walter de Gruyter & Co., Berlin.

⊗ Printed on acid-free paper which falls within the guidelines of the ANSI to ensure permanence and durability.

Library of Congress Cataloging in Publication Data

Schonauer, Klaus.
Semiotic foundations of drug therapy : the placebo problem in a new perspective / by Klaus Schonauer.
p. cm. – (Approaches to semiotics ; 112)
Includes bibliographical references.
ISBN 3-11-013532-9 (cloth : acid-free paper)
1. Chemotherapy. 2. Semiotics. 3. Placebo (Medicine)
I. Title. II. Series.
RM263.S37 1994
615.5'8'01–dc20 93-36818
CIP

Die Deutsche Bibliothek – Cataloging in Publication Data

Schonauer, Klaus:
Semiotic foundations of drug therapy : the placebo problem in a new perspective / by Klaus Schonauer. – Berlin ; New York : Mouton de Gruyter, 1993
(Approaches to semiotics ; 112)
ISBN 3-11-013532-9
NE: GT

Disk conversion and printing: Arthur Collignon GmbH, Berlin
Binding: Lüderitz & Bauer, Berlin
Printed in Germany.

Preface

The practice of using drugs brings forth numerous tales of an inconspicuous nature but with highly individual settings. These tales may give the outside observer – and him alone – some insight into the dramaturgy of the therapeutic confrontation between suffering and healing. This practice is pervaded with rituals. It embodies hoards of sensorily perceptible material. To those involved in this therapeutic confrontation, both of these appear relatively insignificant.

The drug, which has a specific color, an often cryptic name, an aroma of its own and – last but not least – its price, seeks and finds its own place in everyday life, for instance "three times a day after meals" or in accordance with a crisis-prone bodymind that demands "its drops" only as required. And in between times too, the drug is deposited in a special place for safekeeping – in a shoebox, in the top drawer of a writing-desk or in an ivory-inlaid miniature box specially reserved for it and characteristic of the pragmatics of its application but giving food for thought only to an outside observer.

The more a person is concerned with the application of drugs – whether through direct involvement or for professional reasons – the more likely he is to consider the ritual and the esthetic aspect of this application insignificant. And the less consciously he directs his attention to these two aspects, the more likely he is to benefit from them.

"The clinical gaze has the paradoxical ability to hear a language as soon as it perceives a spectacle." (Foucault 1976b: 108). With his *Imaginary invalid*, Molière ([1959]) has staged this clinical as-if esotericism as a real-life drama. His criticism was bound to hit the bull's eye, for medical science in his times had very little else to offer in the way of therapy. But even today, in the age of pharmacologically assured drug therapy, drugs still have colors, shapes, names and smells whose therapeutic – or in some cases noxious – effect has long been empirically proven within the framework of placebo research but – as is to be shown – has undergone virtually no systematic investigation.

In this context, the sensorily perceptible treasures of the drug remain insignificant despite being recognised as no longer unimportant. The question of their meaning in the context of general semiotic theory – one well-tried in this very question – is what this book will endeavour to answer.

The unflagging interest shown in medicosemiotic and patholinguistic problems by a large number of fellow-students and lecturers at the Institute for

General Linguistics of Münster University and in particular the constant encouragement given by my linguistics professor, Edeltraud Bülow, provided me with vital stimuli for the concept of the topic dealt with in this book. Work on putting this concept into practice began in 1985 when I was working in the Department of Psychosomatic Medicine at Cologne University. My sincere thanks are due to my colleagues there, to the medical students and to the staff of the Department of Internal Medicine for their support in filling in my questionnaire, a source of valuable material. Credit for a number of bibliographic references is due to Thomas Bliesener and Elke Trzinski. Norbert Rath followed the work on the manuscript with unbroken personal commitment and supported it with valuable impulses during a problematic phase. Detlev Fock took meticulous care in reproducing the photographs to be used. My thanks are also due to the archivists at Bayer Leverkusen, who assisted me in searching out and processing their extensive material on the history of Aspirin and placed valuable files at my disposal.

The original German version of this book was submitted as a Ph.D. thesis to the Philosophical Faculty of Münster University in spring 1989. My thanks are now due to the Dean for having granted me permission to have it published in a translated version. Anna Carrdus translated Chapter 3 and gave me helpful bibliographical and editorial assistance. Susan Griesbach translated the other chapters and provided valuable incentives in our discussions on terminological problems.

The publication project as such would never have been possible without the support and encouragement of Marie-Louise Liebe-Harkort from Mouton de Gruyter and the editor of the series "Approaches to Semiotics", Professor Thomas A. Sebeok, who was the first to recognize the semiotic potential of the placebo problem.

Contents

Graphic conventions

Certain special graphic signs based on a convention proposed by Eco (1976) have been used throughout this book to lend emphasis to the following differentiations:

Single slashes (/) indicate something intended as an expression or a sign-vehicle. The term enclosed by them is the signifier of a sign or string of signs whose significate need not be known at the time when those special signs are used.

Double slashes (//), on the other hand, designate the object of this sign or string of signs as that signified with the enclosed term. This enables the substance //common salt// to be distinguished from the expressions /common salt/ or /kitchen salt/ and both of them to be given a more clear-cut relationship to the terms /sodium chloride/ and /NaCl/, all of them still referring to the same substance.

Enclosing a sign or string of signs in double guillemets («») is designed to give special emphasis to the fact that this term stands for the significate or content of the sign or string of signs. In everyday language, the use of these special signs would almost invariably be tautological, for any speaker using a lexeme is referring in any case at the moment of that use to its significate. For this reason, these special signs are used only in connection with terms whose position in the lexical system is to be worked out in the course of this study, so that their actual meaning must initially be almost obscure.

Square brackets ([]) usually designate either insertions or comments by the author within quotations, or those quotations that were translated specifically for this book in the absence of any known English edition.

The use of these special signs does not imply that the author is in some way dissatisfied with the opportunities for expression provided by the English language and its hoard of signs. They merely represent additional aids to orientation in those uncertain cases that inevitably occur in the course of a metalinguistic or metasemiotic discussion. The reader can, on the other hand, follow the trend of this discussion even if he totally ignores these special signs.

Registered trade names (trademarks) are not identified in this book by specific symbols or special signs. The absence of such indications does not imply that they are unprotected trademarks.

In those cases where the English editions of works which were originally published in other languages are not only translations but also revised editions, the original and translated versions of those works were used in some instances alongside each other. This applies first and foremost to Umberto Eco's writings (cf. de Lauretis 1981: 91–92).

0. Introduction: Knots in a red thread

> We understand that the English navy has a certain arrangement by which every rope in the royal fleet, from the stoutest to the finest, is spun in such fashion that a red thread runs through it which cannot be extracted without unravelling the whole rope, so that even the smallest piece of this rope can be recognised as belonging to the Crown. Similarly, there runs through Ottilie's journal a thread of affection and inclination that binds everything together and characterizes the whole. It is this thread which turns into the peculiar property of the writer these observations, thoughts, aphorisms copied down, and whatever else is there, and makes them significant for her. Every single passage we have selected bears indisputable testimony to the truth of this.
>
> Johann Wolfgang von Goethe[1]

When a person falls ill, his everyday life is deprived of a fragment of order. The more menacing his experience of this loss of order, the more deeply he is concerned about it. When the illness is of a trivial nature, these concerns will resolve themselves in the comfort gained from the illness, the prospect of being able to rest and be looked after for a while. From a fractured leg onwards, worries about his job, the fear of being unable to complete an important assignment on schedule, of having to give up an enjoyable hobby pursued with ambition, may well cast considerably longer shadows. Chronic progressive or even life-threatening disorders may throw the plans made for a whole lifetime to the winds, sometimes after a long fight, sometimes with a dynamic force that renders the observer speechless.

Apart from the suffering experienced in a direct sensory way, such as pain or nausea, this structural loss resulting from the intervention of the illness in the ill person's everyday life is one of the most important motives for him to consult a doctor. From that moment onwards, he is a patient.

The doctor will examine him and will interpret the symptoms of the disorder as he has learned to. First and foremost, however, he will have to answer as precisely as possible two questions of special concern to the patient: What is the cause of the illness, and how can it be cured as quickly as possible? On the other hand, the negotiating of these questions is determined from the patient's viewpoint essentially by the painful experience of structural loss. If his sole concern were to be cured of his symptoms, then the question of etiology would be of little interest to him. He and his now confused everyday life, however, require as complete and plausible an explanation as possible, for they are now hoping not only for relief from complaints but for a restoration of that order which they now see jeopardised.

From the semiotic standpoint, work on these two cardinal questions flows into the attempt to attain a form of structural gain tantamount in the ideal case to the metaphor of "legibility". Diagnostic interpretation of the symptoms of the disorder is familiar to the doctor – and in a rudimentary form to the patient too – as a sign-processing activity whose methods he does not as a rule consider consciously but which he has nonetheless learnt with care. He is experienced in reading signs of disorders. The patient is aware of this too, for that is his very reason for consulting him. But working out and implementing the therapeutic offer with which the doctor endeavours to answer the second cardinal question will bring into play a whole range of signs, in whose production and reception the doctor and patient are involved to vastly differing degrees from the methodological aspect but to similarly weighted degrees as far as implementation of the process is concerned. Observing these markedly heterogenic – verbal and nonverbal – signs a little more closely and as systematically as possible is the aim of this study.

According to a distinction proposed by Uexküll (1984a: 4), "Eine Semiotik in der Medizin sollte Zeichen untersuchen, welche dem Arzt Hinweise auf die Interaktionen geben, die sich zwischen dem Organismus eines Kranken und dessen Erleben, zwischen dem Organismus und seinen Organen bis hinunter zu den Zellen abspielen" ['semiotics in medicine' should 'examine signs that give the physician indications of the interactions taking place between the organism of a patient and what he is experiencing, between the organism and his organs right down to the cells'] whereas "Semiotik der Medizin ... die Medizin selbst als Zeichensystem, z. B. als Menge unterschiedlicher Fachsprachen, als System von Zeichen, welche die Kommunikation von Ärzten, Laien usw. ermöglichen [zum Gegenstand hätte]" ['semiotics of medicine ... would be concerned with medicine itself as a semiotic system, e.g. as a set of different professional languages, as a system of signs permitting communication between physicians and laymen etc.']

Within the framework of this distinction, this book is assigned relatively clearly to the latter sphere. Sociomedical and psychomedical research carried out during recent decades has shown with some precision that this interaction between physicians and laymen complies with a number of highly context-dependent laws that occasionally promote but far more often impede, delay or even prevent fulfilment of its aim of "communication". The medical practice and the hospital are places at which professional routines and private, highly subjective needs collide in a way implying different levels of competence and power rarely found elsewhere among adults in the civilian sector of democratic societies. The inpatient in particular is exposed during his period of hospitalisation to a "hohes ungeregeltes Sanktionspotential" ['high, uncontrolled sanction potential'] (Siegrist 1976: 33), occasionally even to "Institutionalisierte Zumutungen" ['unreasonable institutionalised demands'] (Raspe 1976), which leave their mark quite distinctly on his communication with the specialists consulted by him. Special credit is due to the relatively new field of research into ward rounds (Coulthard – Ashby 1975; Haberland – Mey 1981; Bliesener – Siegrist 1981; Köhle – Raspe 1982; Bliesener 1982; Hoffmann-Richter 1985) for having recorded and followed up these marks in the concrete example of the ward-round conversation as a specific type of text and communication, so that the extensive empirical material published by these authors can be used to work out concrete proposals for improving the unwelcome situation (Bliesener – Köhle 1986). This empirical material is also of significance in the attempt being made in this book to examine verbal and nonverbal signs in the context of drugs. In a collection of 72 ward-round conversations transcribed in full, Pummerer (1985: 99) found that 8.8% of their text, quantitatively speaking, was concentrated on the subject of drugs.

The fact that many ward rounds lapse repeatedly into a conversation *about* the patient instead of one *with* him is a regular finding in ward-round research based on discourse analysis. This manifestation occurs with notable persistence even when all those involved in the conversation undertake explicitly to avoid such a development and when, for example, exceptionally emancipated patients meet with exceptionally sensitive and self-critical doctors and other medical staff. The frequently contrasting ways in which their knowledge is constituted apparently activate a kind of /automatic divergence mechanism/ for which Mechthilde Lichnowsky (1925: 24) has found in her essay *Der Kampf mit dem Fachmann* [The battle with the specialist] an arithmetical formula: "Fachmänner sind meistens halb, Laien doppelt." ['Specialists are mostly half that, laymen twice that.']

One important cause of this high degree of "asymmetry" (Siegrist 1982) in the doctor-patient relationship may be that some patients are able to profit in a special way from this relationship at that very moment when they are being not only advised but also patronised; for this patronising manner – embarrassing and degrading as it might seem to the outsider – has at least one asset: it provides structure.

In her linguistic analysis subtitled *Untersuchung zur Verständigung von Arzt und Patient in der Visite* (study of communication between doctor and patient in the ward round), Hoffmann-Richter (1985: 38-39) proposes a metaphorical comparison focusing the patient's communicative handicap in the ward-round situation on an analytical – and, metaphorically seen, a spatiotemporal – point: If, despite the proportions contributed to the conversation being formally balanced, the patient does not manage to realise his thematic concern during the ward round, his "red[1] thread" tangles, leaving a "knot" whose unravelling would have been an indispensable prerequisite for the abortive objective of the conversation: "communication". Within the framework of the spatiotemporal confusion of //tangles// – to keep to this metaphor for the time being – //knots// do, however, represent marked states of relative order. They act as a mnemonic device, like the thread given by Ariadne to Theseus, and they offer minor yet tangible experiences of success in the attempt to unravel the //tangle// as a superordinate organisational form of chaos.

In the practical aspect of the doctor-patient relationship, drugs act as "structurators" (Koch 1971: 15) which activate substantial divergences on the one hand but are of central importance to the "shared topic area" (Brown – Yule 1983: 89) of the interacting partners. One important source of both divergent and shared topic areas here is the opportunity open to both interacting partners to understand something highly individual under the drug concerned, to attribute to it a certain degree of idiosyncratic meaning. The two partners avail themselves of this opportunity in very different ways, connected essentially with their roles as layman or specialist. Both have great expectations of each other's method, and both have as a rule the tendency, once a drug has been introduced, to attribute to that drug all changes taking place in the patient's state of health. The possibility of such changes occurring spontaneously or for unknown reasons is suspended for the time being by the compulsive demand for a concrete, controllable and influential parameter to whose introduction both of them have agreed. Charles Sanders Peirce has sharply criticised this tendency from the standpoint of the semiotic logician:

> Nothing, therefore, more pitiably manifests the looseness with which people in general reason than the readiness of nine persons out of ten to pronounce upon the merits of a medicine upon the most limited, the most inexact, and the most prejudiced experience which it is possible to call experience at all. Any old woman who has seen any amelioration of symptoms follow after the administration of a medicine in a dozen cases at all resembling one another, will not hesitate to pronounce it an infallible cure for any case resembling at all any one of the dozen. This is shocking. (Peirce, unpublished Manuscript [Harvard Corpus No.Ms.696] quoted from Sebeok – Umiker-Sebeok 1980: 53).

When a doctor "prescribes" "his" patient a drug, this process constitutes substantially more and is many times more complex than a mere impersonal recommendation to incorporate a specific, pharmacologically defined substance. It is this process that fixes the starting point and the determining factors in the development of an interpersonal encounter from which at least one of the interacting partners, but frequently all of them, will emerge distinctly changed. Balint (1964) rated the significance of the drug so highly in his study – one that was theoretically to set the trend for research into the doctor-patient relationship – that he proposed designating the physician himself as a "drug" – in other words putting a "pharmacomorphic" interpretation on this relationship. The sphere in which this process is executed as a form of "public intercommunication" (cf. Goffman 1971) is so extensively ritualised in numerous details up to that point that the "symbolic mode" referred to by Eco (1985a: 230–238) becomes effective and influential in it as a sign-constituting factor.

This mechanism can be illustrated in somewhat more concrete terms by a superficially trivial phenomenon – one that is, however, still widespread and therefore of importance to the social reality of pharmaceutics: the "three times a day" prescription.

Pharmacokinetically speaking, it seems unreasonable – with few exceptions – to administer any pharmacological substance to a diseased organism three times during the first half of a 24-hour day but not once during the second half of that period. This may result in unnecessarily high, even toxic, cumulative doses taking effect during the daytime, whilst the serum level needed for a therapeutic effect may not be maintained during the night. Yet figures published by Haas (1981: 44) for the reference year 1979 show that 57% of all oral preparations prescribed bore the dosage instruction "three times a day". There is no rational explanation for this phenomenon, one that must seem downright contradictory to an outsider. In the perspective of the semiotic interpretative framework outlined at the beginning of this chapter, however, it appears to be more than comprehensible and suggests a link (although the doctors and patients performing the ritual interaction are certainly not aware of this at the moment of this link being established) with a form of numerical symbolism handed down within a cultural framework (cf. Haas 1981: 45–46). The contradiction might furthermore be resolved within this interpretative framework with the additional statement that the patient's demand for "structural gain" is activated only in his daytime state of wakeful consciousness, being quite literally dormant during the night. For "structural gain" obviously permits "three times a day" to be prescribed with disarming simplicity.

Another, equally widespread, example can be used to illustrate that such interpretations – even when empirically or experimentally verifiable – involve some degree of uncertainty and that the attempt made by them to give a "plausible" explanation to what are, on the face of it, rationally inexplicable findings should not result in an interpretative monopoly: When children hurt themselves, whether by contact with heat or by mechanical traumatisation, many parents resort to a therapeutic instant-measure with which they often succeed remarkably well in intercepting the initial phase of excessive pain: they blow on the traumatised spot or "kiss it better". Justice is by no means done to this "Hush-a-bye, baby" method, however, by endeavouring to explain it completely and plausibly with a link to magic-ritualistic healing practices. Recent fundamental research into the physiology of pain (Zimmermann 1982) has revealed that high-frequency stimuli at the dolorific site may lower the disposition of the body to transmit afferent pain impulses to the central nervous system. The vibration induced on the skin surface and in particular in the hairs anchored in it by the parents' blowing or kissing is capable of generating just such high-frequency stimuli. This mechanism can be put to therapeutic use with so-called "transcutaneous nerve stimulation" in chronically painful disorders by applying electric impulses designed to "oust" the natural pain impulses, metaphorically speaking, from their afferent nerve tracts. This method is based heuristically on a principle that may seem familiar to the semiotically orientated observer: *aliquid stat pro aliquo*. But for the pragmatics of the "Hush-a-bye, baby" method too, it is still of importance in a non-material, meta-physical sense that the blowing or kissing is directed at that very spot at which the source of the pain can be localised visibly by the child and that this blowing or kissing is done not by just anyone but by a caring key person capable of combining a promise of affection and comfort symbolically with this act. This gives rise at the scene of crime, as it were, of a "représentation ontologique du mal" ['ontological representation of sick and evil'] (Canguilhem 1972: 12) to a complementary /représentation ontologique du bien/ that develops a genuine effectiveness even without high-frequency stimulation.

An attempt is now to be made in the following four chapters to work out as clearly and precisely as possible the semiotically significant function of such complementarity as a "modelling of similarity". Regarding this attempt as a prolegomenon to a new subdiscipline of applied semiotics – referred to perhaps as "pharmacosemiotics" – would be a misunderstanding. The aim is rather to observe from an angle that is theoretically unusual, at least in this context, the cultural interdependency of suffering and healing, their place in the manifold "organized artful practices of everyday life" (Garfinkel

1972: 309) as a piece of real-life world that seems to us familiar beyond recognition.

Chapter 1 looks, while keeping as accurately as possible to detail, into those of the many semiotically relevant aspects of "meaning" that prove promising and methodologically accessible for more profound theoretical analysis, based on the paradigm of a ubiquitous drug.

Chapter 2 focuses on the pragmatic aspect of the production and reception of signs in the doctor-patient relationship, in so far as they are connected with the application of drugs. The question of the influence of sensorily perceptible qualities of pharmaceutics (such as their colour, shape, taste, smell and – last but not least – their name) on their effect is identified in this process as an empirical ganglion of this aspect. The methodologically conspicuous finding that the quantitatively substantial significance of such influences in the context of "placebo research" was recognised at a relatively early stage but has yet to be more than superficially researched from the qualitative-systematic standpoint is discussed in some detail. A hypothetical three-factor model is finally condensed from the existing empirical material as an incentive towards bridging this gap in research.

The heuristic aspect of the semiocity of drugs is the focal point of Chapter 3, in which the "modelling of similarity" is worked out as an historically contingent and theory-forming factor in the history of occidental pharmaceutics and chemistry. In the preliminary historical consideration, it is practicable to put the closest possible terminological confines on the complex term /similarity/.

In Chapter 4, two of those aspects of the "meaning" of drugs that were developed and probed with a selected example in Chapter 1 are observed on a more general level, with special attention being paid to empirical data. In this connection an empirical study of my own is first presented, one that attempts to deal with the problem of the "meaning" of drug names, using an empirical instrument developed by Osgood, Suci and Tannenbaum (1957) as the "semantic differential". The second part of that chapter deals with possible influences of the sensorily perceptible qualities of drugs on the empirically extant prescribing behaviour of physicians.

Whilst special attention is paid at various phases of this book to the dual-structured linguistic sign – for instance by examining different specialist language systems, the onomastics of drug names, lexemes in the semantic field /pain/, and the etymology and history of the words /placebo/ and /signature/ – a theoretical monopolistic position in the object range of general semiotic theory is admittedly not assigned to it.

Two object areas that are fundamentally rewarding for the set thematic framework are given only very superficial treatment in this book, considering the wealth of empirical material available on them: on the one hand, the hoard of ritual healing practices compiled in the framework of ethnomedical research, in which the "symbolic mode" develops a basically far more spectacular efficacy, and on the other the two major subject areas "endosemiotics" and "biosemiotics". One important reason for these two omissions is that I do not feel adequately competent in the basic disciplines of "ethnology", "information theory" and "systems theory". As far as the second omission is concerned, the fact that I as a linguist grew up with the convention that at least the receiver – if not even the sender – of signs must by definition be a fully-fledged representative of the "human" species certainly plays an important role. This convention has the advantage of keeping the vast universe of signs within manageable proportions. Axiomatic validity, however, would have to be bought with an anthropocentric scotoma that would amount to the "Annahme einer geistlosen Natur und eines übernatürlichen Geistes" ['assumption of a mindless Nature and a supernatural mind'] being confronted disjunctively with an "Einheit von Natur und Geist" ['unity of Nature and mind'] (Uexküll 1986) – an aspect that I have declared not to be my aim.

The minimum condition of this convention is also an essential component of Eco's sign definition,[2] which deduces from it the practical-methodological restriction that the phenomena of neurophysiology, for example, are not the semiotician's business, but that the neurophysiological information theory derived from observing these phenomena is for its part indeed so (Eco 1975: 35).

In concrete terms, the implication of this for the example already given of "transcutaneous nerve stimulation" would be: The fact that this therapeutic method follows, from the heuristic standpoint, a semiotically describable principle in that it partially ousts – *aliquid pro aliquo* – natural pain signals in the afferent nerve tracts with deceptively similar, artificial electrical impulses does not make it semiotic therapy in the narrower sense.

Yet even this semioticity, reduced by convention to the heuristic aspect, is of immense practical significance to the fact that this therapeutic method exists today, for it makes the method culturally acceptable. One of the reasons for its being used by physicians and patients is that it does not act in accordance with an impenetrable "black box" mechanism but that it models //similarity// quite obviously, because it gives the fascinating notion that the exchange implicit in the Greek root of the word "meta-bolism" applies not only to "matter but" to "information" too. This connection was vividly illustrated by William of Baskerville:

> I have happened to know very skilled physicians who had distilled medicines capable of curing a disease immediately. But when they gave their unguent or

their infusion to the simple, they accompanied it with holy words and chanted phrases that sounded like prayers: not because these prayers had the power to heal, but because, believing that the cure came from the prayers, the simple would swallow the infusion or cover themselves with the unguent, and so they would be cured, while paying little attention to the effective power of the medicine. Also, the spirit, aroused by faith in the pious formula, would be better prepared for the corporal action of the medication. (Eco 1983: 88)

1. Encyclopedic outline of a cultural unit: «Aspirin»

> Ein Mann namens Rotnagel erfand einen neuen Klebstoff, der sehr vertrauenswürdig aussah und nach Oleander duftete, viele Frauen bedienten sich seiner, um angenehm zu riechen. Gegen diese Unsitte kämpfte Rotnagel heftig an – er wünschte, daß seine Erfindung sinngemäß verwendet werde. Gerade da aber bot Schwierigkeiten, denn der neue Klebstoff klebte nichts, jedenfalls nichts Bekanntes. … Darum gab Rotnagel drei Jahre seines Lebens daran, einen Werkstoff zu entdecken, der sich von diesem Klebstoff kleben ließ, allerdings nur von diesem. Nach langem Überlegen nannte Rotnagel den neuen Werkstoff Nihilit.[3]
>
> Kurt Kusenberg

What is the meaning of /aspirin/? Some of the many possible answers to this question are sketched fragmentarily, and others dealt with in more detail, in this chapter. Some of these answers are in contradiction, whilst others complement one another. All of them together are designed to project as precise and realistic a picture as possible of what the sign /aspirin/ in the shape of its significate – as yet to be determined – means. The use of this sign is shown to be imbedded in some markedly differing contexts. The various denotative and connotative references to be reconstructed on consideration of these contexts flow, with differently weighted proportions, into one common concluding reach, contributing in this (inductive-synthetic) way to providing an answer to the initially posed question of the meaning of /aspirin/.

This procedure could also be characterised with a term borrowed by Eco (1976: 71) from geometry as a circumscription of "cultural units in an asymptotic fashion". Its opportunities and risks have been obvious since the discussion stimulated by Feyerabend (1978): concreteness and proximity to the phenomenon on the one hand, heterogenity and a comparison drawn between incommensurables on the other. Those semiotic aspects of the use of pharmaceutical products proving in the course of this introductory consideration to be of outstanding importance and abstractable from the concrete example are then examined in more detail and above all with methodically keener division in the subsequent chapters.The precision and the plausibility with which the initially posed question can be answered is crucial to the final decision on whether it can be meaningful at all to assume the existence of a sign /aspirin/ and to regard this sign as an essential selective aspect of the existence of the medical preparation //aspirin//.

The interest guiding our understanding in the search for the significate of the sign /aspirin/ is determined essentially in this process by a ruling proposed by Eco, which takes up as a definitory key-term Peirce's concept of the interpretant as the "effect of the sign" or as "something created in the mind of the interpreter." (Nöth 1990: 43). Eco writes:

> (a) meanings are cultural units; (b) these units can be isolated thanks to the chain of their interpretants as revealed in a given culture; (c) the study of the signs in a culture enables us to define the value of the interpretants by viewing them in a system of positions and oppositions; (d) the postulation of these systems makes it possible to explain how meaning comes into existence ..." (Eco 1976: 83).[4]

The question to be answered in this chapter is thus, in more precise terms: What is the meaning of /aspirin/ as a cultural unit? Or: How can the content of the interpretant of /aspirin/ be defined with positional and oppositional concepts within semantic systems? Or, in a style based on the graphic conventions of Eco (1976): What is «aspirin»?

1.1. /Aspirin/ as a proprietary name in Germany

/Aspirin/ as a lexeme of modern German language serves the referential designation of a specific medication with a specific chemical composition. As a phonetic structure, this lexeme is arbitrary and unmotivated. From the diachronic perspective, it was coined in 1899 and is nowadays attached – in an even more concrete sense than other propria – like a label, as a quasi artificial *nomen proprium*, to the industrial product bearing its name. At first glance /aspirin/ appears to have no "meaning" in the sense of linguistic semantics, and it is dubious whether it might have a semiotic "significate". "Denn im Grunde bedeuten alle Namen dasselbe: Dies ist ein Einzelding unserer Welt, ecce homo, ecce locus oder ähnlich." ['For all proper names have fundamentally the same meaning: This is an individual object in our world, ecce homo, ecce locus or something similar.'] (Gerhardt 1950: 5).

Leys (1977: 26), on the other hand, has pointed out that "die Eigennamen, so wie sie uns heute erscheinen, letzten Endes auf Appellative oder irgendwelche andere vorpropriale Grundformen zurückzuführen sind" ['proper names, as they appear to us today, ultimately stem from appellatives or any other preproprial basic forms'].

Nomina propria too thus have thoroughly demonstrable correlations with appellative lexemes, at least from the diachronic aspect, so that, as Leys (1977: 26) further defines, "die propriale Funktion ... in diachronischer Hinsicht eine sekundäre Funktion der Wortform [ist]" ['the proprial function ... is, from the diachronic perspective, a secondary function of the word form']. This correlation is vividly illustrated by the derivation of so many surnames from occupational designations, a feature which shows at the same time that propria in current day-to-day use may, in a large number of cases, become completely detached from the appellative past – for instance in all people named /Fletcher/ who are not //fletchers// (and probably have no idea what a //fletcher// might be).

Postproprial aspects of meaning of a more denotative kind arise from lexicalisation of inventors' or discoverers' names. The lexeme /diesel/[5], for instance, denotes a specific fossil energy preparation that can be converted into kinetic energy by a high-efficiency engine with the same lexical designation. The lexeme /Watt/ denotes a defined quantitative unit of comparison[6] with which this energy can be measured in relation to a unit of time as output. In some cases, such lexicalisations even undergo a grammatical transition from *nomen* to *verbum*. Gipper (1978: 126) quotes the examples "to Morse" and "to roentgen" in this connection.

Names of medical preparations bearing an exceptionally distinct component of postproprial connotative significance include, for example, /interferon/, /Contergan/[7] or /heroin/. Eco (1972: 95–97) analyses a comparable process, taking the example of the name of a sweetener whose suspected carcinogenic properties have given rise to heated debate among the general public: /cyclamate/. Clinical jargon occasionally exemplifies postproprial denotative lexicalisation of drug names that succeed in remaining stable beyond a change from one word category to another: For instance, /digitalising/ a patient suffering from cardiac insufficiency means treating him with //digitalis preparations// in accordance with a specific dosage schedule.

Leys (1977) points out at the beginning of the already frequently quoted article entitled "Der Eigenname in seinem formalen Verhältnis zum Appellativ" ['The proper name in its formal relationship to the appellative'] that he is not taking account of "künstlich entstandene Namen (Kodak, Sabena und dergleichen)" ['artificial or synthetic names (Kodak, Sabena and so on)'] (Leys 1977: 26). The conclusion can be drawn from the examples given that "artificial or synthetic" refers above all to those names that have arisen in the industrial context as proper nouns for products, manufacturing companies or suppliers of services. In the initial answer to our question "What does /aspirin/ mean?", this distinction also played an important role. /Aspirin/ was characterised there as an arbitrary, diachronically young, quasi artificial *nomen proprium* without any semantic meaning. But where is the essential difference between so-called genuine *nomina propria* and so-called artificial ones? The latter have arisen in a context that might be characterised for the time being as /techno-industrial/, a term that covers the already quoted examples of /Watt/ and /diesel/ in the broader sense together with proprietary names such as /Aspirin/ in the narrower sense. This differentiation is something of a linguistic reflex resulting from a socio-historical opposition between the natural and the artificial. This opposition has been of special significance in the cultural standing of medical preparations throughout pharmaceutical history. Its linguistic and semiotic traces in the course of this history are thus of special interest to the question under consideration here. Römer, writing on the linguistic aspect of this opposition, states:

> *Kunst*, ... hat jahrhundertelang die Bereiche *ars* (schöne Kunst ...) *artificium* (Handwerk) und *scientia* (Wissenschaft) gedeckt. Als 'Wissen, Können, Geschicklichkeit des Menschen' hatte es von jeher *Natur* als Gegensatz. Das zugehörige Eigenschaftswort *künstlich* mit dem Inhalt 'kenntnisreich, wissend, geschickt, kunstvoll' wurde allmählich auf den Inhalt 'nicht naturgewachsen' ('unnatürlich' wäre zu grob) eingeschränkt, in dem es heute allein noch gilt. ... Damit hat *Kunst* einen neuen Inhalt hinzubekommen: 'technisch, chemisch, synthetisch, in der Fabrik hergestellt', der zwar die alten Inhalte 'Wissenschaft, Können, besondere Fertigkeit' auf unverhoffte Weise bestätigt, dennoch anders verstanden wird, zumal da diese *Kunst* nicht mehr das Vermögen des einzelnen ist, sondern auf die Art der Herstellung in großen technischen Anlagen hinweist. [Art ... has for centuries covered the spheres of ars (fine arts ...), artificium (skill) and scientia (science). As 'expertise, qualification, dexterity of mankind' it has had Nature as its antithesis from times immemorial. The relevant adjective 'artificial' with the content 'learned, knowledgeable, skilled, artistic' was gradually confined to that content 'not deriving from nature' ('unnatural' would be going too far) which represents its sole usage today. ... Art has thus acquired a new content: 'technical, chemical, synthetic, factory-made' which, whilst confirming the former contents 'science, qualification, special skills' in an unexpected manner, is nonetheless understood in a different way, especially as this art is no longer the endowment of the individual but refers to the type of production in large technological plants.] (Römer 1963: 109).

On the other hand, product names in particular are "als Teil unseres Alltags ... Ausdruck bestimmter Verkehrsformen" ['as part of our daily life, ... an expression of specific forms of interaction'] (Lötscher 1987: 282). At the end of a phonological analysis of numerous German proprietary names, Schuhmacher comes to the following conclusion:

Das Vokabularium der Markenartikelnamen ist … nicht das Ergebnis einer zufälligen Synthese von Elementen, sondern ist den gleichen elementaren Gesetzmäßigkeiten unterworfen, die auch das zentrale Feld der Sprache bestimmen. Für die meisten Namen gilt daher: Im Rahmen einer Betonungsstruktur, wie sie im zentralen deutschen Wort anzutreffen ist, wird ein vertrautes phonotaktisches Grundschema durch die Auswahl von Elementen variiert, die im zentralen Feld eine geringe funktionelle Belastung erfahren. [The vocabulary of the brand name is … not the outcome of a chance synthesis of elements but is subject to those same elementary natural laws that govern the central field of language. It can therefore be said of most names: Within the scope of an emphasizing structure, as is found in the central German word, a familiar phonotactic basic scheme is varied by choosing elements that undergo minimum functional strain in the central field.] (Schuhmacher 1969: 72).

According to a differentiation introduced elsewhere by Schuhmacher, the "peripheral" phonetic system of a language comprises those phoneme sequences which, although feasible on account of the phonetic inventory, are – in contrast to the "central" phonetic system – very seldom realised. The introduction of elements of this "peripheral" phonetic system into a "central" accentuating structure might be, at least from the phonological aspect, a *differentia specifica* of proprietary names. One important economic explanation for these *differentia specifica* is probably the need to reduce the "rischio di omonimia" ['risk of homonymy'] (Eco 1975: 126)[8] as far as possible, especially in proprietary names. Schuhmacher writes in this connection: "Die Forderung nach Unmöglichkeit einer Verwechslung zweier Namen zwingt zu einer größtmöglichen Distanz[9] des zu schaffenden Namens zu den bereits existierenden." ['The demand for the impossibility of two names being confused enforces as great a distance as possible on the name to be created from those already existing.'] (Schuhmacher 1969: 70)

Proprietary names depend on a special degree of phonetic distinctivity in view of their proprial function, that of making an individual referent unmistakable. On the one hand they are clearly identified as artificial propria by the use of "peripheral" phoneme combinations. But beyond this they have to remain distinguishable from one another too, through the greatest possible phonetic "distances". This secondary distinctivity is important especially when a number of proprietary articles with an identical use value have to compete with one another on one joint market. It is for this reason that certain other distinctive characteristics of proprietary products, such as their color or packaging, also play an important role with regard to their presentation to the general public, even if these characteristics assuredly have no substantial influence on their use value. In hardly any range of products is this competition and the associated fight for distinctivity so great as on the pharmaceutical sector. The active substance contained in the medical preparation //aspirin//

was, for example, being marketed worldwide in 1984 under 108 different, registered proprietary names, not taking into account the far greater number of compound preparations in which it is also contained (Wissenschaftliche Zentralstelle des Schweizerischen Apothekervereins [Central Scientific Agency of the Swiss Association of Pharmacists] 1984: 11). It may well be due to this urgent need for distinctivity that a departure is being made more and more frequently from the traditional structure of classical names for medical preparations[10] in new applications for registered names.

If the proprial function of proprietary names is given somewhat more precise consideration, it is actually not correct to define them – as has been done above – as the "identification of an individual referent " totally in the sense of traditional personal, place or farmland names. Two fundamental characteristics of proprietary products in the mass production era are in conflict with that and thus also justify the limitation of proprietary names as artificial as opposed to natural propria:

(1) Proprietary names always denote at one and the same time individual consumable products and the entirety of their actual or potential replicas on the market. As such they are also generic names from the very outset.

(2) Some proprietary names, especially those denoting "leading" products or those opening up new markets, moreover develop into generic names of a very special kind, in that they are even lexicalised as a collective term for all articles with an identical use value, independent of their producers. This is illustrated on the consumer goods market, for instance, with vacuum cleaners (/Hoover/) or with ball-point pens (/Biro/).

The issue of generic names, designated by Debus (1977: 4) as "Kernproblem des Verhältnisses zwischen nomen proprium und nomen appellativum" ['the crucial problem of the relationship between nomen proprium and nomen appellativum'] is now to be given somewhat closer consideration, based on the example on which attention is focused here: The active substance contained in //aspirin// was marketed under this very trade name by several different companies in North America after the First World War. The American Bayer Company as original producer thereupon applied for an injunction to prevent the United Rexall Company, as major competitor on that market, from marketing the active substance under the same trade name. The petition was, however, complied with only in part, in a judgement that created a precedent for American (but not for European) jurisdiction and on which Ladas (1964: 419–420) comments as follows:

> Das Gericht kam auf Grund der Beweisaufnahme zu dem Ergebnis, daß die Chemiker und Ärzte, die sich als Hersteller betätigten, und die Drogisten als Einzelhändler Aspirin als eine Marke der Klägerin [= Bayer Company; K. S.]

anerkannten. Das breite Konsumentenpublikum verstand unter diesem Wort dagegen lediglich eine bestimmte Art von Droge. Die Konsumenten konnten diese Droge in Form von Tabletten von verschiedenen Herstellern in Flaschen mit der Bezeichnung "Aspirin" ohne den Namen der Klägerin bekommen. [In view of the evidence, the court came to the conclusion that the chemists and physicians working as manufacturers and the pharmacists as retailers recognized Aspirin as a trademark of the plaintiff [= Bayer Company; K. S.]. The general consumer public, on the other hand, merely understood by this word a certain kind of drug. The consumers were able to obtain this drug in the form of tablets from various manufacturers in bottles labelled "Aspirin" without the plaintiff's name.]

Explaining the reasons for its judgement, the court had raised the degree and the direction of lexicalisation already undergone by the disputed proprietary name at the crucial time of the contentious issue: "The simple question in all these cases is merely one of fact: what do the buyers understand by the word ...?" (quoted from Ladas 1964: 419).

The judgement passed by the court of last resort in 1921 then proved to be a consistent application of this principle: "Das Gericht verbot es dann der Beklagten [= United Rexall Company; K. S.] die Droge unter dem Namen "Aspirin" an herstellende Chemiker, Ärzte und Drogisten zu vertreiben; es wurde ihr aber nicht verboten, an Verbraucher zu verkaufen." ['The court then enjoined the defendant [United Rexall Company; K..S.] from distributing the drug under the name "Aspirin" to producing chemists, physicians and druggists; it was not enjoined, however from selling to consumers.'] (Ladas 1964: 420).

The proprietary name had thus also lost its copyright in the "Verkehrsgemeinschaft" ['social community'] (cf. Leys 1977: 32) in which it had been "socialised" by its proliferation among the masses into a product-independent generic name. Even today /aspirin/ is therefore not a protected proprietary name in North America but an unprotected "generic name" in the same way as the designation for the active substance contained in it.[11]

Although every producer and every consumer of goods is obviously aware that proprietary products are not to be identified as individual objects[12] but occur in large quantities as the outcome of industrial mass production, there are still important types of transaction forming a symbolic link with the practice of pre-industrial bartering in some spheres of public interchange. The question of whether the use of medical preparations can be considered such a sphere is examined in Chapter 4. At this juncture the working hypothesis that semiotics in general provides a methodologically and epistemologically favourable aspect for dealing with this question[13] is merely corroborated with a few brief references.

In contrast to cars or quartz watches, which rely on production in industrial series – but also in contrast to loaves of bread, coins or terracottas, which have been produced in series as long as division of labour has existed – the production, distribution and application of drugs has traditionally been a process in which individuals could find their own identity. The interchange between the physician and his patient, which this process underwent in the three procedural stages comprising "symptom", "diagnosis" and "therapy", is a form of social intercourse shaped by tradition and largely ritualised into routine. In about the sixteenth century this dyad is supplemented by the apothecary, who very quickly develops into a partner of equal status in the "arcane practice"[14] of pharmaceutical therapy. As a result, the physician initially loses his own economic interest in the patient consuming as many medical preparations as possible, whilst the level of trust and familiarity in the relationship between him and the patient is enhanced. Production and distribution of medical preparations are separated from the personnel and institutional aspects. Communication between these two spheres is effected by what is probably the oldest professional notation system still in use today: the medical prescription.[15] Ever since the sixteenth century it has been written out specifically by the physician and dispensed by the apothecary. His products are meticulously executed, one-off creations. The opportunities for series production are limited not only by problems of preservation but even more by the necessity for individual relationships between the producers, distributors and consumers of medical preparations.[16]

With the pharmacist – the modern equivalent of the apothecary – functioning as a distribution assistant rather than as a producer of pharmaceutical products in the second half of the twentieth century when converting into professional action the written instructions set out in prescription form by the physician, the continuity of this original three-way relationship is still most readily assured by the impact-bearing units of this notation system: by names of medical preparations. The service performed by the physician is (as a rule) restricted in this process to selection of a commercially available specialised preparation, which he denotes on the prescription in the form of its proprietary name. Specification of the quantity – formerly a semiotically significant component of the prescribing and of the service involved – is restricted (as a rule) to an integral multiple of the standard pack, noted as an Arabic numeral bearing a capital /N/ as a modifier immediately after the name of the preparation. The service of the pharmacist is restricted (as a rule) to picking out the required specialised product from his stock, which is arranged alphabetically (according to proprietary names), placing it at the disposal of the consumer, and certifying this act on the prescription. This form of public interchange, whose ritualisation extends to a great many details, has not only a large number of practical, purpose-oriented and economic functions but another one besides: the distribution of pharmaceutical products has to be staged as though they had not yet reached the "age of mechanical reproduction" (cf. Benjamin 1970).

The prospect of interpreting the essence of this performance in diachronic and synchronic perspectives by describing it as an interchange of signs would now appear decidedly promising. This aspect is anything but new, at least with respect to the procedural stages of symptomatics and diagnosis.[17] But the procedural stage of therapy too can be described as a process analogous to the first two stages in so far as it includes the use of medical preparations.

Eco (1975: 37–39, 1976: 22–24, 1987: 45–46) describes three stages of development that can make the use of an object for a specific purpose into an act of cultural communication and thus into a rewarding subject of semiotic consideration:

(1) The function of a specific object is discovered and established by a thinking being as use value.

(2) This use value is stabilised as a cultural unit in that the object is called ("denominato") by this thinking being in terms of its function.

(3) The same use can be repeated with other objects similar to the first with respect to this function.

As a fourth stage of development, one admittedly not considered necessary by Eco for the establishment of use value, it could be added that (4) this use is at least recognised by other subjects too in the cultural environment of the thinking being or undergoes a minimum of diffusion in one form or another. It is probably only by this means that a development stage of "cultural coding" (Eco 1975: 257, 1976: 192, 1987: 256) is attained, one that Barthes (1965: 106) has expressed in the disputed formula: "Dès qu'il y a société, tout usage est converti en signe de cet usage" ['No sooner has society emerged than all use is converted to a sign of that use']. Eco refers in fact to the same context when he suggests that an object progresses in the course of the development depicted here into the "concrete sign of its virtual use" (Eco 1975: 39, 1976: 24, 1987: 49).

If such a proto-semiotic model of instrumentalisation of objects from the real-life world is applied to medical preparations as virtual and actual cultural units, it is seen to be a very apt means of describing the invention, the propagation and also the diachronous handing-down of specific principles of pharmaceutical therapy. A weighty argument for the justification of this analogy is the orientation of the therapeutic agents of one medical epoch by the theoretical structure of its diagnostics and symptomatology, which are provedly to be understood in the framework of metatheory first and foremost as semiotically based models. Paracelsus' doctrine of "signatures" (cf. chapter 4.2) and the homeopathic *similia similibus curentur* illustrate this correlation particularly vividly. It can be applied in an equally exemplary though more concise form to late medieval "humoral pathology":

This set of concepts, which was to dominate occidental medicine for many centuries, interpreted numerous syndromes as an imbalance between four cardinal bodily fluids. Its symptomatology described many manifestations with great precision as indexicalic references designed to suggest to the physician a disproportionately high or low presence of one or more of these fluids at a specific location in the unhealthy body. This model, though empirically largely inadequate from current perspectives, was the characteristic "perspektivische Segmentierung der Realität" ['perspectival segmentation of reality'] (Eco 1972: 169) not only for diagnostic interpretation of the symptoms but to the same extent for their therapeutic management too. For the therapeutically applied substances were intended to restore the lost balance by expelling a surplus of or correcting a deficiency in individual bodily fluids. The hypostatised model exerted considerable influence on the social reality of medical preparations and on their synchronous and diachronous propagation as cultural units, as well as on the act of designation[18] (Eco 1975: 37: "denominazione") with its semiotically central status in terms of Eco's model. This influence can be traced through the names designating the groups of therapeutically active substances rather than through those of the different individual substances (e.g. /choleretics/ as /agents expelling yellow bile/; further examples in Schneider 1968).

Further consideration given in this chapter to the question of the meaning of /aspirin/ will reveal that names of medical preparations in current use, as proprial identifiers of individual preparations, also conceal appellative components referring to specific, hierarchically arranged semantic elements. The objective is to show that these elements hypostasise both pragmatic models of instrumental application and heuristic models, permitting their development at a specific time in pharmaceutical history to be codified in cultural terms.

Nomina propria that have arisen in the techno-industrial context perform other important linguistic services beyond their identification function: Within the framework of a "Produktionsöffentlichkeit" ['production publicity'] (cf. Negt – Kluge 1972) made increasingly complex by innovations, they denote very specific, precisely defined methods of production, conversion or measurement. If they moreover attain a minimum of diffusion, they may also denote a specific, culturally codified and distinctive unit of use value , whose extra-verbal object acquires semiotic meaning by becoming the reference of the "concrete sign of its virtual use" (Eco 1976: 24). Finally, at an even higher stage of diffusion, specific *nomina propria* may attain additional, more connotative significance, generally regardless of the original proprial function, as mass-culture phenomena in the vicinity of contemporary events or figures. The borders between these three more appellative functions of artificial propria are admittedly fluid. All of them are the outcome of a process characterised by Eco (1976: 129) as "overcoding", one that could for its part be placed in the context of a process whose historical and sociological dimension has been developed in detail by Habermas (1989) as "structural transformation of the public sphere". Its provisional terminating point can be described most fittingly with a phrase coined by Paul Valéry in an essay on the fundamental conditions of art in the twentieth century: "la conquête de l'ubiquité" ['the conquest of ubiquity'] (Valéry 1960: 1284, 1957-1975, 12: 225). Why this phrase applies so very fittingly to the process outlined here is best illustrated by the introductory passage of an article published in a German pictorial in the 1980s:

> Es ist so alt wie dieses Jahrhundert, so erfolgreich wie Coca-Cola, so unentbehrlich wie das Auto und so billig wie Pfefferminzdrops. Zur Ausstattung einer Weltraumfähre gehört es ebenso wie zu der eines Handschuhfachs. Eskimos nehmen es nicht weniger gern als amerikanische Hausfrauen. Den Ureinwohnern von Tasmanien hilft es so zuverlässig wie europäischen Managern, und in westlichen Krankenhäusern ist es, wie auch in der chinesischen Barfußmedizin, therapeutischer Standard. Schon vor 26 Jahren schlug eine New Yorker Zeitung vor, es dem amerikanischen Trinkwasser zuzusetzen. Dazu kam es nicht. Doch neben Kaffee und Orangensaft etablierte es sich als wichtiges Element des amerikanischen Katerfrühstücks: Aspirin. [It is as old as this century, as successful as Coca Cola, as indispensable as the motorcar and as cheap as peppermint drops. It is equally at home in a space shuttle and in a glove compartment. Eskimos take it just as readily as American housewives. It helps the natives of Tasmania as dependably as it does European managers, and in Western hospitals it is a therapeutic standard, as it is in Chinese barefoot medicine. Even 25 years ago a New York newspaper suggested adding it to the American drinking water. That never came about. But along with coffee and orange juice it has become established as an essential element in the American hangover breakfast: Aspirin.] (de Ridder 1984: 80).

1.2. /Aspirin/ as //acetylsalicylic acid//

In public interchange involving patients and consumers, drugs are usually denoted by their trade names, most of which are protected proprietary names.

The various phonetic and semantic constituents of these proprietary names as well as their copyright are tuned to establishing the most stable exchange relationships possible between producers and consumers of pharmaceutical products along the lines of different distributional institutions (medical practice, hospital, pharmacy, health insurance agency) and influencing factors (advertising, publicity, history, legislation). As was shown in the course of discussion of a provisional answer to the question "What is the meaning of /aspirin/?", these mediation processes can assert an important influence on the social reality of pharmaceutical products. The methodological objective to be attained by working out an answer to this question was outlined as follows at the beginning of that chapter, based on a ruling proposed by Eco (1976: 83, 1975: 120): "... the study of signs ... in a [given] culture" in order to "define the value of the interpretants by viewing them in a system of positions and oppositions [inside of semantic systems]".

The second answer to this question now turns the discussion to another semantic system, whose significance for the social reality of pharmaceutical products and thus for their existence as "cultural units" (Eco) is less of an economic than of a heuristic nature: the formular languages of organic chemistry. As semiotic systems they tend to be closer to "natural" languages than the system of proprietary names. One of these three formular languages has a dual structure as its most important combinatorial principle and is capable of representing consistently an infinitely varying spectrum of natural phenomena with finite means. The "thought styles" (Fleck 1979: 125) of the chemical analytic process could be claimed somewhat provocatively to be governed by a manifestation of dual-structure codes so purely and indisputably potent in its explanatory effect that a comparative metatheoretical consideration of its duality would hardly be worthwhile as it simply has too few problems to offer.

Weissbach (1971) has set out the history of these formular languages and their heuristic significance – which was commonly not reflected upon[19] by their users – in a detailed monograph. He writes: "Diese grundlegenden Zeichen der chemischen Formelsprache sind gleichsam ihre 'Buchstaben'. Sie werden zu 'Wörtern' verknüpft – den Strukturformeln. Für die Art der Verknüpfung gibt es strenge Regeln, die jeder Oberschüler wie das ABC lernt." ['These fundamental signs constituting the language of the chemical formula are at the same time their "letters". They are linked to form "words" – the structural formulae. The type of linkage is subject to strict rules which every senior schoolboy learns like the ABC.'] (Weissbach 1971: 138).

Elsewhere: "So wie die Wörter zu Sätzen werden auch die Strukturformeln zu höheren Einheiten verknüpft. Dadurch entstehen die Reaktionsgleichungen. Das sind die wahren 'Sätze' der chemischen Formelsprache; sie geben das wieder, was den Chemiker eigentlich interessiert und womit er es in Wirklichkeit zu tun hat: die chemische Reaktion." ['In the same way as words forming sentences, structural formulae are also linked to form higher units, resulting in reaction equations. These are the real 'sentences' of the chemical formular language: they reflect what actually interests the chemist and what he is really dealing with: the chemical reaction.'] (Weissbach 1971: 139).

The initial impression that this analogisation is somewhat superficial is due solely to the fact that the line taken by their author in his statements is one of scientific theory but not of semiotics in the narrower sense. The fundamental structural similarity can, however, be shown to fulfil very consistently the similarity criteria of homology. Table 1 shows the individual steps of this analogisation in context and extrapolates them beyond the framework proposed by Weissbach to cover the entire range of linguistic constituent analyses. This figure is now to be given somewhat closer consideration so that the theoretical status and any heuristic effects of the fundamental analogy can then be pursued with maximum differentiation, based on the //acetylsalicylic acid// paradigm. It is not the aim of this consideration to propose a new terminology for any constituents in any field or to establish a new analytical method. The objective is rather to observe existing terminologies and methods with close interest to see how they perform "perspektivische Segmentierung" ['perspectival segmentation'] (Eco 1972: 169) of the realities to which they are exposed. Any parallelism between the continua of language and of organic chemistry revealed by this consideration would be weighty arguments in favour of our endeavour to regard the question of the meaning of /acetylsalicylic acid/ as an eminently semiotic one.

The left-hand and middle columns of Table 1 show the specialised terms taken from organic chemistry and synchronous linguistics for the five most important complexity stages of their respective object areas. The right-hand column parallelises these two terminologies with that proposed by Koch (1971) and Nöth (1985, 1990) as a generally semiotic orientation for conceptualisation of non-verbal, so-called "representematic" codes.

The analogy between /atom/ and /phoneme/ as terms of the smallest distinctive units of the first structural level of our synopsis has its scientific origin in pre-Socratic atomism. Both are elementary fundamental units of each and every attempt at analysis, and neither can be further divided without severe loss of meaning. They are represented essentially in both specialised language systems by the same stock of graphemes: by characters. Harder has drawn attention to the origin of a parallelism between characters and atoms in Ancient Greece: "Lautschrift und Atomistik stammen aus der gleichen

Table 1: Juxtaposition of three scientific fields. Perspective segmentation of reality. Five structural levels of increasing complexity in three scientific languages: analytical chemistry (left- hand column), synchronous linguistics (middle column) and general semiotics (right-hand column). Concepts quoted from Weissbach 1971; van Dijk 1980; Koch 1971 [For the synoptic principle, cf. Nöth 1985: 213.]

Level	Continuum of COMPOUNDS occurring in organic chemistry	Continuum of LANGUAGE	Continuum of REPRESENTMATIC SIGNS
0	Nuclear particles electrons	Location and mode of sound generation	
1	Atom	Phoneme	"Representeme" (Koch)
2	Functional group	Morpheme	"Representomorpheme" (Koch)
3	Molecule "structural formula" (Weissbach)	Lexeme	"Representologeme" (Koch)
4	Reaction "Reaction equation" (Weissbach)	Clause Proposition	"Representosyntacteme" (Koch)
5	Metabolism	Text "Macrostructure (van Dijk)	"Representotexteme" (Koch)

Sehart, einer ausgliedernden Kraft von radikaler Systematik." ['Phonetic writing and atomism originate from a common point of view, a selecting force of radical systematism'] (Harder, quoted from Blumenberg 1986: 37).

The significance of the atomism concept in scientific theory is also the subject of the first scientific paper published by a theoretician whose name was later to acquire special significance in connection with a re-formulation of general semiotics: Charles S. Peirce (1982: 95–100).

/Phonemes/ and /atoms/ are combined at the next structural level to form /morphemes/ and /functional groups/. Both these instances concern constituents which do not so much bear as modify meaning. In contrast to the /lexemes/ (or /monemes/[20]) and /molecules/ of the third structural level, neither can occur autonomously in syntagmas without being supplemented. Whereas "lexemes" and "molecules" rather function as elementary bearers of complex semantic and semiotic units, "morphemes" and "functional groups" are rather modifiers of these units with respect to their ability to be combined into syntagmas.

These syntagmas correspond at the fourth structural level to the /reaction equations/ of the analytic process of organic chemistry on the one hand and to the /clauses/ or the /propositions/ of language on the other. It is at this fourth level that the first major flaw in our synopsis occurs, that all examples – no matter how carefully selected – start to stumble: The combinatorial results of the reaction of "molecules" with "molecules" are invariably new "molecules". These may be more complex than their original constituents, yet certainly in hardly any single case is this increased complexity comparable – with respect to the concentration and the transport of semiotic units – with the qualitative flaw made in combining "lexemes" into a "clause" or a "proposition". The quantitatively exact determination of a "reaction equation" is known in the terminology of organic chemistry as "stoichiometry". As a balancing activity, "stoichiometry" restricts the possibility of laboratory reactions undergoing a general increase in complexity from the very outset: If "atoms" have been added to a "molecule" following a chemical reaction, then they must be missing from another "molecule". The diagrammatic model of the chemical combinatorial process at the fourth structural level is the equation, for which an enclosed system is, in cybernetic terms, a prerequisite. The linguistic "clause", on the other hand, is anything but that. It is open, and both the concentration and the transport of semantic units permitted by it depend on and change with their environments. Its form and the combination of its elementary bearers of meaning, "phonemes", "morphemes" and "lexemes", are admittedly not changed any further by these environments. "Stoichiometry" is committed to an analytic process directed strictly downwards with respect to the degree of complexity, fully in the sense of the atomistic tradition about which Blumenberg writes: "Das griechische *stoicheon* bezeichnet ursprünglich den Laut und den Buchstaben als unselbständige Teile eines Zusammenhangs, als Glieder einer Reihe (*stoichos*), metaphorisch dann das, wovon man für einen Zusammenhang ausgehen muß, auch die Grundlagen eines Beweisgangs und die letzten allgemeinen Begriffe einer Wissenschaft, deren 'Elementarlehre'." ['The Greek stoicheion originally designates the sound and the letters as dependent parts of an association, as links in a row (stoichos), metaphorically then what has to be taken for granted for an association, also the fundamentals of a line of reasoning and the last general terms of a science, its 'elemental theory'.'] (Blumenberg 1986: 37).

The view of the fifth structural level, in other words of the highly complex biochemical metabolism, is blocked with good reason by the visual direction of "stoichiometry"; for it is at this stage of complexity that its combinatorial potential has finally reached the limits of its validity and the proven model has lost its explanatory monopoly. The structure of biochemical macromolecules cannot always be explained in "stoichiometric" terms. Above all, they are connected with one another by intermolecular forces that cannot be explained by the traditional model of "electronic pair binding". This, however, brings the balancing calculating system of "stoichiometry" into disarray. The transition from the fourth to the fifth structural level of linguistics produces analogous difficulties: One fundamental problem confronting discourse analysis in its attempt to expand the focus of grammatical analysis beyond the limits of the clause also derives from the fact that the laws of combination valid below this limit and virtually free from contradiction are no longer applicable above it. Special care is undoubtedly essential when interpreting such segmental parallels between different fields of research with marked methodological deviations from one another, such as chemistry and linguistics – at least at the fourth and fifth structural levels under consideration here. In general and quite superficially, however, it can be stated that the transition from the fourth to the fifth structural level has given rise in both domains to crises and progress as are symptomatic of "paradigm changes" (Kuhn 1962), and that one essential prerequisite can be described for both developments – rather with respect to crises than to progress – namely the challenging of syntagmatic limits, on whose monopoly major parts of traditional theory were based: "electron pair binding" and "clause limit ". The expansion of the analytical focus beyond these limits had some connection in both cases with the development of new technologies. In the sphere of biochemistry it was above all the new "chromatography" procedures and "X-ray structure analysis" that permitted macromolecular compounds too to be depicted in precise detail. Within the framework of discourse analysis, computer-aided "artificial intelligence" research has probably had thoroughly comparable effects (cf. van Dijk – Kintsch 1983).

Let us now return to the starting point of this analogy consideration and thus to the question of whether this interdisciplinary structural similarity as a common foundation has left on general semiotics any heuristic effects that can be reconstructed with the //acetylsalicylic acid// paradigm.

Consideration of the "structural formula" of one molecule of //acetylsalicylic acid// (middle box in Figure 1) shows this to be – in one of the formular languages of organic chemistry – a complete representation of the "lexeme" (in the terminology used by Koch (1971) of the "representologeme") corresponding to the active substance of //aspirin//. The chemical //atomic bodies// constituting the overall //molecule// through a structured layout subject to

Acetylsalicylic acid	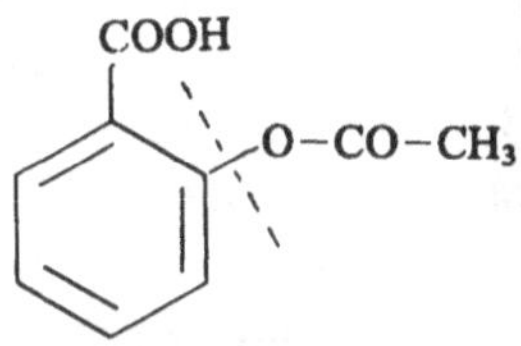	$C_9H_8O_4$
Representomorpheme + Representologeme	Representeme + Representomorpheme + Representologeme	Representeme
= chemical nominal term	= structural formula	= empirical formula

Figure 1: //Acetylsalicylic acid// in the three formular languages of organic chemistry. As to the structural formula: Each corner of the hexagon represents one carbon atom, i. e. is equivalent to /C/. The three lines inside the hexagon represent four hydrogen atoms that 'oscillate' inside the hexagon, i. e. are not consistent in their location. Each line outside the hexagon represents one 'electron pair binding'.

specific selection restrictions, and illustrated in the /structural formula/ by means of Latin letters, correspond as the smallest distinctive units to the /phonemes/ of "natural" languages (or to the /representemes/ of non-linguistic codes in the terminology of Koch). The broken line divides the molecule into two constituents: to the left of the line the //salicylic acid// (the actual /lexeme/ or /representologeme/) and to the right the //acetic acid residue// (corresponding as an attached /functional group/ to the /morpheme/ or /representomorpheme/ from Table 1).

In their development, the script systems of the chemical formular languages have hinged on the native language of their inaugurators. To this extent it is hardly surprising that they bear the structural principles, highly differentiated in part, of Indo-European languages; these were, after all, still available for communication in scientific discourse on those natural phenomena on whose observation the formation of the chemical model was based. The principle of dual structure, comprising columns 1 to 3 of Table 1, is, however, fully preserved only in the system of the /structural formula/ (Figure 1, middle box). The meta-linguistic terminology of organic chemistry, which assigns a noun to each organic compound (Figure 1, left-hand box) is, by itself, the only one incapable of imparting the principles of dual structure: Neither the term /acetylsalicylic acid/ nor its synonym /ortho-acetoxy-benzoic acid/, which is more differentiated in the descriptive respect, indicates which smallest distinctive units constitute one //molecule// of this compound.

Decisive significance for the agglutinating, progressively determining formation of these nouns can be attributed only to the /representomorphemes/ as smallest constituents of chemical compounds; like /morphemes/ of linguistic codes, they are of semiotic significance and may also occur as /lexemes/ or /representologemes/ in their own right. One molecule of //acetylsalicylic acid// consists of one /representologeme/, //salicylic acid//, and one /representomorpheme/, the //acetic acid residue//, which is denoted in chemical nomenclature by the string of characters /acetyl/ (from lat. *acidum acetatum* 'acetic acid'). /Acetyl/ is identified by its introductory position in the progressively determined technical term /acetylsalicylic acid/ unequivocally as a modifying and not primarily a meaning-bearing constituent.

At the lowest structural level, one molecule of //acetylsalicylic acid// is broken down into twenty-one /representemes/ as the smallest distinctive units with no autonomous significance, namely into nine //carbon atoms//, eight //hydrogen atoms// and four //oxygen atoms//.

Finally, a third formular language of organic chemistry takes account only of the type and number of /atoms/ constituting a /molecule/: the empirical formula (Figure 1, right-hand box). It is thus directed exclusively by the bottom level of the dual structure .

This system, which is rooted in the atomism of antiquity, is certainly the oldest of the three formular languages of chemistry presented here. Although the concept of the atom and its representation as a model have undergone very radical changes in the course of scientific history (cf. Lasswitz 1889; Bloch 1919; Gadamer 1968), the conceptual framework was held together at least by Democritus' postulate of indivisibility without loss of meaning until the discovery of radioactivity. The way for the chemical nomenclature (Figure 1, left-hand box) still in use today, a terminology that assigns to each compound a combination of /phonemes/ (and /graphemes/) of natural languages, was paved only at the end of the eighteenth century with publication of the *Méthode de nomenclature chimique* by Lavoisier, Guyton and Fourcroy (cf. Crosland 1962; Goltz 1972). The dual-structure formular system (Figure 1, middle box) was developed another century later, with Kekulé's terminological proposals playing an essential role (cf. Weissbach 1971).

Like the limits between /morphemes/ and /lexemes/ of natural languages, the limits between the individual /representomorphemes/ and /representologemes/ of chemical structural formulae are recognisable only to those familiar with the "semantics" of the underlying system of signs. The broken line in the middle box of Figure 1 is merely an auxiliary line, the outcome, as it were, of a metasemiotic reflection analogous to the separating lines between "prefix", "stem" and "suffix" in a linguistic discussion on the word grammar of one specific language.

The signifier /acetylsalicylic acid/ has so far been dealt with as though the representologeme /salicylic acid/ were, in the same way as the /lexemes/ of natural languages, the actual bearer of its meaning, whilst the representomorpheme /acetyl/ played a more modifying and selection-restricting role within the framework of the overall syntagma. This representation implies a certain hierarchy of meaning between the two elements, one that has previously been founded extremely superficially and demands further concretisation. This concretisation is worked out later in this chapter, based on the objective set at the beginning of the chapter, that of defining the "value" of the "interpretant" of a sign by means of positional and oppositional concepts within the semantic space or system in a given culture (Eco 1976: 83).

The second answer to the question of the significate of /aspirin/ to be discussed here refers to a chemical substance – //acetylsalicylic acid// – denoted by this significant – /aspirin/ – as an artificial nomen proprium of the type exemplified by the "proprietory name". It is now shown, within the framework of the semantic system determined by the formular languages of organic chemistry, that this chemical substance can be divided into further semiotically relevant subunits, that the denotatum of /aspirin/, namely //acetylsalicylic acid//, itself regarded as a sign, may denote further signs. If these subunits have any essential influence on the reality of the chemical substance as a "cultural unit", then those signs representing these subunits may be well worth examining in our objective of delineating "in an asymptotic fashion" (Eco 1976: 71), as it were, cultural units – linking up with the processes of infinite semiosis. As indicated above, the influence of the two main constituents of //acetylsalicylic acid// on the semiotics of this chemical substance is essentially of a heuristic nature and is rooted in the history of science. In order to grasp this influence more precisely, the diachronous development of these two constituents is dealt with in greater detail. Both //salicylic acid// and the //acetic acid residue// could – were each of them to be provided with one additional //hydrogen atom// on the borderline between /representologeme/ and /representomorpheme/ (broken line in middle box of Figure 1) – also exist as autonomous, self-contained, in chemical terminology "saturated", compounds in the same way as /morphemes/ of "natural" languages can become autonomous /lexemes/ when supplemented by additional /phonemes/, as, for instance, in the formation of infinitives. Figure 2 shows the structural formulae of the two resulting compounds.

The "wechselvolle, oft romanhaft anmutende Geschichte der Salicylsäure" ['checkered, often story-book history of salicylic acid'] (Hangarter 1974a: 3)

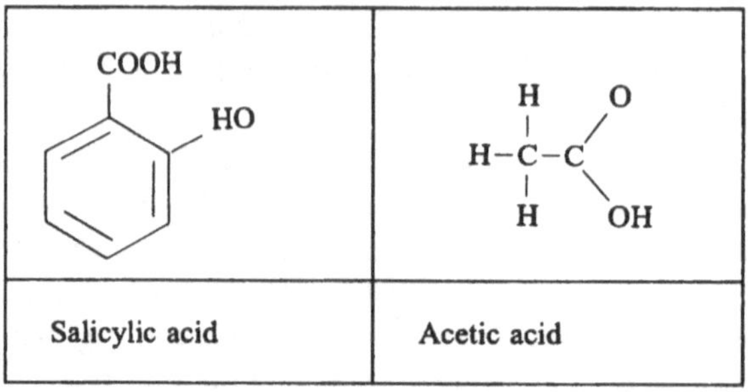

Figure 2: Structural formulae of salycylic acid and acetic acid.

is a very instructive example of the interpenetration of theory formation and practical empiricism and of the modelling of similarities in the real-life world as an outcome of this interpenetration. Its biphasic dynamics could be characterised very fittingly with a formulation by Blumenberg (1986: 199): "Das Sinnverlangen, rational des Feldes verwiesen, ist listiger als die sich selbst zur List ernennende Vernunft." ['Ordered off the field for rational motives, craving for sense is even more artful than Reason assuming the self-appointed title of artfulness.']

The beginning of this history, hardly to be localised in spatial or temporal terms, goes much further back than the beginning of any scientific publication. The infusions and extracts of willow (Latin: *salix*) bark as a febrifuge belong to the established store of knowledge of almost every lore of healing recorded by word of mouth and by personal perception, at least in regions in which this type of tree is widespread. The first publication dedicated solely to this therapy dates back in pharmaco-historical literature to the year 1763, when Edward Stone presented a paper on the influence of willow extracts on the course of malaria, observing 50 case studies, to the then 99-year-old Royal Society of Medicine. These extracts had, in the same way as extracts of cinchona bark, an oily consistency and a bitter taste. They were regarded by some authors as a low-priced alternative to this undoubtedly most potent natural febrifugum that had to be imported in those times, mainly from Peru. Apart from its febrifugal application, the willow bark was also used for all manner of other "indications", with alleviation of pain, however, not playing a major role. Samuel Hahnemann judges its therapeutic value rather with scepticism, with the fusion of empirical competence and authoritarian dogmatics so typical of him, in the second volume of his *Apothekerlexikon* published in 1783:

> Nun ist zwar nicht zu leugnen, daß sie wirklich zuweilen Wechselfieber gehoben hat, allem Ansehen nach aber bloß solche, deren Fortdauer durch gewöhnliche Stärkungsmittel Enzian, Galläpfel, u.s.w. ebenfalls hätte gehemmt werden können. Es fehlt ihr so viel daran, daß diese Rinde mit der wunderns-würdigen Kraft der China übereinkommen sollte, daß sehr sorgfältige Ärzte sie sogar nie eigentlich antipyretisch wirken sahen, und sie wohl zu irgendeinem Behufe, wo gewöhnlich bittere adstringierende Mittel erforderlich sind, vorzüglich zu äußerem Gebrauche, vortrefflich finden, sich aber nie entschließen können, die Stelle der China durch sie ersetzen zu wollen. [Now it cannot be denied that it has indeed occasionally alleviated malaria, though to judge by all appearances only that whose continuance might likewise have been checked by customary restoratives such as bitter-wort, gall etc. This bark is so far from attaining the wondrous power of cinchona that highly meticulous physicians have never truly seen it acting antipyretically; they find it excellent for any purpose for which bitter adstringent agents are commonly necessary, yet can never resolve to substitute it for cinchona.] (Hahnemann 1966: 434)

One outstandingly important framework for the modelling of similarity in late medieval pharmacy is the so-called "doctrine of signatures ", dating back in fundamental aspects to Paracelsus and Jakob Böhme. This is presented in more detail in connection with other so-called /similarity-modelling/ theorems in the third chapter of this book. Its underlying idea "…daß die Natur die pflanzlichen und tierischen Drogen bereits gekennzeichnet hat … [und] … daß für jede Krankheit in der Welt ein bestimmtes Heilmittel zu finden ist, dessen Wirkung der suchende Arzt aus der Signatur erschließen muß" ['… that Nature has already given drugs of plant and animal origin their distinguishing mark … [and] … that for every illness in the world a specific remedy is to be found, whose effect has to be concluded by the searching physician from the signature'] (Haas 1948: 295), has certainly not lacked influence on the history of willow bark as a remedy.[21] The preferred habitats of the most frequent types of willow are damp locations: riversides, ditches, marshes. It is precisely there, however, that almost all infection-transmitting parasites and microorganisms find exceptionally favourable conditions. From the perspective of the medieval herbalist, this important febrifuge was thriving, as it were, in the breeding-grounds of fever. It is not altogether easy for the modern mentality, but essential for a clear understanding of the associations depicted here, to imagine what teleological temptation must have emanated from this association on the formation of a theory by any physician, no matter how empirically disciplined.

In 1828 the Munich chemist Buchner succeeded in purifying willow extract by removing certain vehicles and tanning agents. He called his product /Salicin/, a name that was taken over by the French pharmacist Leroux, who continued work on perfecting the chemical concentration method in 1830. In

1832 the Prague clinician Krombholz published a report on initial therapeutic results obtained with the new substance. Within the scope of his attempt to explain its favourable influence on feverish processes, he writes (quoted from Hangarter 1974b: 1968): "... da die Weide feuchte und sumpfige Gegenden liebe, bestätige sich wieder 'Ubi morbus ibi remedium'" ['... as the willow loves damp, marshy regions, "*Ubi morbus ibi remedium*" is confirmed once again'].

In 1835 the Berne pharmacist Pagenstecher extracted from //meadow-sweet// (*Spiraea ulmaria*) a volatile oil whose main constituent is now assumed to have been chemically identical with the substance isolated by Buchner and Leroux from the //white willow// (*Salix alba*). The Zurich chemist Löwig, continuing work on Pagenstecher's production method with a view to simplifying the molecule, obtained in 1835 a compound that is designated in current nomenclature as /salicylic aldehyde/ but to which he gave the name *spiroylige Säure* 'spiroyligous acid' with reference to the //*Spiraeae*// as carriers of the raw substance. The two Swiss researchers were unaware, however, that they were contributing in this way to a further development of a *febrifugum* or *antipyreticum*. Nor were they put on this trail by the fact that many //*Spiraeae*// – and especially those with which they had been working – flourish, like the willow, most profusely in moist habitats. It was only some years later that it was taken up, and then as a result of a frequently underestimated mode of informational diffusion: travel[22]. Although all previous authors specified with great precision the original products and the production methods of their substances as well as some of the chemical characteristics, they were not capable of determining the location, type and number of their smallest distinctive units.

In the mid-nineteenth century it was by no means unusual to experiment, within the scope of general pharmacological interest, with substances of unknown composition, even if these were low-molecular, in other words relatively uncomplex, substances. Even if the relevant technical facilities had been available, analytical theory formation had not yet reached a level that would have permitted systematisation of the many analytical steps needed to clarify the structure. There was, above all, no empirically based theory on the spatial – or, in more general terms, on the structural – organisation of atoms into molecules and their consequently deducible tendency to form bonds with one another. This framework was to be established only in the last third of the century, as an outcome of / carbon chemistry/.

In 1838, the Neapolitan Rafaele Piria was continuing work on the //salicin// produced by Buchner and Leroux. His series of tests yielded an acid which crystallised at normal pressures and temperatures and which he named */acide* *salicylique/*. This was the first instance of the substance denoted by the /representologeme/ of //acetylsalicylic acid// being synthetised. Piria even succeeded in determining its empirical formula, in modern-day terminology: /$C_7H_6O_3$/. A short time later, while travelling in Berne, his Parisian teacher and laboratory supervisor Dumas chanced to meet Pagenstecher, who introduced him to Löwig's //spiroyligous acid//. In 1840, prompted by Dumas, Liebig's pupil Ettling compared the two substances: he then described the *//salicin//* extracted from the willow bark as being fundamentally identical with the //spiroyligous acid// obtained from meadowsweet. In 1843, Cahours and Procter discovered a plant from which Piria's //salicylic acid// could be extracted in far greater quantities: the //teaberry// (*Gaultheria procumbens*), a member of the wintergreen family, whose main habitat is North America. Eventually, in 1859, Kolbe had a breakthrough in the fully synthetic production of //salicylic acid//. A new compound, whose composition had been clarified at least to the extent permitted by the contemporary state of the art, which had a known relationship with fundamental pharmacological expertise, and which moreover could be synthetised, had become available in an unexpectedly short time.

The consequences of this constellation remained remarkably few for a remarkably long time. The therapeutic application of //salicin// or //salicylic acid// was initially restricted to a few single cases. Hangarter writes in his monograph: "Die neuen Stoffe begegneten damals allseitig großem Interesse, ohne daß die spätere eminent große Bedeutung der Salicylsäure vorauszusehen war." ['The new substances aroused great interest on all fronts at that time, without the later, outstanding importance of salicylic acid being predictable.'] (Hangarter 1974a: 4). With reference to //salicylic acid// and the inventor of its synthesis, Hermann Kolbe, Schlenk writes:

> Zwar kannte man noch keine Verwendung für die jetzt leicht zugängliche Säure, aber in kluger Voraussicht ließ sich Kolbe seine Erfindung in den einzelnen deutschen Staaten und im Ausland durch Patente schützen, und in dem zusammenfassenden DRP 426 (1877) sprach er die Hoffnung aus, daß "der Salicylsäure wie den ihr isomeren und homologen Verbindungen, im großen hergestellt, ein würdiger Platz in der chemischen Technik wird eingeräumt werden müssen. [Although no application was known at that time for the now easily accessible acid, Kolbe, with prudent foresight, had his invention patented in the individual German states and abroad, and in the summarizing "German Reich patent" DRP 426 from 1877 he expressed the hope that "salicylic acid and its isomeric and homologous compounds in mass production will have to be assigned a worthy place in chemical technology.] (Schlenk 1947: 9).[23]

What Kolbe originally had in mind – according to Schlenk – was its application as a preservative. He did, however, induce the Leipzig surgeon

Thiersch to use //salicylic acid// as a local antiseptic in clinical trials. 38 years after its initial production in pure form by Piria, //salicylic acid// was used for the first time for therapeutic purposes. This was done in studies by Stricker, who introduced it into the Berlin Charité hospital as a method of treating arthritic pain, thus initiating a development that was summed up provisionally by Schlenk in 1947 in the following words: "Es dürfte wenige Krankheiten geben, zu deren Heilung während der unterdessen vergangenen 70 Jahre nicht da und dort Salicylsäure versucht worden wäre." ['There can be only few disorders where salicylic acid has not been tried out here and there as a remedy during the 70 years that have now elapsed.'] (Schlenk 1947: 246)

At Kolbe's suggestion, the Dresden chemist von Heyden set up the mass production of //salicylic acid// in Radebeul in 1874. The quantity produced in the first year by the "*Salicylsäurefabrik Dr. von Heyden*" was 4 tonnes; four years later it was 25 tonnes. On the one hand, //salicyclic acid// was a long-desired miracle drug: it kept under control the often excruciating pains of phlogistic arthritic processes, a syndrome whose development was frequently progressive. On the other hand, its application also induced quite considerable side-effects such as nausea and stomach-ache, which could certainly be more excruciating than the pains they were supposed to be controlling. Their direct tissue-damaging effect could moreover result in serious ulcers on the mucosal lining of the alimentary tract. They also had a agonizingly nauseating taste.

Even in the nineteenth century there was hardly one single instance of pharmacological therapy where it could be stated with certainty whether the diseased organism would be influenced more by the desired main effect or by an adverse side-effect. The uncertainty had two vital consequences for medical theory formation: On the one hand, it encouraged the "therapeutic nihilism" that had originated in the Viennese school at the turn of the century and which sought "im Expectare die allein nützliche therapeutische Handlung" ['in expectation the only useful therapeutic activity'] (Haas 1948: 290) in its efforts to do as little harm as possible. On the other hand, the therapeutic uncertainty once more led to the metaphorisation of medical therapy as a "fight" against evil. This interpretation saw the pharmacological side-effect as an indispensable battle-cry in the difficult and inevitably destructive extirpation of the disease: No (therapeutic) gain without pain. Old as the side-effects problem was at the end of the nineteenth century, so unexpected and new was the impending solution. Since the introduction by Kekulé and others of electron pair binding and the representation of carbocyclic compounds into the formular language of organic chemistry, scientists had learnt to think in terms of structures and to associate the phenomena of the *attractio electiva* of Torbern Bergman ([1968]; cf. chapter 3.3) theoretically with these struc-

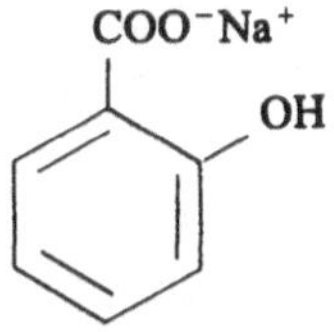

Sodium salicylate

Figure 3: Structural formula of //sodium salicylate//

tures. This was the outset of a development that ultimately suggested that the undesirable side-effects might be "decocted" through targeted chemical changes to the molecule, and which culminated in the production of synthetic medical preparations. From 1877 onwards, the //sodium salt of salicylic acid// was used by See for therapeutic purposes without, however, inducing a substantial decrease in the rate or intensity of the side-effects (Figure 3).

The "change of paradigm ", that was decisive as we see it today, took place in 1897 when Felix Hoffman attached an //acetic acid residue// to the //OH-group// of //salicylic acid// at the *Farbenfabriken*, formerly *Friedrich Bayer und Co.* in Elberfeld. The literature repeatedly presents the anecdote of Hoffmann having had this /change of paradigm / for personal reasons too, because his father was suffering from severe rheumatic complaints and had an extremely poor tolerance level to //sodium salicylate//. He was by no means the first chemist to synthetise //acetylsalicylic acid//. This had been attempted with some measure of success in 1853 by the Strasbourg chemist Gerhardt[24], in 1859 by Gilm, and in 1869 by the Hanoverians Prinshorn and Kraut. In 1895, pharmacological trials had even been performed with it, though without spectacular success, at von Heyden's *Salicylsäurefabrik* in Radebeul. Hoffmann was, however, probably the first chemist capable of producing the new substance in an adequately pure, stable form. Even more important, he was the first to attach the //acetic acid residue// as a modifying /representomorpheme/ to the /representologeme/ with the intention of reducing the side-effects of //salicylic acid//.

Just why he chose //acetic acid// is unclear and, for reasons dealt with in more detail below, still a matter of dispute. But he really had no choice in the true sense of the word: although the structure of such elementary bases could meanwhile be grasped theoretically, the pharmacological principle of its efficacy could not. One possible explanation is that it was simply in vogue in pharmaceutical research at the turn of the century to use //acetic acid residues// for modification purposes, to "acetylate".

The elementary significance of Hoffmann's work on salicylic acid in the development shown here is that its procedure uses an instructive example to present the heuristic function of the dual structure of the chemical structural formula for the industrial era of medication research: It was due solely to this – primarily speculative – differentiation between those molecular constituents representing in elementary terms the main pharmacological effect of a substance and those merely modifying it, possibly destroying or supporting it with side-effects, that new medical preparations could be synthetised purposefully, without any basic biochemical or pathophysiological expertise. The discovery of representologemes such as /salicylic acid/ as bearers of the main pharmacological effect, which always had to precede a systematically modifying research process of this kind, was the direct outcome of a functionalistic or utilitarian concept only in those rare cases in which the discovery could link up with the wealth of experience passed down by the lore of healing. It was much more frequently the outcome of a "durch scharfe Naturbeobachtung veredelten Zufalls" ['coincidence refined by keen observation of Nature'] (Hofmann 1920: 274) or of a pharmacological assiduity that examined at random all possible synthetisable substances for possible biological effects. From this perspective, today's development in therapeutics can be described very fittingly as a discontinuous process, during the course of which systematic research projects are constantly being induced by more or less fortuitous "changes of paradigm " (Kuhn 1962[25]) in a particularly literal sense. In this process, it was quite possible for more than one main effect to be discovered in one single representologeme during the course of its history, resulting again and again in such an induction.

Mutschler (1982) has illustrated this with the example of //sulfachrysoidine// – developed, like so many parent substances,[26] from an industrial dye – which played an important part in the early stages of development of /sulfonamides/ by Domagk on account of its bacteriological properties. The /sulfonamides/ later acted in their turn as /representosyntactemes/ for the development of an important group of /diuretics/ and for the most important group yet of /oral antidiabetics/.

An economically rather than heuristically significant cause of the morphematic modification of representologemes emerged as the pharmaceutical industry underwent further development. Attaching some – therapeutically inconsequential – representemes to an already proven representologeme enabled flourishing markets to be penetrated with a new, patentable preparation. Fritz Hofmann described this practice as "schofle Analogieschusterei" ['paltry analogy-cobbling'] as early as 1920. This pharmacologist, who had long been engaged in research work at the Elberfeld *Farbenfabriken* (and who was not related to his Elberfeld colleague Felix Hoffmann, who had discovered the chemistry of //acetylsalicylic acid//), presented a paper on the development of medical preparations to Breslau Chemical Society in July 1920. This was published with the subheading *Erinnerungen aus den Praxis* [Recollections from experience]. Referring to the incipient production of medical preparations, he writes: "Wie neue wirksame Arzneimittel zu machen waren wußte damals eigentlich niemand. Ob man es heute weiß?" ['No one really knew at that time how new, effective drugs were to be made. Do we know now?'] (Hofmann 1920: 274).

A somewhat longer passage is now to be quoted from his paper; this reflects much of the atmosphere of the pioneering period, whose most successful outcome can still today be regarded as //acetylsalicylic acid//. This passage also mentions the proprietary name of another substance (/Heroin/) that resulted from the "acetylation" of a previously known base, //morphine//. With its preproprial, denotative constituents, this proprietary name may link up with the "battlefield metaphorics" referred to above. Its postproprial connotations, related to a side-effect of this substance that long went virtually unheeded – their vast addiction-producing potential – should be sufficiently known:

> Gestehn wir es nur offen: die Herren haben damals eine feine Nase gehabt und "Instinkt ist eine große Sache", sagt schon Falstaff. Wirklich hervorragendes haben sie mit ihrer simplen Acetylierung geleistet. "Heroin" – als Diacetylmorphin chemisch schon längst bekannt – wurde als Sedativum besonders der Respirationsorgane durch Dreser so eingeführt und erfreut sich noch heute der Wertschätzung, und ganz besonders brachte uns diese Arbeitsrichtung das Aspirin. Unreine Acetylsalicylsäure war einst in den 60er Jahren [des 19. Jahrhunderts, K. S.] als Doktorpräparat von Prinshorn, dem nachmaligen Direktor der "Continental" in Hannover im Krautschen Laboratorium zuerst dargestellt worden. Ihre Bedeutung aber hatte niemand erkannt. Felix Hoffmann aus Elberfeld bereitete die Säure aufs neue, diesmal aber rein und machte sie der pharmakologischen Prüfung zugänglich. Der Stamm des Namens Aspirin ist der gleiche wie in Spiräa. In Spiräenblüten sind ja schon sehr früh Salicylsäurederivate gefunden worden. Diese Erinnerung wollte man in Aspirin verewigen. Sie kennen alle das Aspirin zur Genüge, und ich brauche deshalb mit seinen Eigenschaften und unleugbaren Vorzügen bei Ihnen nicht hausieren zu gehen. [Let us admit it quite frankly: the gentlemen used their sixth sense at that time and "Instinct is a great matter" is one of Falstaff's statements [Shakespeare: King Henry IV, Part I, II, IV; K. S.]. What they achieved with their simple acetylation was truly outstanding. "Heroin" – long known in the chemical field as

diacetylmorphine – was thus introduced by Dreser as a sedative for the respiratory organs in particular and is still esteemed today, and most important of all it was work in this direction that brought us Aspirin. Impure acetylsalicylic acid was first produced in the 60s [the 1860s; K. S.] as a medical preparation by Prinshorn, the subsequent director of "Continental" in Hanover, in the Kraut laboratory. Its significance went unrecognised, however. Felix Hofmann from Elberfeld produced the acid anew, but this time in pure form, and made it accessible for pharmacological testing ... The name Aspirin has the same root as Spiraea. Salicylic acid derivatives were found at a very early stage in flowers of Spiraea. This evocation was to be immortalised in Aspirin. You are all so familiar with Aspirin that there is no need for me to go peddling its characteristics and undeniable advantages to you.] (Hofmann 1920: 274; accentuations removed).

Hofmann thus gives in his lecture an explanation of the preproprial constituents of what subsequently became a proprietary name: /acetylsalicylic acid/. With this interpretation he links up with a chapter from the history of /salicylic acid/ already referred to here. Heinrich Dreser, manager of the pharmacological laboratory of the *Farbenwerke* at the turn of the century, explains the nomenclature as follows: "Die Bezeichnung Aspirin ist abgeleitet aus "Spirsäure" = alter Name der Salicylsäure und A = Acetyl; statt acetylierte Spirsäure, kurzweg "Aspirin"." ['The name Aspirin is derived from "spiroyligious acid" = former name of salicylic acid and A = acetyl; instead of acetylised spiroyligious acid, condensed to "Aspirin".'] (Dreser 1899: 30).

It is not quite clear to whom credit is due for the proprietary name of the new substance. According to Gordonoff (1965), it was a proposal put forward by the then manager of the pharmaco-scientific department of the *Farbenfabriken*, Arthur Eichengrün. The smouldering hierarchy conflict that possibly developed between the departmental managers, Dreser and Eichengrün, with regard to its clinical testing and introduction may well – as is shown below – also have a significant bearing on its proprietary name.

In spring 1899, German and international patents were applied for to protect the proprietary rights of /Aspirin/[27]. The mass production of //Aspirin// was accompanied by what was then an extremely costly and time-consuming production of demand for Aspirin[28]. Within the scope of an international advertising campaign, the new product was boosted as a "substitute for salicylates " (cf. de Ridder 1984), even though it too – at least from the pharmacological viewpoint – was a salicylate, though one that admittedly stood out against the older salicylates on account of its sensationally good tolerability. The development in demand and the accompanying conquest of ubiquity gained breathtaking momentum and very soon resulted in the name losing its copyright – as already stated – on some markets. As early as 1928, 3000 tonnes of //acetylsalicylic acid// were being produced worldwide. De Ridder (1984) estimated worldwide annual production in modern times at 50,000 tonnes. Application of the new remedy was initially restricted, like the older //salicylates//, to symptomatic antipyresis and the alleviation of rheumatic complaints; it then expanded, however, attaining its broadest scope between the two World Wars, until eventually, as Schlenk (1947) states in his monograph on //salicylic acid//, there were virtually no disorders that had not been treated with it at some time or another. In 1911 a doctor writing in a reputed German scientific journal enjoined "Menschen zwischen 50 und 60 Jahren … chronische Salicylesser zu werden, und aber besonders jede frische Infektion sofort energisch mit diesem Medikament zu behandeln" ['people between 50 and 60 years of age to become chronic salicyl takers and yet to treat each fresh infection in particular with this drug immediately '] (quoted from Hangarter 1974a:8).

There are some indications that //aspirin// and /aspirin/ now and then had the standing enjoyed by universal remedies and longevity enhancers throughout social history, that they may even have become an acme of a hope, typical of that epoque, of further advances in bringing Nature under control. In 1950, an anthology of eyewitness reports on the political culture of the USA between the Prohibition and /Pearl Harbor/ was published in London. Its title was The Aspirin Age[29]. The substantiation of this choice of title in the publisher's preface shows clearly how this culmination of hope came about and how macabre it must have appeared to the observer in retrospect, some five years after /Hiroshima/: "We seem to have fluctuated between headaches: sometimes induced by prohibition, more frequently by the fevered pace of the time. During these throbbing[30] years we searched in vain for a cure-all, coming no closer to it than the aspirin bottle. Hence: The Aspirin Age." (Leighton 1950: XI).

The great extent to which the range of indications and the frequency of side-effects also hinge on culture can be observed very vividly in contemporary American culture, in which /aspirin/ has crossed the threshold between use of and indulgence[31] in products with a platitude otherwise unusual for medical preparations by becoming an essential part of the hangover breakfast (cf. Cornfeld – Edwards 1985). With a higher pro capita consumption and higher single doses, side-effects are probably less prevalent in the USA than in Central Europe (Hangarter 1974b: 1976).

The phases of the interdependent disciplines of natural history and the social history of //acetylsalicylic acid// so far covered in this chapter have shown how accurate observation of natural phenomena has given rise, by mediating various similarity models, to a natural remedy with limited application and then – through a leap forward in quality, designated here as a "paradigm change" (Kuhn 1962) – to a synthetic remedy with apparently almost unlimited application. The distinction drawn here between /natural/ and /synthetic/ is admittedly largely arbitrary; for at least when the definitory difference is to be settled by reference to the production method, it very soon becomes clear that all synthetic basic and intermediate compounds of the //acetylsalicylic acid// synthesis must at some time have been natural products. But what is synthetic is above all the chemical, atomistic – or, in more general terms, the representematic – concept in Felix Hoffmann's project dating from October 1897. The outstandingly important point is that this project originated at a time when elementary factors of algophysiology and ways and means of influencing it were still largely uninvestigated. This delineation is more a speculative similarity mosaic than the utilitarian outcome of an equation with only one unknown quantity.

In the course of discussing a third answer to the question /What is the meaning of aspirin?/, it is now to be shown how remarkably close to the ars naturam imitandi from the early period of human control over Nature the production and application of "analgesics" have been drawn again by some more recent results of research into pain.

1.3. /Aspirin/ as an analgesic

A search in dictionaries for the lemma /aspirin/ will reveal either no entry, most likely the paraphase /analgesic and antipyretic/, and possibly a reference to //acetylsalicylic acid//. This appears to characterise adequately the "state-of-the-art" lexicalisation of its everyday usage as well as its status in the positional system of medical preparations and of compounds occurring in organic chemistry. Within the scope of the considerations set out above and with the objective of forming a precise definition of the meaning of /aspirin/ as the significate of a cultural unit, it now seems possible to trace back the history of this lexicalisation systematically in diachronous perspective. /Systematic/ means here, in more precise terms: based on three important stages of development of the psychobiological event "pain" and the degrees of human control over nature reflected in these stages. The individual stages are:

(1) The secularisation of pain in the seventeenth century.

(2) The consumability of /analgesia/ through the introduction of /aspirin/.

(3) The discovery of //prostaglandins// (and //endorphins//) as a link with the *ars naturam imitandi* in the "fight" against pain.

It was in the first decade of the twentieth century that the development of //acetylsalicylic acid// led for the first time in pharmacological history to the mass production of an analgesic suitable for self-administration. As a "concrete sign of its virtual use" (Eco 1976: 24), /aspirin/ radically deposed pain as an ontological admonisher from a specific stage of its diffusion onwards. Consideration of the prerequisites for this deposition and of the events leading up to it shows it to be extremely surprising for two reasons:

(1) //Acetylsalicylic acid// was neither the first nor at that time the most potent analgesic in the pharmacopoeia of occidental medicine[32]. Pain as the limit to human control over Nature had, after all, outlived the discovery of morphium (1803), the introduction of anesthetic nitrous oxide (1844) and anesthetic ether (1846). The //opium poppy// as a natural base of all pain-killing opium alkaloids is moreover recorded in pharmacopoeias dating from antiquity and has been identified, at least as an important cultivated plant, at the margin of neolithic lake-dwelling settlements (Valentin 1950: 7). The /catalyst function/ of /aspirin/ in social history as reflected in the twentieth century rationalisation process can obviously not be explained by its pharmacological properties alone.

(2) //Acetylsalicylic acid// was not developed as an analgesic but as an antipyretic, and possibly as an antirheumatic agent with better tolerance than //salicylic acid derivatives//. The pain-killing properties of //salicylic acid// in the treatment of rheumatic diseases were described as early as 1876 by Stricker, but only in close conjunction with this group of syndromes. Initially, however, these pain-killing properties had virtually no influence on classification within the semantic system of medical preparation designations. The historical encyclopedia of pharmacological drug groups published by Schneider (1968) makes no mention of today's customary group designation of /analgesics/ for the entire nineteenth century. Salicylic acid is listed there (Schneider 1968: 32) only as an "antirheumatic agent". It would have been unlikely to occur even to Felix Hoffmann to use //aspirin// for fighting pain outside the rheumatic sphere, such as for the relief of headache or toothache, as is customary today.

The deposition of pain as an ontological admonisher, which resulted from the consumability of /analgesia/, can be understood as an interaction of at least three factors:

(1) the development of a pharmacologically efficient substance,

(2) its new utilitarian interpretation as an outcome of everyday use, and

(3) the diffusion of this re-interpreted use in the wake of a dynamic multiplication of economic interchange relationships, leading to mass consumption.

This mass consumption has in its turn set another re-interpretation in motion, one that can only be touched upon here.[33] As we have seen, one of the factors to which acetylsalicylic acid owes its popularity is the virtual absence of those undesirable side-effects that had occurred with all other salicylic acid derivatives. The proliferating consumption of aspirin resulting from this popularity led, on the other hand, to another development that has brought to light new side-effects of this substance, some of them ominous, that would certainly have long gone undetected had consumption remained at nineteenth century levels. Yet mass consumption makes rare phenomena quantifiable too. De Ridder quotes – though without acknowledging his source – the annual incidence rate of severe salicylate poisoning (due mainly to allergic side-effects) in the USA at 10,000 cases with a total annual consumption of 36,000,000,000 tablets containing acetylsalicylic acid (de Ridder 1984: 82). In quantitative terms, the influence of this re-interpretation on the cultural unit is admittedly – in view of the underlying side-effects – negligible.[34]

Let us now consider the earliest of the three diachronous stages of development of the cultural event /pain/ that play a special role within the framework of interpreting the significate /aspirin/ as an analgesic: the secularisation of pain in the seventeenth century.

Fabrega and Thyma (1976) have made a detailed diachonic analysis of the use of the four major pain-related lexemes /pain/, /ache/, /hurt/ and /sore/ from their Greco-Roman or Indo-European roots up to present-day language. Their study illustrates quite clearly that a stable semantic system for designating different qualities or locations of pain has never been formed, that it is only the intensity of pain that could be differentiated with any invariance (Fabrega – Thyma 1976: 365). The authors highlight the collocative proximity of various preliminary stages of /pain/ and /ache/ to the semantic field surrounding suffering, punishment, wrongdoing and justice. Their comment on this finding is guarded: "One is left to speculate whether a folk theory of natural or prenatural causality may have underlain this theme." (Fabrega – Thyma 1976: 365)

Toellner has published a survey of the various re-interpretations of pain as "Zeichen für den allgemeinen Mangel der Natur" ['a sign of the general deficiency of nature'] (Toellner 1971:39) up to its decisive re-interpretation by Descartes. He identifies one characteristic peculiarity of the problem of pain in the fact "daß derjenige es gar nicht zu Gesicht bekommt, der versucht, sich zu dem Schmerzproblem wertneutral zu verhalten" ['that he who endeavours to adopt neutral values in his attitude towards the problem of pain never sets eyes on it'] (Toellner 1971: 37). The history of pain is unfurled consistently as a sequence of evaluating attitudes anchored in various contexts:

> Ob dieser Mangel nun verstanden wird als Disharmonie unter den Elementen und Qualitäten des Kosmos, wie bei den hippokratischen Ärzten, oder als notwendig defizienter Modus alles Daseienden in seiner Vielfalt wie bei den Neuplatonikern und den Gnostikern; ob dieser Schaden verstanden wird als Folge der schlechten, unzureichenden Arbeit des Demiurgen, wie bei den Manichäern, oder – wie bei den Christen – als Folge des Sündenfalls, immer liegt die Auffassung zugrunde, daß die Natur der Dinge wesenhaft verderbt und daß dies letztlich die Ursache für Schmerz und Tod sei. [Whether this deficiency is understood as disharmony among the elements and qualities of the cosmos, as it was among the Hippocratic physicians, or as a necessarily deficient mode of everything existing in its diversity, as it was among the Neo-Platonics and the Gnostics; whether this damage is understood as a consequence of the poor, inadequate work of the demiurges, as it was by the Manichees, or as a consequence of the fall of man – as among the Christians – the fundamental concept is always that the nature of things is corrupted in its substance and that this is ultimately the cause of pain and death.] (Toellner 1971: 37)

As long as association with pain remained restricted to the ontology of /why?/, the idea of fighting pain had of necessity to find itself in hopeless conflict again and again with respect for the "Erbübel der gefallenen Schöpfung" ['stigma of the fallen creature'] (Toellner 1971: 40). This constellation may have succeeded in conserving so much self-consciousness and caution far beyond the secularisation of pain that "trotz Kenntnis narkotisierender Mittel dem Versuch der Schmerzausschaltung so wenig Beachtung geschenkt worden ist" ['despite knowledge of narcotising agents, so little attention was paid to the attempt to eliminate pain'] (Toellner 1971: 40).

Whilst the re-interpretation of pain originating with Descartes in the seventeenth century did bring about a radical change in the sign of traditional valuations, it nevertheless resisted any temptation to idealise its conquest. The consequence of a rationalisation of the body was that pain was promoted from "penance" to welcome protector of life, to alarm system or – if the process is observed from the aspect of profanation – even to watchman over biological integrity. And yet it created one important prerequisite for the consumability of analgesia in the twentieth century: Pain not only lost its spell but was simultaneously deprived of its soul, cut off from the significant world of fear and awareness of guilt, as whose significate it had been so reliably established and for whose residues Descartes had set up a reserve in the pineal gland ("epiphysis"):

> Weil Descartes das Bewußtsein, als das erkennende Subjekt, von der Gegenstands-, der Körperwelt, als dem erkannten Objekt, und damit den Leib von der Seele trennt, kann er jetzt den entseelten Körper als technischen Apparat, als Automaten verstehen. Auf das Schmerzproblem angewandt, bedeutet dieser Entwurf, daß der Schmerzvorgang zu einem rein körperlichen wird, die

Schmerzreaktion zu einem Reflex. Der Körperschmerz löst Schutz- und Abwehrreaktionen aus, die allesamt auf Nervenbahnen ihren Weg über die Epiphyse nehmen. Erst in der Epiphyse als dem Sitz der Seele entsteht das Schmerzerlebnis, aus dem die Seele lernt, das Schädlichste zu vermeiden. Der Schmerz ist gut, weil er zweckvoll ist, weil er nützt. [Because Descartes detaches consciousness, as the perceiving subject, from the concrete, bodily world, as the perceived object, he can now understand the inanimate body as a technical apparatus, as an automaton. Applied to the problem of pain, this outline means that the pain process becomes a purely physical one, and the reaction to pain a reflex. Physical pain triggers protective and defensive reactions, all of which make their way on nerve tracts by way of the epiphysis. It is only in the epiphysis as the seat of the mind that the experience of pain occurs, an experience from which the mind learns to avoid what is most harmful. Pain is good because it is purposeful, because it is beneficial.] (Toellner 1971: 41).

By dissecting the event /pain/ analytically into anatomical and morphological components and giving them a functionalistic interpretation, Descartes reifies a previously abstractly threatening event into a spatiotemporally limited process. This process begins with the pain-triggering impulse at the periphery of the body and ends with a central representation that can be located in the brain. From this point onwards, physiological and chemical – and to a high degree anthropological – research into pain is focused primarily on the spatiotemporal connection between these starting and finishing points of the Cartesian program. Pain is consequently grasped as a mediation, modification and transfer of something that might be designated /information/ in the broadest sense of the word. Within the scope of a "dialectic between codes and messages" (Eco 1976: 161), pain is thus experienced as interesting for a long time to come, principally on the part of the codes: "The perceptual experience of pain is viewed as identical to a state of the brain; more generally as the accompaniment or representation of a state of the nervous system as a whole." (Fabrega – Thyma 1976: 350)

With respect to the degree of control over Nature permitted and explained by it, the second and third diachronous stages of development of the event /pain/, which are now to be examined, can be understood only as an outcome of this perspectival ruling. Closer consideration of /acetylsalicylic acid/ first leads to the starting point of Descarte's program, to the periphery of the human body: it shows how pain is interpreted in the course of its biochemical research as a significant signal of a lesion in organic material and what role is played by /acetylsalicylic acid/ within the context of this interpretation. A subsequent excursus deals with one chapter of pain research not directly related to /acetylsalicylic acid/ but representing a prolific example of an approach to the artefact issue in the context of control over Nature through the fight against pain. The setting for this chapter from pain research is at the finishing point of the Cartesian program, at the location of centralised representation of pain in the human central nervous system.

Around the beginning of the second third of the twentieth century, fundamental research into organic chemistry shifted the focus of its interest from the systematic consideration of low-molecular compounds to far more complex "macromolecules" that might be composed of thousands, even tens of thousands, of single atomic bodies and were hardly to be conceptualised in terms of traditional double-coded "structural formulae". Within the framework of the sequence of different complexity stages of organic chemistry (compared in Table 1 with different complexity stages of synchronous linguistics), this implies a shift of interest from the fourth to the fifth structural level or – in more precise terms – from the formulation of "stoichiometrically" exact reaction equations to a description of the biochemical metabolism based on systems theory and enriched with new speculative elements. This advance towards the phenomena of life was bought at the expense of customary analytical precision. For a long time, the existence of many hormones, vitamins and enzymes was substantiated solely by observation of their effect and not by precise knowledge of their structures.[35] It was for this reason that biochemical macromolecules, though relatively well researched, were far from being synthetisable. These substances were, however, hardly suited to pharmacological /application/ even beyond the eventual clarification of their structure; for although synthesis was consequently possible in individual cases, it once again remained economically unviable over a long period on account of the high costs involved[36]. The special role played in pharmacology by modern biochemistry was initially due not so much to its having permitted new remedies to be produced as to its having helped explain the mechanism of action of already proven remedies. This in its turn led to a change – though at first only in the circles of those professionally involved with it – in the cultural status of these remedies, for the clarification of their mechanism of action released them in a fascinating way from the odium of artificiality and in many cases substantiated the naturalness of their use in retrospect. Any drug is of necessity far less suspect as a cultural unit if its effect can be explained as a simulation of natural biological processes; its status as an instrument of control over Nature then appears legitimated once and for all. The effect of this re-interpretation is now to be analysed in more detail, based on the /acetylsalicylic acid/ paradigm, even though it certainly has to be admitted that the significance of this effect in the cultural status of this remedy is probably negligible. For a semiotic approach, however, it is of special qualitative significance, for the basic semiotic structure permitting this effect is the modelling of similarity.

In 1933 and 1934, Goldblatt and von Euler (reference taken from Samuelsson 1965) isolated from human seminal fluid and from the seminal vesicle of the ram a substance capable of stimulating smooth muscle cells and blood vessels on direct local exposure. The two authors had hardly any precise concept of the "structural formula" of the new substance. Because of the topographical proximity of their tissue of origin to the prostate gland, they called it /prostaglandin/. It was eventually shown to comprise a group of different substances, which were given the collective designation of /prostaglandins/ as a heuristic framework concept. In the course of time, numerous biological effects of these substances were discovered, starting with their close association with the metabolism of vitamins and hormones and culminating in their connection with the biochemistry of the event /pain/, which is to be dealt with in more detail below. In 1972, a scientific journal dedicated solely to the prostaglandins was founded; this journal meanwhile enjoys a good reputation and high circulation figures.

Vane (1971) proved in an in vitro experiment that a marked fall in the synthesis rate of prostaglandins in pounded organic extracts from guinea-pig lungs was induced by adding acetylsalicylic acid. This discovery had trend-setting effects for a biochemical concept of the biological integrity of organic material, and it paved the way to the first well-founded explanation of the possibility of relieving pain by means of //acetylsalicylic acid// in peripheral body tissues. Varying as the effects and characteristics of the different prostaglandins were, so unexpectedly mutual was their highly concentrated presence in damaged tissue, no matter what the cause of this damage might be. Vane then inflicted the greatest possible mechanical damage on the guinea-pig lungs examined by him by homogenising them, in other words by mincing and pulping them, using a standardised method. The addition of acetylsalicylic acid to the homogenate resulted in a distinct, dose-related reduction in the expectedly high concentration of prostaglandins. Acetylsalicylic acid thus prevented the formation or the release of substances linked spatiotemporally with the influence of tissue damage. Very little was known at that time about a direct link between the event pain and the prostaglandins. This trail can be said to have been followed systematically only as a result of Vane's experiment. In the meantime it has been established (Stacher 1984) that damage to the membrane of any tissue cell triggers off a cascade-like synthesis of prostaglandins. Some of these prostaglandins lead, through a largely unknown mechanism, to a significant reduction in the pain threshold, to what is known as hyperalgesia (Ferreira – Nakamura 1979). Whilst not inducing any pain, they do enable the nervous system to detect otherwise non-specific events as significant stimuli for perception of pain. The influence of acetylsalicylic acid stops the synthesis of these prostaglandins, interrupting the related signification process. This procedure is explained in essentially hypothetical terms by the model of /enzyme inhibition/:

Enzymes are /biocatalysts/ essential for the conversion of biochemical substrates into living organisms. They induce the sudden increase in biochemical reactions between substrates that are to be changed by these reactions, whilst themselves remaining unchanged. The achievement of these enzymes, as demonstrated by the model, is in their specificity. They are equipped with receptors enabling them to identify the substrate needed for the reaction to be catalysed. The specific affinity between enzymes and their substrates is a modern realisation of the *attractio electiva* (Bergman [1968]) which is constitutive of chemical theory and which is dealt with in greater detail, based on further examples, in Chapter 3. The catalysing function of enzymes can – as provided for by the model – be cancelled by being confronted with /pseudosubstrates/ so similar to the genuine substrate as to bind to them despite their unsuitability for the reaction that is to be catalysed. This reaction is thus inhibited by having its catalyst misled by a "pseudosubstrate". The affinity of the "pseudosubstrate" with the genuine substrate is one of subtly calculated similarity: It has to be just great enough for the pseudosubstrate to be identified by the enzyme but not enough for the reaction of significance to the enzyme to take place too.

The experimentally substantiated interpretation of acetylsalicylic acid as a "pseudosubstrate" of prostaglandin synthesis sees the effect of a pharmacon as a deception permitted by calculated similarity. /Aspirin/ appears in this interpretative context as an artefact outwitting[37] the organism by cancelling the validity of one of its codes at a decisive point. The "pseudosubstrate" /acetylsalicylic acid/ is a heuristic link in the "chain of interpretants" of «Aspirin».

The diachrony of /aspirin/ as a lemma of contemporary language with the meaning /pain-killer/ or /analgesic/ thus turns full circle: Pain as an ontological admonisher, as a real-life recollection of the "Erbübel der gefallenen Schöpfung" ['stigma of the fallen creature'] (Toellner 1971: 40), but also as a psychobiological event expressing sorrow and depression, has been deprived of a major part of its cultural significance in the course of a rationalisation process initiated by enlightenment and completed by the precise analytical methods of the natural sciences. This process of deposing, perhaps even outwitting, pain is accompanied by the rise of /aspirin/ to the status of a mass-consumption analgesic. An outstandingly important factor here is that this discovery coincides, at least temporally, not so much with the discovery of appropriate substances as with its explosive diffusion by industrial production and marketing. It was during the most intensive phase of this development, in the industrialised society between the two World Wars, that the influence of /aspirin/ as a universal remedy and potential longevity enhancer had peaked, to stand for a time as a promising symbol of human control over Nature. In the "chain of interpretants" of «Aspirin», this is a monumental, still effective link from the most recent past, a link that may give the postproprial connotative constituents of the proprietary name /Aspirin/ their essential direction. If "... eine Gesellschaft, die Gesundheit als höchstes Gut feiert, Schmerzlosigkeit höher als den Konsum setzen muß" ['... a society that acclaims good health as the supreme good has to set freedom from pain higher than consumption'] (Ridder 1979: 5), then what may the very consumption of analgesia mean to it?

In the early 1970s, biochemical research into pain brought to light a discovery that was to turn the traditional concept of artificial pain-killing upside down: the discovery of /endorphins/. Mutschler (1982: 16) has designated it "eines der interessantesten Kapitel der Arzneimittelforschung der letzten Jahre" ['one of the most interesting chapters of drug research in recent years']. As the distinction between /natural/ and /artificial/ has a special status in semiotic discourse, this chapter of research is to be dealt with briefly at this point, based on a summarised presentation by Herz (1982), although it has no direct bearing on the analgesic mechanism of action of //acetylsalicylic acid//:

Since the discovery of //morphium// by Heinrich Sertürner in 1803, knowledge of the narcotic, euphorising, cough-suppressant – and above all the analgesic – properties of this "opium alkaloid", prepared from juice of the opium poppy, had gradually spread. Based on this heterogeneous constellation of effects, it was very soon hypothesised that this substance must develop its essential effect not in the peripheral tissue but at the location of central control and coordination, in other words in the central nervous system. Morphological location of this effect was not feasible, however, until radiolabeling of substances passed into the body permitted even long-term determination of their location, at least when they were enriched in high concentrations at specific sites.[38] In 1973, three research groups working independently of one another (survey in Herz 1982: 60) succeeded in proving with this method the existence of highly selective opiate enrichment sites in the central nervous system, above all in the so-called "periventricular" brain centers adjacent to the ventricles of the brain and in the //gelatinous matter// of the spinal cord, a structure of immense importance in the processing of peripheral pain signals (Melzack – Wall 1982). The observation that local enrichment of radiolabeled opiates underwent no further increase in these enrichment centers from a specific threshold dose onwards suggested that an infinite number of receptors had to be present in these centers, all of which were saturated on attainment of this threshold dose. This pharmacodynamically straightforward explanation for the dose-dependent saturation of the enrichment centers was, however, problematic, since "... es war unwahrscheinlich, daß der Organismus sozusagen "zufällig" spezielle Haftstellen für normalerweise nicht in ihm vorkommende Substanzen besitzen sollte". ['the organism was unlikely to have "by chance", as it were, specific binding points for substances not normally occurring in it".] (Herz 1982: 70).

It was this discovery that gave rise in its turn to a major teleological-heuristic temptation: If the human organism contained site-bound structures that had a complementary similarity relationship with an artefact (viz. the //opiates//), then it was indeed probable that there had to be a substance at least very similar to this artefact inside the organism as a product of the endogeneous metabolism – in other words, "natural" opiates were being produced, possibly as a constituent of pain-processing by the central nervous system. This hypothesis induced an intensive search for this substance, a search whose driving force was obviously the hope that the problem of pain might one day lose its spell once and for all to techno-scientific solutions, with a natural /analgesic/ developed from the teleological plan of evolution and therefore free from side-effects. Although the search for such substances was highly successful, the hope attached to it proved illusory. From the mid-1970s onwards, several so-called /endorphins/ were isolated; subsequent clarification of their structure permitted them to be synthesised or at least enriched in high concentrations as a prerequisite for therapeutic application. In pharmacological testing, the /endorphins/ proved to be highly potent /analgesics/, which differed in absolutely no way, however, from the artificial //morphines// with respect to the risk of addiction as the most important side-effect. Herz (1982: 73) comments in his survey on this "disappointing result" as follows: "Dieses enttäuschende Ergebnis umfangreicher Tierversuche mag im Hinblick auf das physiologische [= hier: /natürliche/] Vorkommen der Endorphine im Organismus zunächst überraschen. Dieser scheinbare Widerspruch ist wohl dadurch zu erklären, daß die Opiatrezeptoren normalerweise nicht oder nur vorübergehend mit ihren natürlichen Liganden besetzt sind, d. h. daß kein nennenswerter endorphinerger Basaltonus vorliegt." ['This disappointing result of extensive testing on laboratory animals may first be surprising in view of the physiological [here: /natural/; K. S.] occurrence of endorphins in the organism. This apparent contradiction can, however, be explained by the fact that the opiate receptors are normally not or are only temporarily equipped with their natural ligands, i. e. there is no significant endorphinergic basal tonus present.']

If this interpretation is extended to the analogy of the artefact problem, then it means that the organism has at its disposal not only the opportunity for endogenous morphine production but also an endogenous /Dangerous Drugs Act/ as a micro-economic means of preventing this production from getting out of hand.

In a semiotic respect this finding means, in clear terms, that the production of medical preparations as an outcome of creative observation of nature theoretically resulted again and again in an interpretation of human intervention as an /imitation of Nature/. Some of these have been discussed in the course of this chapter: the */ubi morbus ibi remedium/* of antiquity, Paracelsus' (1928a) doctrine of signatures, Hahnemann's (1978) *simila similibus curentur* and finally the discovery of /prostaglandin synthesis inhibition/ and the /endorphins/. A more detailed observation of their historical and semiotic contiguity is the subject of Chapter 3.

1.4. /Aspirin/ as a generator of intersubjectivity – a possible inscription on Wittgenstein's "/beetle box/"

The perception of pain is an individual experience. If pain has a body-related material correlate, then this correlate is exposed only in an indirectly effective way to the individual concerned as a psychophysical unit. If pain has a history, then it affects with its formidable, actualising presence only that individual who has developed along this history. If pain has a meaning, then this is evolved in a highly individual way within the framework of a private structure comprising denotations and connotations. Pain is threatening above all in that it isolates, makes the natural limit of subjectivity appear /painful/, barely surmountable. Yet by this very fact it motivates the often desperate endeavour to surmount it despite everything. Communicating pain is virtually impossible yet simultaneously almost vital. In his "Philosophical Investigations", Wittgenstein used a simile quoted by von Morstein (1964: 133) explicitly in connection with his "investigations into the word pain":

> Suppose everyone had a box with something in it; we call it a "beetle". No one can look into anyone else's box, and everyone says he knows what a beetle is only by looking at his beetle. – Here it would be quite possible for everyone to have something different in his box. One might even imagine such a thing constantly changing. – But suppose the word "beetle" had a use in these people's language? – If so it would not be used as the name of a thing. (Wittgenstein 1967: § 293).

This fundamental paradox is the mutual starting point of some philosophical (von Morstein 1964), sociological (Ridder 1979), linguistic (Ehlich 1985) and psychological (Melzack – Torgerson 1971; Röth – Lehrl 1973) approaches to treating the "language of pain" as the subject of scientific investigations.

The already mentioned diachronic investigation by Fabrega and Thyma (1976) on the linguistic differentiation of pain is supplemented in a synchronic perspective by studies by Melzack and Torgerson (1971) and by Röth and Lehrl (1973). These authors confronted various proband groups with attributes of pain listed in their native language and asked them to assess these attributes with respect to their ability to differentiate between different qualities and intensities of pain.

Melzack and Torgerson first divided the attributes of pain into three main categories: "sensory words", "affective words" and "evaluative words" (Melzack – Torgerson 1971: 52). These they differentiated into thirteen further subcategories to which they had the individual attributes allocated by healthy probands. They then calculated the proportion of conforming allocations in the total proband population for each pain attribute.

Röth and Lehrl (1973) had a similar list of attributes assessed by probands who themselves were affected by a painful disorder. Their proband population was thus more heterogeneous with respect to different qualities of pain, as well as more competent because of its higher proportion of personal experience. The probands were asked to assess the degree of conformity between the offered attributes and their own pain on a six-point scale. Subsequent factor-analytical processing of these data revealed that 72% of the total variance of these allocations was to be explained by 10 main components.

The distinct conformity revealed by the two studies[39] between the individual probands supports the hypothesis that lexicalisation of an attributive differentiating system in the semantic field /pain/ has indeed occurred to a certain degree both in English (Melzack – Torgerson 1971) and in German (Röth – Lehrl 1973), although no consistent allocation of specific attributes of pain to specific qualities of pain (in English) is to be detected in the diachronic analysis by Fabrega and Thyma.

Empirical analysis thus reveals for the language of pain a degree of intersubjectivity probably not quantifiable out of hand on lexicographic principles alone.

Ehlich (1985: 180) has differentiated "three types of expressing pain" with respect to the aspect of linguistic action : "... crying and groaning, pain interjections and pain descriptions".

He shows that pain may well be an important object of both verbal and nonverbal communication, that expressing pain may perform social – in other words /contact-priming/ – functions: "Whereas pain has appeared as one of the most outstanding solipsistic phenomena in philosophical analysis, from a linguistic point of view, pain is primarily an interactional phenomenon, not a solipsistic sensation." (Ehlich 1985: 180).

Nevertheless, the language of pain is often little more than a /painfully/ unsatisfying device with respect to its theoretical potential for imparting information. Within the framework of a confrontation with Wittgenstein's point of view, Ehlich writes on the type of "pain description" expressed by himself: "The vagueness or even absence of words hinders a clear verbalisation; the underdevelopment of the semantic field of expressions for pain forces S ['the speaker'; K. S.] to speak with unclear metaphors." (Ehlich 1985: 185). And: "The addressee of a description of pain easily gets lost when he demands preciseness on the part of the speaker." (Ehlich 1985: 185).

Now the language of pain is probably confined to the digressions of metaphors in a similar way to that used to describe other sensations; what is specific to the problem of pain and its linguistic management, however, is the confusing, multidimensional linking of the experience of pain to thoroughly concrete nonverbal references. And it is this very line that Wittgenstein has taken up in his simile. Pain comprises in a much more concrete sense than joy, hope or fear also a distinct portion of a *res extensa*. Whilst not necessarily visible, this portion is at least present in the perception of pain as well as in any attempt to communicate it. Pain has been associated with it down into everyday consciousness ever since Descartes. This material or at least morphological portion of pain embodies (in a decidedly non-metaphorical sense) and augments the threat posed by the event of pain by assigning to it a spatiotemporally limited extension. One essential message of this threat is the certainty "daß dieser Leib in demselben Maße, in dem er zu mir gehört, mir wesentlich unverfügbar ist" ['that this body, to the same extent as it belongs to me, is essentially not at my disposal.'] (Ridder 1979: 12–13; accentuations removed).

The processing of pain is initiated with such a step of being stemmed by embodiment and augmentation. It flows into a process described by Ridder (1979: 1) as "Konstruktion von Kausalität" ['construction of causality']. Communication about pain is determined – in so far as it is intended to be a processing of pain too – by reference to its location, its temporal sequence and its mainly hypothetical causes. The metaphorics of describing pain may therefore often be determined by a "mechanistic" theme expressed with special clarity in the participial constructions of /piercing/, /throbbing/, /stabbing/ or /searing/ pain. If the general communicability of pain is considered from this aspect, it is these that appear among the sensations as those most suitable for embarking upon interactions anchored in the physical world.

In search of closeness, many people may therefore find it easier and possibly more promising to complain of pain than to display emotions. Pain thus becomes a "symbolische[s] Medium sozialer Interaktion und Kontrolle" ['symbolic medium of social interaction and control'] (Ridder 1979: 18): "in dem Maße, in dem Schmerzsymbole routinisiert werden, können sie Ressourcen von korrespondierendem Wert erwartbar mobilisieren" ['to the extent to which symbols of pain are routinised, they are capable, as would be expected, of mobilising resources of corresponding value.'] (Ridder 1979: 12–13; accentuations removed).

It is precisely at this point that /analgesics/ perform a function of importance to their cultural status: They are *//res extensae//* that demonstrably play a part in the processing of pain. From a specific moment in their diffusion onwards they serve – wherever pain is the topic under consideration – inter alia also to structure what has been ominously unstructured. In the language of pain, /aspirin/ is accordingly a lexeme permitting order and orientation; metaphorically one might refer to: /a hard currency of the commensurable/ or, metaphorologically: "Das Paradies war: für alles einen Namen zu haben und durch den Namen sich geheuer zu machen" ['Paradise was this: having a name for everything and dispelling the sense of unease through that name'] (Blumenberg 1957: 269).

For the significance of /aspirin/ as an instrument of control over Nature, this function is hardly of less importance than its specifically pharmacological effect. A pain inducing the use of an analgesic is accorded at that very moment a status denotable by the name of this analgesic in a gradually developed, perspectival system of varying intensities and qualities. The analgesic moreover acts for the pain as a visible and therefore extra efficiently communicable memento of its morphological correlate. By using /aspirin/, the exterior of the /beetle box/ at least is given something like a label, an intersubjective decor and thus perhaps a semblance of transparency suggesting to many an addressee the gestalt inside another person's box.

The linguistic aspect of fighting pain presented here can be illustrated vividly with the two quotations below. Both of them originated as written texts in non-fictitious intent. Both reflect the characteristics of reference to time, place and hypothetical causes of experienced pain emphasised here, they reify its being vanquished as a search for both the linguistically and the extra-linguistically commensurable. Both texts were written in the early years of the golden age of /aspirin/ as an instrument of control over Nature by man. A special appreciation of language as a medium of communication and reflection and an exceptionally intimate command of it can be attributed to the authors of the two texts:

(1) Thomas Mann: Entry in his diary dated 4. 4. 1919:
Währenddem zunehmender Katarrh, scharfer, schmerzlicher Husten, wehe Luftröhre. Heißer Punsch that wohl. Fieber. Fand nach dem Schlafengehen lange keine Ruhe, der Zustand der oberen Luftwege quälte und beängstigte mich sehr. 38,4°. Aspirin beruhigte. Etwa 1/2 3 eingeschlafen. Morgens 37° und die Brust weniger scharf. [Meanwhile worsening catarrh, sharp, painful coughing, sore throat. Hot punch did me good. High temperature. Remained restless long after going to bed, the state of the upper air passages was very distressing and alarming to me. 38.4°. Aspirin brought relief. Fell asleep around 2.30 a.m.. Next morning 37° and my chest less severe.] (Mann 1979: 185)

(2) Franz Kafka: Letter to Felice Bauer dated 20. 12. 1912:
I don't exactly get a sore throat every time you have one, but when I hear about it, or suspect it, even only fear it, I suffer from it no less than you, in my own way. And I suffer even more from your exhaustion, and more still from your headaches. And if you then take some aspirin, then I too feel physically sick. All last night, that is from 3.30 to 7.30, and into the early part of the morning, I felt a strange kind of pressure inside myself such as I never remember feeling before in the thirty years of my life; it emanated neither from the stomach, nor from the heart, nor the lungs, but perhaps from all the three together. It subsided in daylight. If you took some aspirin yesterday, then I am sure it was due to that; if not, to the previous aspirins. (Kafka 1978: 223–224)

1.5. /Aspirin/ as a recipe for success for //aspirants//

Drug advertising is one of the disputed phenomena inherent in mass culture. It is difficult to have any relationship to it other than either an "apocalyptic" or an "integrated" one (cf. Eco 1964). For the semiotic determination of pharmaceutics as "cultural units", it is more than important. In line with the inductive-synthetic perspective of this chapter, however, it is dealt with here only superficially – in more precise terms, only to the extent that this can contribute towards answering the question of the meaning of /aspirin/. This aspect is dealt with in more detail and more systematically in Chapter 4.

//Aspirin// is available both on prescription and over the counter. Anyone wishing to use it can decide for himself whether to consume it within the framework of an interchange relationship or to be treated with it on professional recommendation and at the expense of his health insurance agency. The two economically fundamentally different worlds of "self-medication" on the one hand and "medical prescription" on the other converge in the use of aspirin. The protagonists of these two worlds are the patient as an enlightened master of Nature on the one hand and the doctor as an overqualified consumer counsellor on the other.

Both worlds are to some extent residues of the late medieval arcane practice in dealing with medical preparations and of a division between the economic interests motivating their production and their use respectively. They may furthermore also be connected with the early medieval division between /use/ and /indulgence /; this is not, however, to be pursued in greater detail at this point.[40] The first division at least has still today a certain direct influence on the distribution of drugs in some domains of "pharmacological therapy" in Germany, for instance. In those areas in which its has lost its validity in practical terms, its influence on the distribution of drugs is more indirect in that it has to be presented in public interchange as though this division still existed. In other words: Advertisements for self-administered drugs in Germany are like those for consumer goods – ubiquitous. Drugs subject to prescription – "ethical drugs" – are advertised in a form adapted to the residues of the division between producer interests and consumer interests, i. e. only in selected areas of distribution publicity such as surgeries and medical journals. These areas are designated and more closely specified in paragraph 2 of the law governing the advertising of medical preparations in the Federal Republic of Germany (Heilmittelwerbegesetz).[41] The doctor is analogously a free but primarily passive-receptive participant in this distributional public, as is the self-administering patient. Besides specific functions such as the exercising of governmental control authority, the restriction of advertising to selected areas is designed to create the impression that the doctor is making an autonomous therapeutic decision when prescribing any drug not available over the counter.

According to Oberender (quoted from Klinkenberg 1985), the advertising of drugs among the general public has a number of valuable functions, for "... sie bedeute für den Verbraucher mehr Markttransparenz, stärke die Souveränität des Konsumenten, erleichtere die rationale Kaufentscheidung und fördere auf der ganzen Breite den wünschenswerten Wettbewerb, sowie dadurch bedingt die Innovation". ['... it implies increased market transparency for the user, fortifies the consumer's supremacy, facilitates a rational purchasing decision and promotes desirable competition and consequently innovation along the whole line".] (Klinkenberg 1985: 7).

The implementation of this and possibly of other functions of drug advertising is now given closer consideration in the light of an advertising campaign for /Aspirin/, which is, as stated in Chapter 1, a proprietary name in Germany. This consideration is focused on the theme of this book by being confined to two fundamental questions:

What is the role played by verbal and non-verbal signs in performing these functions? And: What influence have these signs on the reality of as a "cul-

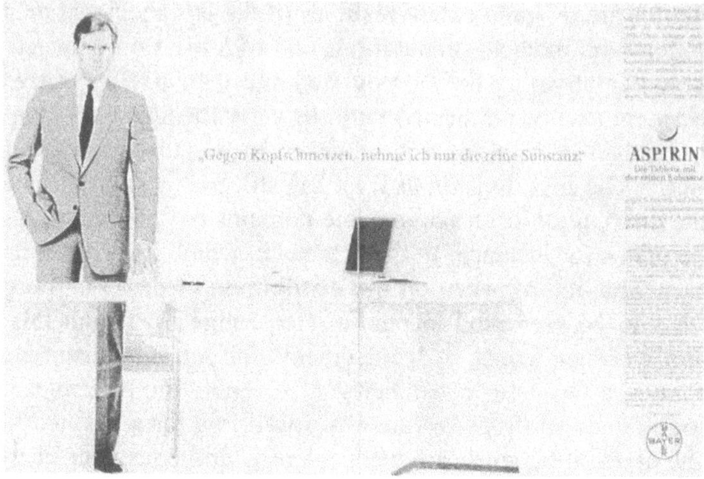

Figure 4: (Reproduced by permission of Bayer AG, Leverkusen).

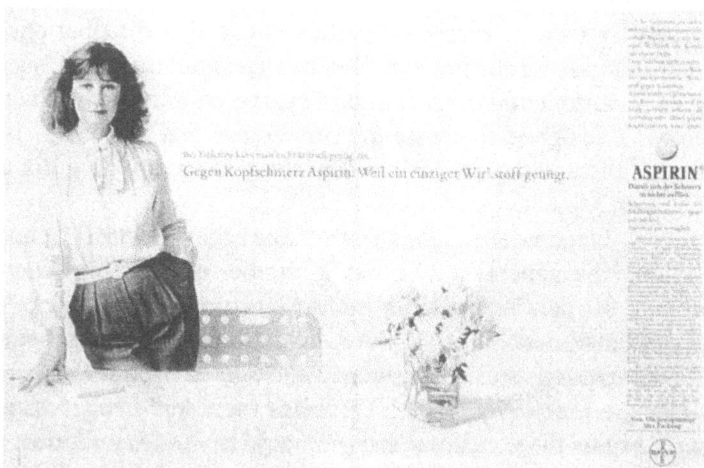

Figure 5: (Reproduced by permission of Bayer AG, Leverkusen).

tural unit"? Do they perhaps flow into one isolatable interpretant of /aspirin/ with a significant affinity with those interpretants already described?

Let us deal first with Figures 4 to 7. These are small-scale reproductions of a series of advertisements published in 1983 in the mass-circulation German pictorial *Der Stern* (vols. 10, 38, 44 and 46):

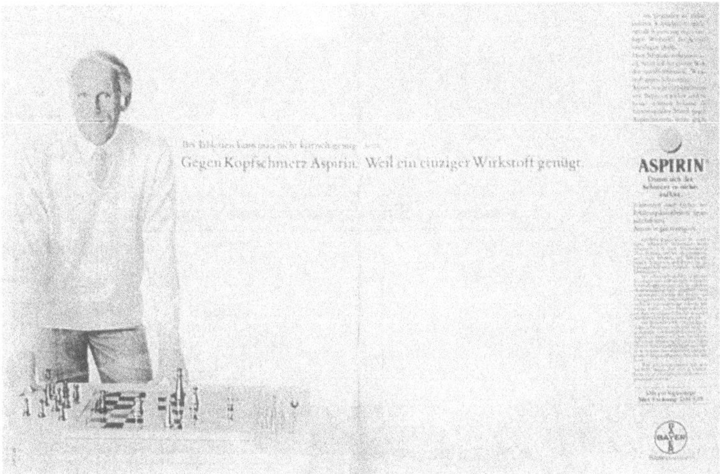

Figure 6: (Reproduced by permission of Bayer AG, Leverkusen).

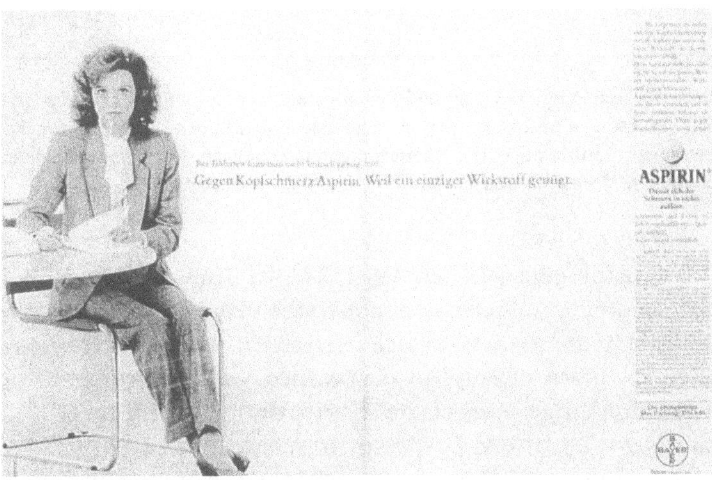

Figure 7: (Reproduced by permission of Bayer AG, Leverkusen).

A synoptic consideration of these four advertisements permits their joint semiotic structure to be described as an invariant composition of a relatively small number of constant elements, an aspect of interest in more profound analysis. So there is much to be said for describing these elements initially according to their allocation to Eco's "Register" ['registers'] of "Reklame-

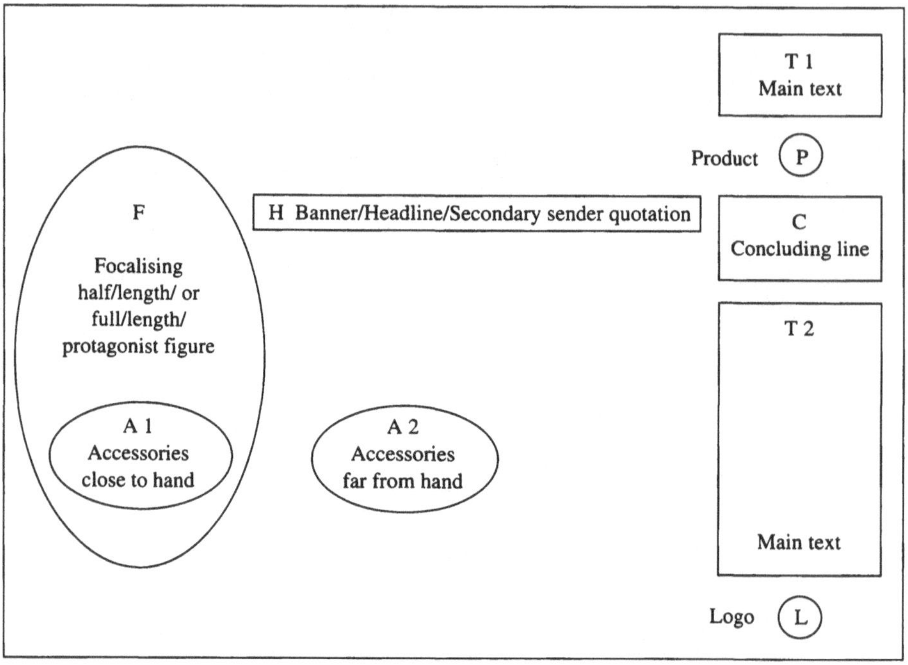

Figure 8: Rounded and angular. Visual and verbal elements of a recipe for success for aspirants. The wording of H and C means, translated into English: (C: "Aspirin. So that pain vanishes into thin air.") (H: "Aspirin against headache. Because one active substance is enough.") For the translation of T1 and T2 see note 43.

codes" ['advertising codes'] (Eco 1972: 271)[42]. They are tabled in Figure 8 and marked according to their allocation to the visual or the verbal "register".

With respect to the use of linguistic elements, all four advertisements can be characterised more closely, in accordance with a distinction drawn by Sowinski as "dreiteilige Werbetexte" ['tripartite publicity texts']. He refers to these in his survey of composite structures in advertisements as the most common form (Sowinski 1979: 70–71), defining them as follows: "Der Text besteht hier in der Regel aus einer Schlagzeile (head-line), einem längeren Zwischentext, den wir wegen des größeren Umfangs Haupttext nennen wollen, und einer Schlußzeile, meistens mit einem abschließenden Slogan, oft zusammen mit einer erneuten Produktnennung, oder allein aus dieser." ['The text here consists as a rule of a headline, a longer intermediate text which we shall call the main text on account of its greater scope, and a concluding line, mostly with a concluding slogan, often repeating the product's name, or of that alone.'] (Sowinski 1979: 71).

Those text sections that can be discriminated by means of this distinction are placed in equivalent positions and executed with the same graphic media in all four advertisements (cf. Figure 8). The sequence of these text sections is determined unequivocally by the graphic media, and in particular by the reading direction from left to right or from top to bottom, an essential characteristic of visual text reception. In the advertisements reproduced in Figures 4, 6, and 7, the headline /H/ consists in each case of two subunits and can be perceived as a "Sekundärsenderzitat" ['secondary sender quotation'] (Sowinski 1979: 71) on account of its topographical proximity to the figure of the protagonist; in advertisement 5 it is identified as such by having its different wording placed in inverted commas. The "main text" consists in all four advertisements of two subunits /T1/ and /T2/.[43] The wording of /T1/ deviates again slightly in Figure 5 from the otherwise conforming execution in Figures 4, 6, and 7. /T1/ and /T2/ are separated from each other by the concluding line /C/ which incorporates the two main elements of Sowinski's definition: concluding slogan and renewed product designation. The fact that /C/ is sited in the direct extension of the reading direction of /H/ permits these two text elements to focalise each other reciprocally within the framework of the overall composition.

On critical consideration of the advertisements, the demarcation of these four text sections may appear to be arbitrary or even an interpretative distortion. Two questions in particular are raised:

Why are /T1/ and /T2/ regarded as two related text sections distinguished from /C/ instead of all three elements being regarded as one textually homogeneous graphic unit presented in one joint graphic block? And why is /C/ designated as "concluding line" in accordance with Sowinski's theory whilst another important and extensive text element, /T2/, still follows in reading direction?

Both these questions can be answered conclusively in material-immanent terms, and this answer reveals a semantically and graphically effective punctuation phenomenon of importance to the syntagmatic structure. The discontinuity between /T1/ and /C/ and between /C/ and /T2/ is implied on the one hand by the selection of different typefaces and above all by /T2/ being connected syntactically directly with /T1/ and representing a grammatical conclusion to the sentence started there. In the further course of /T2/ there is first a brief, assertive sentence that is clearly distinguished syntactically from the previous paratactic construction and whose essential purpose is obviously to transgress the hiatus caused by /C/ between /T1/ and /T2/. /T2/ is then continued, after another indentation, with another change of typeface and with complex grammatical constructions to the very end. This typeface is so small as to be virtually indecipherable in the reproduction. At least from the graphic point of view, then, the continuation of /T2/ in its turn forms a self-contained unit after the indentation.

What is of outstanding significance for the punctuation phenomenon to be demonstrated here is the fact that this continuation of /T2/ contains nothing but that information about the product on offer that is stipulated in paragraph 4, section 1 of the law governing the advertising of medical preparations in the Federal Republic of Germany .[44] With regard to the advertising function of the text as a whole, this information is either inconsequential or – in so far as it refers to risks and side-effects of the product on offer – even detrimental. What /T2/ accordingly sets out to do is essentially to meet a statutory requirement that is in conflict in some respects with the advertising function of /H/, /T1/ and even /C/. /C/ is thus the text section designed to draw the actual advertising text to a distinct conclusion within the framework of the overall syntagma, once /T1/ has satisfied and possibly exhausted any interest that may have been taken in the small print.

At the iconic level, in other words with respect to the visual "register" (Eco 1972: 271), a distinction can be made between five elements that are executed with a certain degree of variation in the individual advertisements. The fine degrees of this variation, however, indicate the very consistency of the significance of these elements within the scope of an overall composition of iconic signs. Again in the sequence of reading direction, they are as follows (cf. Figure 8):

The total length and one quarter of the width of each of these advertisements is taken up at the left-hand margin by a focalising protagonist figure /F/. In Figures 4 and 6, these are half-length figures; in 5 and 7, they are full-length figures divided or delimited by desk-tops. At the lower end of each of the half-length figures (in Figures 4 and 6) and at the dividing level of the full-length figures (in 5 and 7) there are several accessories /A1/ sharing a topographical continuity with at least one hand of the protagonist figure. Likewise within the range of gesticulation of the protagonist figure, but not in any direct spatial relationship to it, there are additional accessories /A2/ in Figures 4 and 5. The text block at the right-hand margin is interrupted by two further iconic elements lending support to the punctuation of the text elements: by illustrating the offered product /P/ in the form of an //Aspirin tablet// in the hiatus between /T1/ and /C/ and by reproducing the logo /L/ of the company offering the product. In Figure 4, /P/ and /L/ are the same shape and size. In 5, 6, and 7, on the other hand, /L/ is somewhat larger than /P/.

With this total of nine delimitable elements, of which – according to Eco's distinction (1972: 271–275) – four are to be allocated to the "verbal register" and five to the "visual register", the semiotic structure of all four advertisements can now be described with sufficient accuracy as an invariant syntagmatic composition of constant elements:

The viewer's attention is first directed by the focalising protagonist figure /F/ to the banner /H/ and moved on from there in a direct extension of the reading direction to the concluding text /C/ and the product illustration /P/ adjacent to it. The elementary constituents of an advertising text as outlined by Sowinski (1979) are thus already prescribed, even if the viewer's attention is then distracted from the two-page spread, an inevitable occurrence in many cases. All the other elements deviate topographically from the horizontal central line and are in some respect mere appendages, corroborative but dispensable specifications of this elementary message. Within the framework of Peirce's trichotomy, the effect of the linguistic signs of this advertising message is primarily "symbolic", and that of the visual elements primarily "iconic". The reading direction as an elementary structure of visual text reception and the relations of spatial contiguity among the visual elements have accordingly a primarily indexical function[45]. The elementary advertising message follows the propositional pattern: Something about /P/ is stated by /F/ in /H/.

But now back to one of the starting-points of our discussion, to the question of whether this product message with its very clear structure and its conspicuously discreet presentation as compared with product advertising in general has any influence on the cultural unit . The only rhetorical figure in the text elements of the advertisements is the metaphor used in the concluding text /C/ of Figures 4, 6, and 7: "Aspirin – damit der Schmerz sich in nichts auflöst" ['Aspirin – so that pain vanishes into thin air']. The suggestive aggressiveness of the banner /H/, conceivable as a "secondary sender quotation" in Figures 4, 6, and 7 and even identified as such in 5, appears rather on the reserved side when compared with the average advertisment. A further conspicuous point is that the secondary sender quotation is preceded in Figures 4, 6, and 7 by an apparently consumption-critical text element: "Bei Tabletten kann man nicht kritisch genug sein" ['With tablets, you just can't be critical enough']. Obviously the advertisement presented here succeeds at first glance in performing, in a highly exemplary way, at least two of the four beneficial functions of publicity in the pharmaceutical field specified by Oberender (cf. Klinkenberg 1985: 7): reinforcing the supremacy of the consumer and promoting a rational purchasing decision. A significant contribution is also made towards facilitating "market transparency":

//Aspirin// contains only one single active pharmacological substance, //acetylsalicylic acid//; it thus differs from the large number of analgesic com-

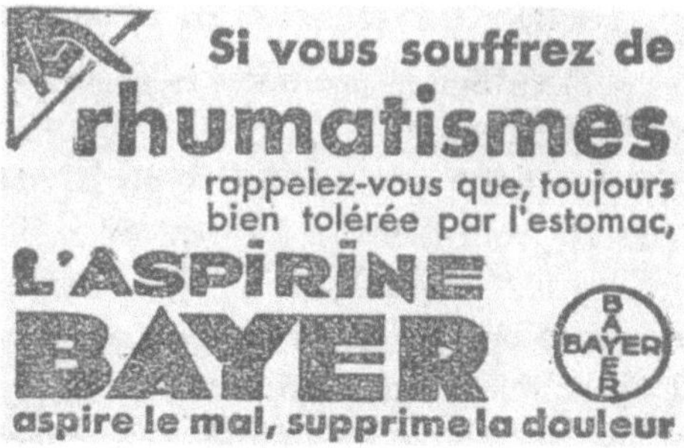
Si vous souffrez de
rhumatismes
rappelez-vous que, toujours
bien tolérée par l'estomac,
L'ASPIRINE
BAYER
BAYER
aspire le mal, supprime la douleur

Figure 9: Prepropial constituents of proprietary names as an advertising medium: classified advertisement from "Les Annales" dated 15. 4. 1931, p. VIII.

pound preparations whose market share in the Federal Republic of Germany is about three times that of "monopreparations" (Langbein – Martin – Weiss – Werner 1983: 42). As the risk of side-effects is often greater in "compound analgesics" than in "monopreparations" but their efficacy the same, the recommendation being made by the protagonist /F/ is indeed a constructive proposal for the critical consumer.

Who, though, are the men and women depicted in the four advertisements? Whom or what do they represent, and on what is their impressive supremacy based, a supremacy that they themselves recommend emulating? Since the focus here is on the semiotic aspect of drug advertisements, this question is to be followed up by consistent application of the principle *aliquid stat pro aliquo*. The figure of the protagonist deserves a separate analysis here, not only because it represents a special focus within the framework of the advertisement but also because consideration of it reveals, at least hypothetically, a possibly surprising connection with prepropial constituents of the proprietary name /Aspirin/. Figure 9 illustrates such a connection between proprietary name and prepropial root, using another, somewhat more obvious, example.

This is a reproduction of a classified advertisement from the French pictorial *Les Annales* published on 15. 4. 1931. In this case /Aspirin/ is recommended in one single grammatical sentence, one that is produced with very simple graphic resources in comparison with our contemporary advertisement and flows into the concluding text: "L'Aspirine Bayer aspire le mal, supprime la douleur." ['Bayer Aspirin absorbs sickness and suppresses pain.'][46]

In the case of the contemporary series of advertisements, any connection with prepropial constituents of the substantive /Aspirin/ is far less obvious and hardly an integral part of the intended advertising message. And yet a clue is given to such a connection by an iconological analysis of the protagonist figure. In his survey of semiotic aspects of advertising analysis at the iconographical level, Eco distinguishes two essential "codification types":

> Wir haben zwei Codifizierungstypen. Eine Codifizierung 'historischen' Typs, wodurch die Reklamekommunikation Konfigurationen benutzt, die in einer klassischen Ikonologie auf konventionalisierte Bedeutungen verweisen (von der Aureole, die Heiligkeit anzeigt, bis zu einer bestimmten Konfiguration, die die Idee der Mutterschaft suggeriert, bis zur schwarzen Binde auf dem Auge, die Pirat oder Abenteurer konnotiert usw.). Die andere Codifizierung ist publizitären Typs, wo z. B. das Mannequin-Sein von einer bestimmten Art, mit überkreuzten Beinen dazustehen, konnotiert wird. Die Gewohnheit der Reklame hat konventionalisierte Ikonogramme in Umlauf gesetzt. [We have two codification types. One codification of an 'historical' type with which advertising communication uses configurations referring in a classical iconology to conventionalised meanings (from the halo indicating sanctity to a specific configuration suggesting the idea of motherhood, to the black eyepatch connotative of a pirate or desperado etc.). The other codification is of a publicistic type where, for instance, being a mannequin is implied by a certain manner of being depicted with the legs crossed. The standard practice of the advertisement has put conventionalised iconograms into circulation.] (Eco 1972: 272)

The configuration formed by the representation of the four protagonist figures evidently joins the two codification types into one discreet and therefore exceptionally effective overall composition: At the level of the publicistic type, these people are occupants of the executive suite – elegant, their eyes fixed self-confidently on the viewer, refined from head to toe, and worldly-wise. The word that springs instantly to mind is "yuppy", though the figure in 6 is precluded from this label by his seniority. The way in which the accessories are dealt with in Figures 4, 5, and 7 indicates that these people gain an essential part of their personal fulfilment from performing work processes but that their leisure-time sphere (/A1/ in 6) too is determined with a high degree of rationalism and perspicacity. They thus connote success and social prestige in a manner that is widespread in the field of consumer goods advertising and whose codification has already been the subject of relatively detailed publications within the framework of semiotic advertising analysis (Barthes 1965; Koch 1971; Eco 1972, 1987b; Dorfles 1974; Nöth 1975, 1990).

If the representation of the protagonist figure is compared at the level of the historical type with some essential stations in the development of iconography in occidental portraiture, certain structural similarities with an outstandingly distinct reference to the type of "state portrait" that evolved during the sixteenth century can be detected. In her monograph on this type of portrait, Jenkins has pointed out that, even at an early stage of its development, "certain poses and gestures came to be employed for much the same purpose.

Finally, carefully chosen material accessories were often supplied to serve as clues to the intellectual and occupational pursuits of the subject, or to indicate the associations that conditioned his acts and thoughts" (Jenkins 1947: 11).

One exceptionally influential compositional formula within the framework of this development is the half-length or full-length portrait in which the potentate is holding one hand close to his body or braced on his hip while the other is resting on an external object, often a piece of furniture (cf. Jenkins 1947: 12, 14, 16, 18, 24, 26). This formula, whose historical roots can be traced back primarily to Tizian, was given renewed topicality and some degree of explosiveness at the end of the eighteenth century in the wake of civil revolution, when many artists were confronted with the task of portraying commoners as the new representatives of a constitutionalised state power. On the one hand they were dependent on the iconography of the feudal potentate portrait, the only one codified and therefore the only one available. On the other hand, the introduction of new iconic elements was a special, quite historic, challenge. /Authority/ had to be both indicated and simultaneously withdrawn, since it could be legitimate in the hands of its new representatives only as a delegated authority. The three reproductions at the top of Figure 10 show approaches of a more traditionalistic nature to this dilemma:

10.1: Portrait painted in 1792 by Jean-Luis Laneuville (1748–1826) of Barère de Vieuzac (1755–1841), a member of the National Convent. The portrait depicts him "im ... Moment seines größten politischen Triumphs ..., als er auf dem Nationalkonvent den Kopf Ludwigs XIV forderte" ['at the moment of his greatest political triumph when, from the platform of the National Convent, he demanded the head of Louis XIV'] (Bock – Grosshans 1980: 189).

10.2: Portrait by Jean-Auguste Dominique Ingres (1780–1867) of Napoleon Bonaparte as self-appointed first consul.

10.3: Portrait painted in 1812 by Thomas Sully of Captain James Stewart (1768–1836), an American naval officer.

All three portraits unite the obvious continuity of pose and gesture of the feudal state portrait with the introduction of new, bourgeois elements evident in particular in the clothing and in the accessories grouped around the supporting hand. Those portrayed have their eyes fixed on the observer with the same cool, slightly condescending detachment as the protagonists in Figures 4 to 7. They have exchanged regalia and imperial insignia for the frock-coat and above all for their writing materials. Like the protagonists in 4, 5 and 7, they command the art of writing in an outstandingly literal sense. Even more strongly than those protagonists they represent a specific – in roughly simplified terms bourgeois – type of successful person.

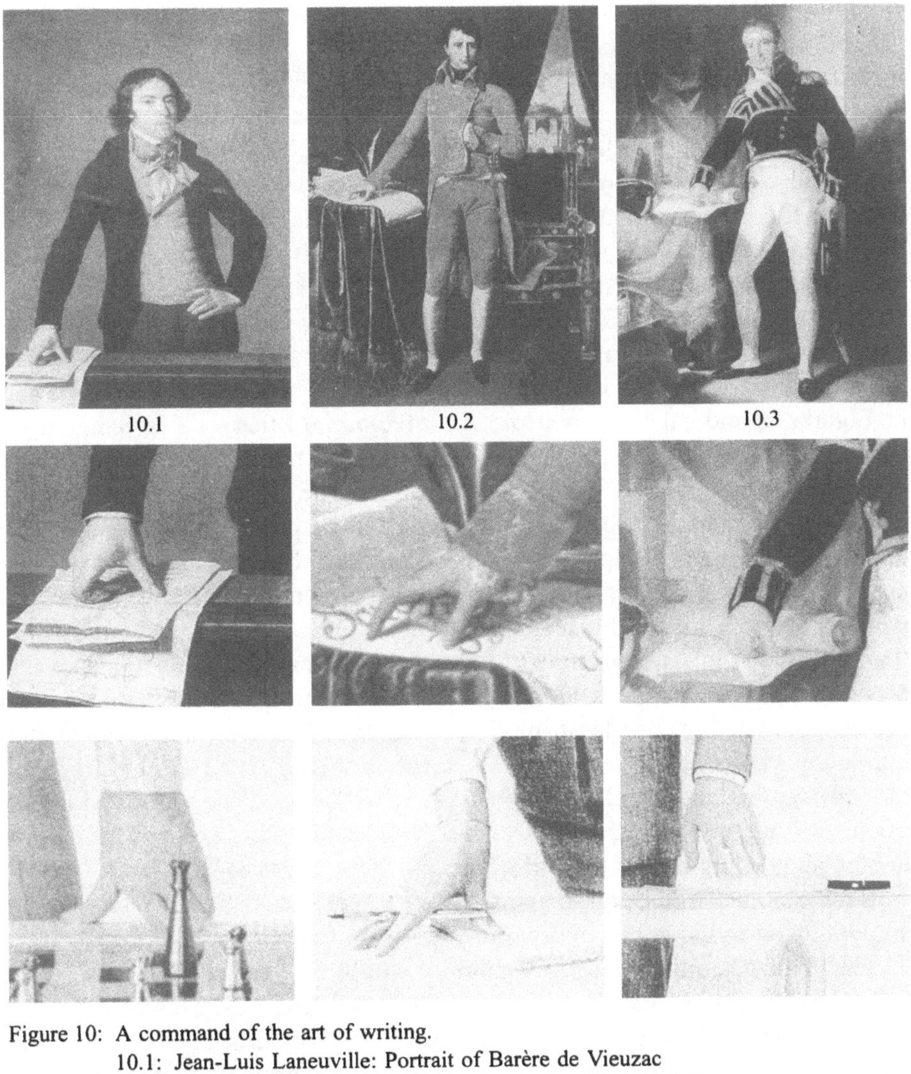

Figure 10: A command of the art of writing.
10.1: Jean-Luis Laneuville: Portrait of Barère de Vieuzac
10.2: Jean-Auguste-Dominique Ingres: Portrait of Napoleon Bonaparte
10.3: Thomas Sully: Portrait of Captain James Stewart
Enlarged details from Figures 10.1 to 10.3 (middle row) and 4 to 6 (lower row).
(Reproduced by permission of Städtische Kunsthalle Bremen [10.1], Musée des Arts Modernes Liège [10.2], National Gallery of Arts Washington [10.3].)

Their social ascent is not only iconographically implied but also biographically documented. It is important to bear in mind at this juncture that, whilst all three had reached a peak of such an ascent when their portraits were painted, an end to or a break in this ascent was far from being in sight, indeed further gains in power and influence seemed likely: For Vieuzac an influential position on the Vigilance Committee (not attained by him because of his arrest following the overthrow of Robespierre), for Napoleon the emperorship (which he conferred upon himself in 1804), and for Stewart receiving command of the brig *Argus* at the outset of the struggle with Great Britain. The three men portrayed are thus not only representatives of social success but also //aspirants// to even more success. There are, of course, problems involved in basing conclusions about a contemporary constellation on this historical constellation and its iconographic representation merely because the means used to represent it are strikingly similar. This similarity goes so far in Figures 4 and 10.1, even in details of clothing, that one is tempted to suspect iconographic plagiarism. A conclusion on the historical //aspirants//, drawn from the contemporary protagonists, may be allowed at least in complete awareness of its speculative character: If the protagonists in Figures 4 to 7 can be claimed to represent not only successful persons but also //aspirants// to a certain objective, e.g. a specific room in the executive suite, on which their eyes are fixed just as firmly as on the reader of the advertisement, then a relationship is determined to a possible preproprial constituent of the proprietary name /Aspirin/. However intricate, subtle and speculative it may be, this relationship is at least implied in the advertisement, not at the verbal but solely at the iconic level. In this sense, Eco's (1972: 145–151, 1987b: 61–64) "ambiguous" and "autoreflexive" message could be translated into a linguistic slogan, along the lines of the 50-year-old classified advertisement quoted above (Figure 9): "Aspirin: a recipe for success for aspirants."

Such a slogan would fail to approach the effectiveness of the purely iconic solution used in the series of advertisements for two essential reasons:

Firstly, absence of linguistic ambiguity would take the spellbinding effect from the visual message. The effectiveness of different degrees of arbitrariness in a carefully poised equilibrium would be jeopardised by making the reader aware at the linguistic level of the iconically implied connotative connection between the product on offer and social or professional success. Secondly, the lexeme /aspirant/ in the sense of /qualifier, applicant for a post/ is outdated in contemporary usage or confined to limited circles. An additional factor is that it may be encumbered with derogatory connotations such as /slogger/, /opportunist/ or /careerist/, so that it hardly lends itself to use as an attribute for a progressive, publicising identification figure. Schulz' German dictionary of foreign words, *Deutsches Fremdwörterbuch* (Schulz 1913 [1974]: 54) was still listing it as a lexeme of contemporary German usage.

According to this source, it was taken from the synonymous French lexeme /aspirant/ and first registered in Campe's dictionary (cf. Campe 1801 [1970]: 130). The *Grand Larousse* (1971: 271)[47] quotes */candidat/* as a synonym, paraphrasing it as: "Personne qui désire obtenir un poste, un titre" ['Person who desires to obtain a post or title']. The first spheres in which it was lexicalised – according to the historical examples given in *Larousse* – were the estates of the realm and the academic ("aspirant à la maîtrise", Larousse 1971: 271) and military fields. In his *Illustriertes Lexicon der deutschen Umgangssprache* (illustrated dictionary of colloquial German), Küpper (1982: 189) lists the compound word */Aspirinaspirant/*, giving the meanings 'junior doctor in the armed forces' and 'soldier reporting sick'. 14 of the other 15 compound words based on /Aspirin/ and listed by Küpper are rooted in the military field. Lötscher (1987: 24–25) gives in his lexicographical collection of proprietary names three suggested interpretations for the lemma /Aspirin/: (1) as a composition of a privative /a/ and the Latin root spira, meaning 'perspiration', "womit wohl angedeutet werden soll, daß dieses Mittel von Fieberschweiß befreit" ['which is intended to indicate that this remedy gives relief from feverish sweating'], (2) like the Larousse, as a compound of a privative /a/ and /spiric acid/, and (3) as "...überlappende Bildung aus Asparaginsäure und Spirinsäure ...; neben der oben erwähnten Spirinsäure wird damit auch auf die ähnlich fiebersenkende Asparaginsäure angespielt, die früher aus Spargeln (lat. asparagus) gewonnen wurde. Am plausibelsten dürfte wohl diese Deutung Nr. 3 sein" ['an overlapping formation from aspartic acid and spiric acid ...; in addition to the above-mentioned spiric acid, an allusion is thus made to the similarly febrifugal aspartic acid[48] which used to be obtained from asparagus ... This third interpretation has to be considered the most plausible.'] (Lötscher 1987: 25)

Where, though, is the connection between the product on offer, //Aspirin//, the strategy of its presentation to the public and these preproprial constituents of its proprietary name? Is it perhaps merely a coincidental, unmotivated, semiotically meaningless, phonetic and graphemic similarity?

Considering that the proprietary name was originally created to draw attention to the synthesis of the active substance from //salicylic acid//, also designated /spiroyligous acid/ (German: *Spirsäure* or *Spiersäure*), this does seem almost to be the case. What, then, has /Aspirin/ to do with //aspirants//? An interesting answer to this question – though one that cannot be verified with certainty from historical sources – is to be found at the very outset of the story-book history of aspirin. It thus relates to a time when the pharmaceutical industry was just developing into a factor of economic importance in the capitalistic system and thus a possible representative of its attitudes and one in which the lexeme /aspirant/ may still have been a lexicalised element of contemporary German usage. It is embodied by three //aspirants//: Arthur Eichengrün (1867–1949), Felix Hoffmann (1868–1946) and Heinrich Dreser (1860–1924).[49] All three had been called by Carl Duisberg into the research team of the Elberfeld enterprise in the 1890s, at a time when its expansion had taken on breathtaking proportions.

Hoffmann, who had studied pharmacology and chemistry in Munich, joined the *Farbwerke* in 1894, one year after being awarded a doctor's degree in chemistry. On 10. 10. 1897 he recorded in his laboratory journal a new method for synthetising acetylsalicylic acid. He had been looking into the problem of how to free the sodium salt of salicylic acid – which was already being used to treat rheumatism – from its unpleasant side-effects, in particular its corrosive effect on the gastric mucosa and its revolting taste. At this juncture he could do no more than suspect that he had already solved this problem by attaching an acetic acid residue (as a representomorpheme) to the body of the salicylic acid (as a representologeme). How he came to attempt it with an acetic acid residue in particular has never been fully explained, though in those times it was undoubtedly in vogue to work with acetic acid residues, to acetylate. Double acetylation of //morphine//, for instance, had resulted in //diacetylmorphine//, which was later to gain extensive popularity as a cough remedy until its addictive side-effects were recognised. Just three years earlier, a probatory agent against diarrhea, /Tannigen/, had been developed in Elberfeld by acetylating //tannic acid//. The synthetisation of acetylsalicylic acid was to remain Hoffmann's only coup at the *Farbenfabriken*. As he was granted the American patent rights for the production of acetylsalicylic acid from 1900 onwards, however, this development also brought him a considerable measure of economic success. He turned his attention mainly to commercial and organisational matters in the two decades preceding his retirement, and then studied history of art, living as a bachelor on his private income at a Lausanne hotel.

About two years elapsed between initial synthetisation of acetylsalicylic acid and initial clinical testing, an exceptionally long period for those times. The official presentation of the new substance to the scientific world was made by Heinrich Dreser with an article in *Pflüger's Archiv für die gesamte Physiologie* not long after initial, consistently positive, clinical results obtained with aspirin had been published. In this article Dreser, who had resigned the chair of pharmacology at Göttingen university on being appointed manager of the pharmacological test laboratory at Elberfeld in 1896, gives a survey of the most significant chemical and physical characteristics of acetylsalicylic acid, summarises the most important results of the bioassays carried out in his laboratory and also mentions self-administration performed by him. In the same essay he attributes the name /Aspirin/ to a combination of the two roots /acetyl/ and /spiroyligous acid/ (German: *Spirsäure*). Dreser is described by one biographer as an "echte Gelehrtennatur, eine etwas kantige, originelle Persönlichkeit. Nicht sehr umgänglich hielt er sich von seinen Fachkollegen fern und war nur schwer zu bewegen, hin und wieder einmal deren Versammlungen oder sonst einen Kongreß zu besuchen. Frei von jeglicher Pose, für seine Person einfach und anspruchslos, legte er auf Äußerlichkeiten keinen Wert" ['a genuine scholarly being, a somewhat sharp-edged, original character. ... Not very approachable and sociable, he kept his distance from his professional colleagues, and it was hard to persuade him to attend one of their meetings or some other congress now and again. Free from any pretence, simple and undemanding for a person like him, he attached no value to external appearances'] (Lomnitz 1925: 81). From the economic aspect, the introduction of Aspirin was to be profitable for him in all events, as his contract provided for automatic participation in the profits made on any drugs introduced during his employ, no matter whether they could be patented or not. Dreser was also responsible for //diacetylmorphine// being introduced as a cough remedy. In 1914 he left the Bayer company as a wealthy man in his mid-fifties, living on his own private income in Liège, Düsseldorf and Zurich and devoting the rest of his life to pharmacological research, untroubled by any economic or hierarchical pressure.

Arthur Eichengrün had come to Elberfeld in 1896 at the age of 28 as manager of the pharmaceutico-scientific department that was to be newly established there. He had spent the five years since being awarded a doctor's degree working successfully in academic and industrial research in Geneva, Ingelheim and Bonn. In an autobiographical note he writes of the initial period at Elberfeld:

> Nachdem die Einrichtung des neu geschaffenen Laboratoriums der pharmazeutisch-wissenschaftlichen Abteilung beendet war, nahm ich mit 10 meist frisch von der Universität gekommenen Chemikern die Arbeit auf. Diese führte im Laufe der beiden nächsten Jahrzehnte zur Auffindung einer großen Zahl neuer Medikamente für neue Indikationen. Von ihnen hat sich ein erheblicher Teil als recht wertvoll für die Therapie erwiesen, wie z. B. Protargol, Alypin, Mesotan, Novocain, Luminal, Autan, Citarin, Helmitol, Glycosal, Jodipin, Sajodin, Heroin, Coryfin u. a.. [Once the installation of the newly created laboratory of the pharmaco-scientific department was completed, I began work with 10 chemists, most of them fresh from university. This led in the course of the next two decades to the discovery of a large number of new medical preparations for new indications. A substantial proportion of them has proved to be of major therapeutic value; these include Protargol, Alypin, Mesotan, Novocain, Lu-

minal, Autan, Citarin, Helmitol, Glycosal, Jodipin, Sajodin, Heroin, Coryfin etc..] (Eichengrün 1949: 582).

Equally at home in technical and pharmaceutical chemistry and in patent law, he was probably by far the most ambitious of the three – from both the scientific and the economic aspect. Numerous new developments in which he also had financial interests – though restricted to the use of patent rights – took place under his auspices. His most effective genuine discovery as far as progress in industrial chemistry is concerned was the development of a process for large-scale acetylation of //cellulose//. //Acetylcellulose// was eventually to become the "parent substance" of a number of important synthetics, among them the first //artificial silk// and //Cellon//, to which he himself gave the name. //Cellon// was a valuable substitute for //celluloid// whose high inflammability had until then made the projection of motion-pictures so hazardous and consequently unsuitable for mass audiences. Eichengrün was neither an opportunist nor an intriguer; he was, however, extremely hierarchy-conscious and observed meticulously the code of honour of the hierarchy to which he belonged. When one of the chemists directly subordinate to him[50] attempted to implement a project of his own behind Eichengrün's back, he wrote a strongly worded disciplinary letter to the management. An internal Bayer memorandum describes him, after first emphasizing his exceptional productivity and loyalty, as follows:

> Neben all diesen Verdiensten geht nun aus den Unterlagen und Akten für die Persönlichkeit Eichengrüns hervor, dass er nicht etwa nur rein ideell zu seinem Schaffen stand, sondern – in ausgeprägtem Maße ehrgeizig, von seinem Können überzeugt, äusserst berechnend und stets seinen Vorteil im Auge – ängstlich auf seine Sicherheit bedacht war. Es zieht sich dies wie ein roter Faden durch all die Jahre seiner Tätigkeit in den Farbenfabriken ... Seine Publizistik ist gewandt, scharf, vielseitig, kämpferisch. [Besides all these merits, it is now revealed by the documents and files relating to the figure of Eichengrün that he did not stand for his work out of pure idealism but – markedly ambitious, convinced of his ability, extremely shrewd and always with an eye to his own advantage – was anxiously mindful of securing his position. This aspect runs like a red[1] thread through all the years of his employment at the Farbenfabriken ... His writings are fluent, perceptive, versatile, militant.'] (Bayer Archives: Eichengrün file).

With all these biographical data – presented here in condensed form – in mind, it is time to return to the original question of what /Aspirin/ has to do with //aspirants//: On 23. 1. 1899, an internal circular was drawn up in the course of business at the Farbenfabriken, proposing "den Körper $C_9H_8O_4$, dessen chemische Bezeichnung ist: Acetylsalicylsäure unter dem Namen Aspirin beim Kaiserlichen Patentamt zum Wortschutz anzumelden" ['to register the substance $C_9H_8O_4$, whose chemical specification is: acetylsalicylic acid, under the name Aspirin as a protected name at the Imperial Patent Office".] (Alstaedter 1983: 28–29; reproduced there in facsimile form).

The initiator of this proposal is not stated in the circular; nor did an evaluation of all files relevant to the history of Aspirin in the Bayer archives reveal his name. In the vast store of literature relating to the history of Aspirin, only one author, Gordonoff, takes up this point with the following statement: "und es wurde beschlossen, das Präparat unter dem von Eichengrün vorgeschlagenen Namen Aspirin einzuführen" ['... and it was resolved that the preparation should be introduced under the name proposed by Eichengrün: Aspirin.'] (Gordonoff 1965: 46)

Gordonoff unfortunately fails to quote any sources in his article. Closer consideration of the circular reveals that the name /Aspirin/ for //acetylsalicylic acid// was by no means undisputed at Bayer but had to compete with the name /Euspirin/ which – as is conclusively shown in the circular – had been suggested by Dreser. In the circular the objection is raised against /Aspirin/ – though not by Dreser – that the name might mistakenly be assumed to derive from the verb *aspiriren* 'to inhale', in other words blurred from the semiotic aspect by "preproprial" constituents (which is precisely what has happened in the advertisement reproduced in Figure 9). The syllable /Eu-/ was in widespread use in those days as a quasi-"qualifying" prefix in names of medical preparations. The only opposition raised on the circular to Dreser's proposal originates from Eichengrün, who added the following comment on initialling it: "Bin für Aspirin, da Eu- im Allgemeinen zu Geschmacks- und Geruchsverbesserungen benutzt wird." ['Favor Aspirin, as Eu- is generally used for improvements to flavor and smell.'] (Quoted from Alstaedter 1983: 29).

What is quite remarkable here is that Eichengrün's argument is totally invalid with regard to its substance, since the improvement in flavor was one of the essential advantages of //acetylsalicylic acid// over //sodium salicylate//. With this in mind, Eichengrün should rather have put forward a reason why the new preparation ought all the more to have been called /Euspirin/. If this was not the reason, then why was he so emphatically against Dreser's proposal? Possibly for the very reason that it was Dreser's proposal. This would make sense, especially if the proposed name /Aspirin/ did indeed, as claimed by Gordonoff, initiate from Eichengrün.

Whoever it was that invented the name, the atmosphere of the epoch in which it was being sought and of the circumstances in which it was being discussed were characterised by the dramatic events heralding the foreseeable birth – certainly hoped for by those involved – of a "new megamachine"

(Mumford 1971: 263): the pharmaceutical industry. The introduction of //acetylsalicylic acid// in 1899 as a mass-consumption analgesic can in all events be specified in retrospect precisely and indisputably as the date of its birth.[51] On 1. 1. 1901 it had an initial concrete consequence for the //aspirants// Eichengrün, Dreser and Hoffmann: All three were vested with full commercial powers of attorney by the *Farbenfabriken* on one and the same day.

The biography of Arthur Eichengrün illustrates with great clarity the "elbowing aspect" of this /aspiration/, which he himself may have immortalised by a proposal for a name and which is reputed to have had a difficult internal relationship[52] with that contemporary development to which he, as a Jew, eventually fell victim.

Eichengrün left the *Farbenfabriken* in 1908, his request for a contract of participation similarly lucrative to that concluded with Dreser having been turned down. His militant publications resulted in libel actions being brought against him in 1908 and 1909 by manufacturers whose products he had criticised. He then worked on a freelance basis, doing research on his own initiative and with some degree of success in the field of technical chemistry, registering new patents and founding in Charlottenburg his own flourishing production enterprise. In 1933 the Fascist authorities began making life more and more difficult for him as a self-employed Jewish entrepreneur who was easily goaded into retaliation. By exhausting all possible legal channels, he managed again and again to postpone individual anti-Semitic actions – compulsory sale of his factory, loss of civil rights – but not to prevent them. Even in the early 1940s, he was still petitioning officially for restoration of his civil rights because of his services to the development of the German chemical industry.[53] His arrest came in 1943; in spring 1944, at the age of seventy-six, he was sent to Theresienstadt, which he survived. Immediately after the war, he set up an improvised laboratory and resumed his research work. He died in December 1949 in Bad Wiessee. In an autobiographical profile written in Theresienstadt, he claimed that it was he who had instructed Felix Hoffmann to work on the synthetisation of acetylsalicylic acid. Dreser had long resisted clinical testing of the new substance, initially believing it to be cardiotoxic. He, Eichengrün, had eventually carried it through by stubborn insistence, high-dose self-administration and unofficial preliminary clinical testing (Eichengrün 1949). Despite exhaustive investigations carried out at Bayer, no evidence was found to support this claim. In fact, Felix Hoffmann was found to have circulated a similar version among his fellow-workers, the only real difference being that he presented himself instead of Eichengrün as a resolute opponent of Dreser (Bayer Archives: Eichengrün file).

What is of importance to the connection discussed here, however, is not so much the history of the invention of //aspirin// as the history of the invention of /Aspirin/. It is, after all, quite feasible – though of course not verifiable – that the competitive, hierarchy-based controversy between the three //aspirants// Hoffmann, Dreser and Eichengrün left a significant mark on the nomenclature. To assume a direct internal connection between their aspirations and the way in which the eyes of the protagonists in the contemporary series of advertisements are fixed on the executive suite would be overstretching this hypothesis, for the same strategy is used today to advertise numerous products with a far less eventful history. It is rather the historical constellation and the topical advertising message that are connected by a *tertium comparationis*, whose outlines and profile circumscribe them asymptotically as links in a chain of interpretants: the cultural unit «aspirin».

1.6. Charting a common approach: What is «Aspirin»?

In an essay on the "structure" of the advertisement, Walter A. Koch writes: "Die Tatsache, daß ein im Zentrum der Massenkultur stehendes Etwas etwas tut, hat, sagt, löst im allgemeinen eine in den Einzelheiten noch schwer verständliche, in den groben Auswirkungen aber unübersehbare Kettenreaktion von Werthaltungen aus." ['The fact that a something located at the centre of mass culture does, has, says something triggers off in general a chain reaction of valuations that is still difficult to grasp in detail but cannot be overlooked in its broad effects.'] (Koch 1971: 238)

The attempt presented here to work out the meaning of a ubiquitous signifier along a chain[54] of different interpretants, whose content is for its part to be defined "by viewing them in a system of positions and oppositions" (Eco 1976: 83), directs the focus of the investigation – with what must often be a bewildering interest in detail – again and again to the level of what Koch refers to as "still difficult to grasp in detail". The main reason for this bewilderment is that, whilst the end of the chain is known, the effect of the chain reaction is "unclear". The special advantage of this procedure, however, is that it reveals some surprising constituents of an overall interrelationship that seems familiar to us beyond all recognition.

/Aspirin/ is probably above all – but with certainty not only – an //analgesic// or //febrifuge//. It is an //analgesic// or //febrifuge// above all – but with certainty not only – because it contains //acetylsalicylic acid//. This reference to the pharmacological component, and thus to a specific position in the semantic system for designating organo-chemical compounds, is probably the primarily denotative meaning of /aspirin/. Nonetheless, this reference alone fails to explain the meaning of the underlying cultural unit even in approximate terms. The empirical test on the significant residue can be presented in terms as simple as they are impressive:

If ten members of a cultural community in which /aspirin/ is diffused take, for pain-killing purposes, a tablet resembling an //aspirin tablet// with respect to all describable and semiotically relevant qualities (name, colour, shape, taste, packaging) but containing no //acetylsalicylic acid// and no other pharmacologically active substances, three to four of them will experience a distinct, quantifiable and objectifiable improvement in their subjective symptoms as a result.

Together with the //aspirin tablet// containing an active ingredient, such a tablet – referred to in modern drug research as an /aspirin placebo/ – forms a semiotic minimal pair. Its effectiveness, which attains approximately one-third of the analgesic potency of the preparation containing the active substance (cf. Moertel – Ahmann – Taylor – Schworton 1972; Peters – Bruce – Fraim – Masel 1983), is the most important empirical clue to be followed up by anyone wishing to learn to understand the drug as a sign. This clue can be illustrated in very simplified form with the following arithmetical equation:

/aspirin/ – //acetylsalicylic acid// = aspirin placebo

or, in more general terms:

/drug/ – //active substance// = /placebo/.

Whereas it was mainly the left-hand side of this equation that was examined in detail in Chapter 1, it is the historical, the pragmatic and – last but not least – the semiotic dimension of the placebo model that are dealt with in Chapter 2. The very fact that the placebo experiment is so simple and simultaneously so important to the effectiveness of pharmacological substances has meanwhile made it an indispensable component of any innovative drug research. So-called placebo effects can be detected not only in the field of pain relief but fundamentally in all pharmacological effects. It is in connection with pain, however, that they occur with exceptional frequency and have been the subject of most thorough empirical research.

From the metatheoretical aspect, the placebo model is something like a reservoir for pharmacologically inexplicable or contradictory, so-called /non-specific/, effects of drugs. Yet the modelling of similarity, which permits this model to be presented from the semiotic perspective, is highly specific. This specificity is one that cannot be illustrated with the structural levels of analysis applied in organic chemistry but can be made experiencable through perspectival segmentation of semiotics in general as a culturally consistent quantity. Demonstrating this with a concrete example has been the object of Chapter 1. According to this, /Aspirin/ is:

(1) an /analgesic/ or /pain killer/; (2) //acetylsalicylic acid//; (3) an /antipyretic/ or /febrifuge/; (4) a pharmaceutical proprietary name; (5) a /pseudosubstrate/ of //prostaglandin synthesis//; (6) an instrument of /control over Nature/; (7) a generator of intersubjectivity towards pain; and (8) a /recipe for success/ for //aspirants//.

All these interpretants of «Aspirin» have been considered in this chapter with respect to their positions within structured semantic systems, some of them hierarchical. All of them are applications and pragmatic concretisations of the principle *aliquid stat pro aliquo*. The sequence in which they have been named reflects an intuitive assessment of their quantitative significance for the cultural unit of the significate. Interpretants (1), (2), (3) and (5) can be combined into one common hierarchy of provisionally so-called /specifically pharmacological/ constituents, whilst interpretants (4), (6), (7) and (8) represent the most important results of an initial endeavour to analyse in more detail the specificity of those constituents that were combined more or less at random in the placebo model. If these interpretants are visualised as tangents of a hyperbola, in other words as projections of the direction in which they run in an observation window with a perspective approaching zero, then the meaning of the cultural unit corresponds to the asymptote of this hyperbola (cf. Eco 1975: 104, 1987a: 105, 1976: 71). With regard to its interpretants, «Aspirin» is barely less than the sum of these parts, but also barely more than part of this sum.

With reference to Katz and Fodor (1964) and to Quillian (1968), Eco (1976) has proposed a "revised semantic model" that might permit an analytical overview of the common finishing course covered by those interpretants presented here of the signifier /aspirin/. This model, like its predecessors, is certainly in dispute within the scope of linguistic semantic theory. Its empirical base is flimsy and actually offers, in hermeneutic dealings with language, only one advantage over traditional models such as the "semantic field" paradigm or Saussure's "Sémiologie": it dissects the complex concept of /meaning/ into a "two-dimensional" or "monoplanar" relational structure (cf. Nöth 1990: 192). The validity of this dissection and its implied priority of the relation over the element always comes up against an early limit, however, if subjected to empirical examination. If this limit is taken consciously into account in the context referred to here, then the benefit to be derived from applying Eco's model appears at this juncture to be essentially a hierarchisation of hypotheses.

/Aspirin/

syntactical characteristics: substantive, neuter, singular

«Aspirin»

denotation d1: /pain-killer/ – denotation d2: /febrifuge/.

connotation c1: /instrument of control over Nature/
connotation c2: /aid to generating intersubjectivity/

context con a: /consumption/

denotation d3: /proprietary name/

connot. c3: /recipe for success for aspirants/

context con b: /pharmacology/

denotation d4: /acetysalicylic acid/

connotation c4: /pseudosubstrate of prostaglandin synthesis/.

Figure 11: What is «Aspirin»? Common finishing course of a chain of interpretants of the signifier /Aspirin/. For diagrammatic principle cf. Eco 1975: 152 ff., 1987: 153.

The systematic consideration of "connotations" and "contexts" in Eco's model seems to be an essential expansion of those put forward by Katz and Fodor and by Quillian. Eco writes: "The Revised Model aims to insert into the semantic representation all coded connotations depending on corresponding denotations as well as contextual and circumstantial selections." (Eco 1976: 105).

The relational structure set out in Figure 11 for the common finishing course of the interpretants of «Aspirin» is based on the notation proposed by Eco. According to the terminology used by Eco (1984b: 80–84), this relational structure is a cutout, a "partial tree", taken artificially from the "rhizome" (cf.Deleuze – Guattari 1977) of the encyclopedically formatted universe. At a purely metaphorical level, this cutting activity is suggestive of the actual technique or activity denoted by the professional title traditionally given to gatherers of medicinal herbs in Ancient Greece. They were known as /*rhizotomoi*/, in English: /root cutters/.

2. The semiotic specificity of the pharmacologically nonspecific: the placebo problem

> On the magical plane, dream and image were not mere signs for the thing in question, but were bound up with it by similarity or names. The relation is one not of intention but of relatedness... Like science, magic pursues aims, but seeks to achieve them by mimesis – not by progressively distancing itself from the object (...). In general, the name – to which magic most easily attaches – is undergoing a chemical change...
>
> Theodor W. Adorno – Max Horkheimer

To twentieth century pharmacology, which had at last been successfully anchored in the analytic methods of organic chemistry, it appeared both fascinating and threatening when laboratory experiments revealed that a small, round, white tablet containing a pharmacologically inert substance such as //lactose// had on an organo-morphological malaise a measurable effect that could in some cases be just as great or even greater than that achieved with the pharmacologically specific therapy of choice. The experimental analgesic effect of an //aspirin placebo// outlined at the end of Chapter 1 illustrates this process as what is now in all probability the most frequently reproduced example within the framework of experimental placebo research. To the semiotically interested observer, the most fascinating aspect of this experiment is that characteristics such as /small/, /round/ and /white/ apparently play a greater role in the observed effect of the //aspirin placebo// than the virtually tasteless //lactose// contained in it and that all these characteristics flow into one definitive similarity relation to an //aspirin tablet// containing //acetylsalicylic acid//. Within the framework of his typology of modes of sign production, Eco (1975: 285–327) has classified this similarity relation as that of a dummy or "campione fittizio".[55]

Now all surprising events which, whilst experimentally reproducible, are inadequately explicable within the scope of the traditionally "normal" (Kuhn 1962) scientific interpretative framework, obviously generate for practical scientific research the exceptionally prolific combination of interest and threat alluded to above, a combination that lends special urgency to a comprehensive explanation of what is as yet unexplained. Systematic research into this phenomenon, one that had probably been known since the eighteenth century, was accordingly not taken up until this combination of interest and threat was first able to take effect. The question: 'Why is a small, white, round tablet that looks like an //aspirin tablet// effective even when it contains no //acetylsalicylic acid//?' assumed a theoretically interesting and threatening aspect only for a pharmacological system that was capable of associating the effect of drugs systematically and exclusively with the substances contained in them. Systematic placebo research starts only at that moment in which the placebo effect becomes problematic for pharmacology. That was initially the case in some approaches in the 1920s (cf. Kleinsorge in: Hippius – Überla – Laakmann – Hasford (1986): 20); there is conformity among all authors, however, in dating the real beginnings of placebo research back to the publication of Pepper's article "A Note on the Placebo" in the *American Journal of Pharmacology* in 1945.

2.1. Historical background: pre-1945 etymology

Before we continue our chronological consideration of the placebo problem to help provide overall clarity, the history of this term around which this book revolves and some empirical determinants of the effect designated with it will be covered on in somewhat closer detail. First to the early etymology:

Placebo is the first person singular of the future indicative of the Latin verb *placere* 'to please'. The earliest evidence that has been handed down to us of this somewhat unusual verb form is to be found in Psalm 116 in the *Vulgata*, Hieronymus' Latin translation of the Old Testament. Verse 9 of this psalm is worded: *Placebo domino in regione vivorum* 'I will please the Lord in the land of the living'. Westermann (1977: 76, 1984: 136–141) classifies Psalm 116 in his typology of the psalms as a "berichtender Lobpsalm" ['recording psalm of praise']. In Luther's translation of the Bible, it is preceded by the paraphase "Dank und Gelübde für die Errettung aus großer Lebensgefahr" ['Thanksgiving and avowal for being saved from mortal danger']. In his concordance of the Old Testament, Fischer (1977) has 238 entries for the verb *placere*, the already quoted Verse 9 of Psalm 116 being the only place in the entire Old Testament in which it occurs in the form of interest to us at this juncture – first person singular of the future indicative.[56] The decisive factor in the further history of the etymon *placebo* appears to be the use of this Verse 9 in the vespers for the dead in the late medieval Christian church. Shapiro has looked into this history in more detail than any other placebo researcher, referring in the process to some primary sources. He claims that the lexeme *placebo* as a Latin derivative first appears in English usage in the twelfth century, where it denoted 'Christian vespers for the dead'. One possible explanation for this unusual denotative shift might be that the corresponding passage from Psalm 116 (in which the subjects of /death/ and /resurrection/ also occur) may have played an important role in contemporary Christian vespers for the dead.[57] Shapiro writes:

> The placebo took on a secular meaning in the fourteenth century, and its connotation gradually became decisive during the next several centuries. It was used to describe a servile flatterer, sycophant, toady, and parasite. This usage derives from the deprecation of the professional mourners who were paid to "sing placebos" at the bier of the deceased in substitution for the family, whose role it was originally. (Shapiro 1964: 53).

The first mention of the word /placebo/ in English usage and simultaneously in a medical context was discovered by Shapiro in Motherby's *New medical dictionary* which was first published in 1795 and contains the following entry under the word /placebo/: "A commonplace method or medicine calculated to amuse for a time, rather than for any other purpose." (quoted from Shapiro 1964: 53).

A new medical dictionary published in 1803 by Joseph Fox restricts the placebo definition to the medical context for the first time in written English usage, defining it as "an epithet given to any medicine adapted more to please than benefit the patient" (quoted from Shapiro 1964: 53).

The definition proposed by Shapiro to fulfill historic and heuristic criteria states: "A placebo is defined as a therapeutic procedure ... which is given deliberately to have an effect, or ... which unknowingly has an effect on a patient, symptom, disease or syndrome, but which is objectively without specific activity for the condition being treated." (Shapiro 1964: 57).

Kissel and Barrucand refer in their placebo monograph to some sources in late medieval French poetry in which the secular meaning of /placebo/ outlined by Shapiro recurs in literary contexts. They summarise what their research reveals to have been the widespread colloquial usage of /placebo/ as follows: "Bref, en langage courant, le mot placebo a plusiers sens, fréquemment employés jusqu' au XVIIIe siècle il peut désigner les vêpres des morts, la flatterie, le caractère flatteur, le courtisan, ou l'intrigant, enfin il signifie parfois un effort de conciliation ... ." ['In brief the word placebo has several meanings in colloquial language; often used until the eighteenth century it can denote vespers for the dead, flattery, a flattering character, a courtier or intriguer, finally it sometimes means an attempt at conciliation.'] (Kissel – Barrucand 1964: 6).

In the diachronic dimension the chequered history of the etymon /placebo/ is reminiscent of an empirical characteristic of the preparation used as a //placebo// in the synchronic dimension: The word /placebo/ and the physical object //placebo// are "floating signifiers" (Levi-Strauss 1987: 63). The transformation from a liturgical concept to the term used in experimental pharmacology in the diachronic dimension corresponds in the synchronic dimension to the versatility of use value of empirical //placebos//, which can be applied as pain relievers, laxatives, cardiovascular agents – on principle in any conceivable sphere of indications.

Tables summarizing a wealth of information on placebo efficacy, divided according to indication fields, target organ (-system) and independent physiological variables, are provided by Haas, Fink and Härtfelder (1959: 331–454); Kissel and Barrucand (1964: 35–41) and Beecher (1968: 28, 31). Although the picture presented by the quantitative and qualitative data published by these authors is anything but uniform, the following interrelations can be provisionally – and following the secondary literature – formulated as a working hypothesis:

(1) The effectiveness of placebo therapy undergoes greater quantitative variations from study to study than from organic system to organic system or from syndrome to syndrome. In other words: The effectiveness of placebo therapy depends to a great, possibly decisive, extent on the situational factors surrounding this therapy.

(2) Nonetheless, typical and empirically extremely well researched domains of placebo therapy do exist. These are pain relief and the generating of stimulative or sedative effects within the scope of psychopharmacology

(3) In quantitative terms, the frequency of distinct placebo effects in the different proband groups is about one-third. In other words: Roughly every third proband displays the desired reactions when given a //placebo//.

(4) On average, healthy probands display weaker reactions to placebo therapy than those that are unwell.

(5) In studies comparing the effects of placebo therapy with those of standard pharmacological therapy, the former effects are about half as great as the latter, but with greater variance.

(6) To date, there has been virtually no empirical investigation into the longitudinal time constant of the placebo effect in individual probands (cf. Janke 1986: 160–162).

The //placebo// as a pill, as an injection, ointment or enema gets its curative power from the long and partly obscure history of confrontation between sufferer and healer. The history of the etymon /placebo/ at least suggests that the attitude of the healer is still closely linked with that of the professional mourner in late medieval times. If this hypothesis is followed up, then the semiotic *aliquo* of any possible effect of medication that can be accounted for by the placebo model can be expressed in concrete terms as follows: It is the assurance of an empathic service, of emotional assistance, that relies on a head start in professional experience. From the very moment in which a doctor gives a patient a pill, an injection, an ointment or an enema, he associates himself in a professional capacity with the sorrow, anger, fear and hope to which the onset of an affliction or of an illness has given rise in the patient's world. Or, in more general terms: The application of medical preparations of any kind implies the execution of culturally codified work on the patient's emotions.

2.2. Empirical factors: post-1945 placebo research

Before resuming our chronological consideration of the placebo problem to help provide overall clarity, we shall look in somewhat closer detail into the empirical determinants of the placebo effect. Our main interest will be focused on the question of whether the process of cultural codification, which permits and controls the execution of work on the feeling of being ill described above, can be described in more precise terms than was previously possible.

The empirically examined determinants of the placebo effect can be described in part as sensorily perceptible qualities of pharmaceuticals. These are of interest in the present context especially as the systematic observation of sensorily perceptible qualities often provides very reliable clues leading to precise descriptions of culturally codified connections (cf. Barthes 1985; Greimas 1976; Panofsky 1979). To an extent that is less interesting for our purposes but of greater empirical significance, they are connected with behavior-priming factors that cannot be consciously perceived by those involved nor by disinterested parties at that moment in which they are revealed.

In her article *Systematik der am Placeboeffekt beteiligten Faktoren* [Systematics of factors involved in the placebo effect], Netter makes a fundamental distinction between "causal factors" and "situational influencing factors":

> Das Medikament M in Form eines Placebos P oder einer Substanz X oder Y wirkt unter gleichzeitiger Anwesenheit verschiedener Bedingungsfaktoren … und zusätzlicher Einwirkung situativer Einflußfaktoren … auf den Organismus der Versuchsperson … Unter den Bedingungsfaktoren sind Attribute des Präparates wie Farbe, Form, Größe, Anzahl und Geschmack zu verstehen, sowie

auch Dosis, Dauer, Applikationsart und zugehörige Instruktion, um welche Art von Präparat es sich dabei handelt. Die situativen Einflußfaktoren ... umfassen Faktoren des Behandlungsmilieus wie Krankenhaus, Allgemeinpraxis, Familie, Merkmale des Therapeuten, Einnahmebedingungen (allein oder in Gruppen) und soziale Einflüsse der zur Behandlung und zum Patienten positiv oder negativ eingestellten Menschen. [The medical preparation M in the form of a placebo P or a substance X or Y acts, under the simultaneous presence of various conditioning factors ... and the additional effect of situational influencing factors ..., on the organism of the test person ... The conditioning factors are to be understood as including attributes of the preparation such as color, shape, size, number and taste as well as dose, duration, type of application and relevant instruction about the kind of preparation concerned. The situational influencing factors ... comprise factors relating to the therapeutic environment such as hospital, general practice, family, characteristics of the therapist, conditions of administration (alone or in groups) and social influences of those persons with a positive or negative attitude towards the therapy and towards the patient.'] (Netter 1986: 62).

As the "causal factors" of Netter's model are most closely related to sensorily perceptible qualities – in this context, to semiotically exceptionally relevant characteristics – of the drug, consideration is given first to the possibilities and limitations of their investigation. The "situational influencing factors" are discussed later in this chapter in the course of further consideration of placebo research from the aspect of scientific history, as knowledge of the theoretical constructions used in their operationalisation is a prerequisite for examination.

In a closer examination of the influence of sensorily perceptible qualities of drugs on their effect, the question of primary interest at this juncture is: Can the structure of this influence be described in semiotic terms within the framework of a code model? It is absolutely crucial to bear in mind here that any codes that might help describe or even explain the structure of this influence are not stabilised by administrative and purpose-motivated conventions (such as the Morse code or semaphore) but by essentially variant processes of sign interchange, whose iterative fulfilment generates as time goes by a relational structure that is permanently unstable and thus permanently jeopardised. The question of whether such an interrelational structure can be described adequately and with sufficient precision with semiotic code models will be the focus of our interest in the further course of this second chapter.

One special case of such an interrelational structure that has been the subject of exceptionally detailed discussion within the framework of semiotic considerations and in conjunction with sensory everday experience is certainly "inference" (cf. Sebeok – Umiker-Sebeok 1980), about which Eco writes: "We are able to infer from smoke the presence of fire, from a wet spot the fall of a raindrop, from a track on the sand the passage of a given animal and so on. All these are cases of inference and all our everyday life is filled with a lot of these inferential acts." (Eco 1976: 17).

These acts are – as Eco then qualifies, however – genuine semiotic processes only when the contexts and associations implied by them are "culturally recognized and systematically coded" (Eco 1976: 17). This qualification is applied in the further course of the semiotic presentation of the placebo problem undertaken in this chapter as an orientating criterion for the adequacy of code models in interpreting the so-called "causal factors" (Netter) of placebo effects.

Another special case of such an interrelational structure that is to play an important role in the course of this chapter in conjunction with the "situational influencing factors" (Netter) of the placebo effect is the concept of "attribution" (Heider 1958) developed in the contexts of learning theory and social psychology and defined as follows by Six (1983: 122): "Attribution läßt sich als jener Interpretationsprozeß der Erfahrungswelt definieren, durch den der Einzelne sozialen Ereignissen und Handlungen Gründe bzw. Ursachen zuschreibt." ['Attribution can be defined as that interpretation process of the world of experience through which the individual ascribes reasons or causes to social occurrences and actions.']

The recommendation by Kissel and Barrucand (1964) that //placebos// prescribed as laxatives should be brown and taste salty but that soporific //placebos// should taste bitter gives preliminary access to an interrelational structure between sensorily perceptible qualities of placebos (and other drugs) and their physiological effects. If this recommendation is to be meaningful, then it implies the assumption that patients deduce possible effects from specific sensorily perceptible qualities when taking drugs and that these deductions, whether made consciously or unconsciously, inferentially or attributively, must for their part have an influence on the actual effects. As this recommendation is evidently based, however, more on personal attitude than on systematic observation, it can hardly be used as a basis for further empirical examination. Table 2 gives a survey of some fragmentary results of experimental investigations into the connection between sensorily perceptible qualities of placebos and other drugs and their action.

Whilst not claiming to be complete, this summary is the outcome of perusal and bibliographic processing of nine important monographs on the placebo problem.[58] From a stock of more than a thousand original works published in secondary sources, it is obviously only a very small portion that focuses on the connection between sensorily perceptible qualities of placebos and their effect; most of these were published prior to 1967, in other words

Table 2: Synopsis of empirical placebo research.

Authors	Independant Variable	Dependant Variable	Measuring Methods	No. of Probands	Result	Sensory Quality	Remarks
Schindel (1967)	1. Admin. of placebo in proband's previously determined favourite color 2. Pseudoplacebo (vitamin tablets) in uniform color	Relief of 1. sleeplessness 2. indigestion 3. menorrhalgia 4. hypertension 5. angina pectoris	Subjective self-rating	155 f = 88 m = 67 14−83 y	Subjective improvement greater with favorite color than with uniform color	Color	Quantitative results and statistical parameters not documented
Gowdey, Hamilton, and Philps (1967)	1. Admin. of 1 green and 1 yellow gelatine capsule comp. with: 2. Admin. of 1 red and 1 white gelatine capsule	Concentration and problem-solving behaviour > Occurence of 'side' effects −	Mathem. abilities before and after intake. Subjective self-rating	24 (medical students)	With red/white combination significantly ($p = 0.05$) poorer performance in mathematical problems	Color	Only color combination taken into account
Lienert (1956)	Admin. of 1. Coffein or 2. bitter placebo, both given with instruction: "You have been given coffein equivalent in effect to 1 large cup of mocca." 3. Coffein or 4. bitter placebo, both given with instruction: "You are being given a placebo."	Occurrence of stimulating effects	Subjective self-rating acc. to list of symptoms	1.: 67 2.: 52 3.: 69 4.: 52 (psychology students)	1.: 58% 2.: 48% Frequency of occurrence of subjectively stimulating effects in % 3.: 36% 4.: 17%	Taste	Taste taken into account only as confounding variable with actual target variable (type of instruction)
Kissel & Barrucand (1964)	Admin. of placebos and soporifics in different colors	Sleep yes/no	Casuistic	1	Proband slept only after yellow preparations, no matter whether placebo or verum	Color	Case study

Shannon & Isbell (1963)	4 treatment stages: 1. Injection of local anaesthetic into the oral mucosa (by dentist) 2. Physiolog. saline injection 3. Needle inserted without injection 4. Only notification and preparatory ritual of injection 5. no treatment	Blood cortisol level before and after treatment (as biochemical indicator of 'stress')	Enzymatic in laboratory	1.: 52 2.: 50 3.: 50 4.: 54 5.: 60	In stages 1–4, highly significant increase ($p < 0.001$) in serum cortisol level; between groups 1–4 no significant difference In group 4 no increase in cortisol	Injection ritual	No double-blind approach possible in stages 3–5
Lasagna, Laties & Dohan (1958)	Once per day for 7 days admin. of a yellow tablet, declared as "appetite inducer" and "invigorator"	Appetite, energy	Subjective self-rating scale	34 (hospitalised tuberculosis patients)	Linear increase in subjective well-being as treatment continued > cumulation	Quantity	Result was replicated in 2nd group with non-selected disorders
Morris & O'Neal (1974)	Admin. in placebos 1. with well-known drug names 2. with imaginary names	Concentration, manual skills	Test battery	64 (male students)	No significant differences between 1. and 2.	Name	Imaginary names were made to sound like drug names
Kuschinsky (1975)	Admin. of 1 or 2 blue, 1 or 2 pink capsules, all with instruction: sedative or stimulating effects are possible	Degree of activity	Subjective self-rating	Number and sex not reported	Blue capsules had more sedative, pink more stimulating effects; this varied in line with quantity	Color, quantity	Study is written without bibliographic references

in the first two decades of placebo research. If consideration is given to the epistemological early history of modern placebo research outlined at the start of this second chapter, a plausible explanation can be formulated for this research desideratum: The thematising of the correlation between sensorily perceptible qualities of placebos and their physiological effects is diametrically opposed to a traditional fundamental prerequisite of placebo research. This fundamental prerequisite is connected with the epistemological rooting of placebo research in pharmacology and states in effect:

"Placebos are, since they contain no specific pharmacological components, completely non-specific in other aspects too. Their appearance, taste or name is therefore of no consequence and is unworthy of any systematic examination."

This point continues to be treated with a correspondingly casual attitude in experimental clinical research. Although all placebo researchers consider the greatest similarity possible between the //placebo// and the //verum// containing the active substance to be methodologically important, there is, for example "… hinsichtlich des Geschmacks meist keine Übereinstimmung zwischen dem Medikament und dem entsprechenden Placebo zu erreichen ist, mitunter gar nicht erst versucht wird" ['… with respect to taste, no conformity to be attained in general between the drug and the corresponding placebo'], furthermore ['sometimes not even an effort is made'] (Gross 1984: 10).

Blumenthal, Burke and Shapiro (1974) subjected this methodological inexactitude to experimental examination: They filled various containers with six different drugs together with the respective "identical matching placebos" intended for clinical testing. Uninformed test persons were then found to be capable of separating the //verum// preparations from their "identical matching placebos" again on account of differences, some of them very subtle, in such factors as granulation, edging finish, thickness and shade.

The results reported in Table 2 show very clearly that so-called "non-specific" qualities such as colors, taste, forms and location of administration, ritualisation, quantity of material and possibly (though without experimentally based confirmation in the work reported on) naming may well have important influences, quantitively speaking, on effects of drugs. These factors, however, are far from providing an adequate answer to the question that is of primary interest at this juncture, that of cultural codification of these influences. Yet three elementary factors, though not totally independent of one another, can be identified on the basis of these relatively scanty results. These factors are obviously paramount in determining the influence of these semiotically highly relevant qualities on the effect of drugs. This influence depends on whether and to what extent:

(1) A specific drug confirms through its sensorily perceptible qualities the previous apprehension of the patient in direct or indirect dealings with drugs. The average consumer of tablets or dragees, for example, will expect his preparation to be round and to have one color, to be sold in packaging that is simple compared with other consumer goods, and to have a name following the unwritten rules for composing drug names (cf. Schuhmacher 1969; Martino 1986; Lemay 1968). He will furthermore assume that intravenous applications are of value only in cases of severe illness but are more efficient, and that sleeping tablets tend to be small, but antibiotics or tablets against indigestion large in diameter.

(2) A specific drug permits the modelling of similarity or at least the generation of a complementary structure between the pathological process and the drug. The reason for a brown tablet – as recommended by Kissel and Barrucand (1964) – being an especially good laxative is that its color is in a barely disguised similarity relationship to the desired effect. An exceptionally good pain-relieving efficacy of the placebo injection *in loco dolente* as compared with the systemic intramuscular injection in the study by Traut and Passarelli (1959) might also be due to this factor. The development of healing rituals in tribal medicine is very often based on this principle.

(3) The totality of the sensorily perceptible qualities of a specific pharmacon is pleasant, desirable and esthetically satisfying to the patient. This relationship is confirmed most impressively by the marked efficacy of oral placebo application in a capsule with the previously determined favourite color of the patient in comparison with a standard color (Schindel 1967).

It is, however, important to emphasise that the efficacy of these three factors develops even if (or, rather, especially when) the fulfilment of their prerequisites is not perceived consciously by the patient. The sequence of the three factors is also meant to be a hypothetical assessment of the extent of their significance in the influencing of the effects of medication. This provisional hypothetic assessment is substantiated in further detail in a discussion on some examples of conflict cases between the three factors, summarised once again in Figure 12.

One vivid example of a conflict between factors 1 and 3 is the "bitter" pill. Although a bitter taste is generally rated as unpleasant in occidental culture, it cannot necessarily be concluded that it has to have an unfavourable effect on the efficacy of a drug, as would actually be expected from the sole influence of factor 3. On the contrary – it is rather a favourable influencing of efficacy that is to be expected, since a bitter taste is indeed recognisable as an outstandingly typical characteristic of outstandingly efficient drugs in accordance with the effective connection in factor 1 in occidental culture and

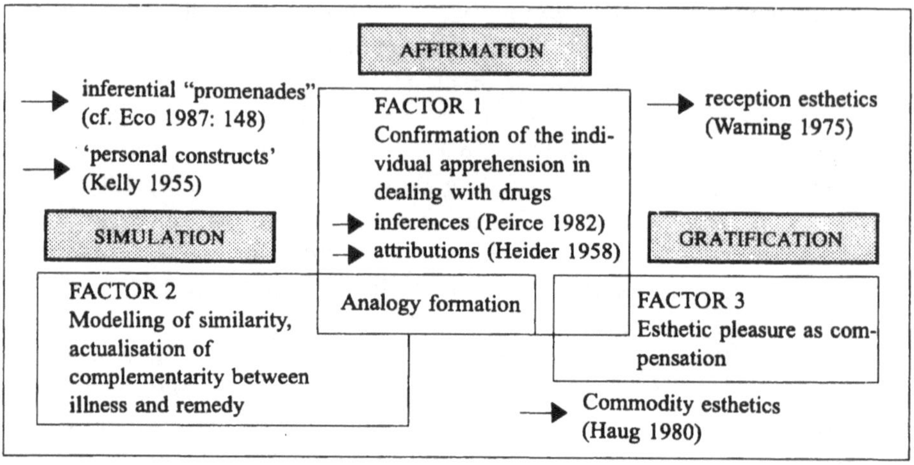

Figure 12: Diagrammatic representation of the three semiotic factors of placebo response.

thus in the apprehension of sick members of this culture. The same applies to the even more unpleasant injection pain as – from the patient's point of view – an inferential indicator of the special efficacy of intravenously applied drugs and of the entire field of "placebo surgery" (Beecher 1968: 33–34).

A conflict between factors 1 and 3, whose outcome goes in favour of factor 3, is the introduction of "commodity-esthetic" innovations in the design of new pre-packed drugs (e.g. in color-speckled cardiovascular drugs introduced in the Seventies). In radically simplified terms, this conflict can be said to have become increasingly frequent during the past few years, the more the design of drugs has approached the commodity esthetics of other consumer goods. The historical starting-point of this development can be surmised when the difficulties confronted in the introduction of aspirin are brought to mind. It was because of the then unaccustomed tablet form – //antipyretics// had previously been available mainly in powder form – that aspirin, according to Eichengrün (1949), had apparently been accepted only very hesitantly by German consumers during the first months.

In his study, Schindel details some further observations that once again illustrate very clearly, though unsystematically, the interaction of the three factors outlined here, based on the example of color effect:

> Interessant waren Erfolge der Behandlung klimakterischer Blutdrucksteigerungen mit Reserpin: Nach Verabreichung des Präparates in der bevorzugten Farbkapsel war durchschnittlich eine größere Blutdrucksenkung nachweisbar,

als in einer Kapsel, deren Farbe als unsympathisch bezeichnet wurde. Bei Menstruationsbeschwerden wurden rote Placebo-Kapseln meist abgelehnt, auch wenn rot zu der bevorzugten Farbe gehörte. Auch bei intestinalen Beschwerden fand rot wenig Anklang, während bei anginösen Beschwerden rot gerne akzeptiert wurde (vielleicht weil Nitroglyn eine rote, Nitroglycerin enthaltende Tablette mit prolongiertem Effekt, eine häufig verordnete Tablette darstellt). [Successes recorded in the treatment of climacteric hypertension with reserpine were interesting. Following administration of the preparation in the favored colour capsule, a greater reduction in blood pressure was recorded on average than with a capsule whose color was described as unpleasant. Red placebo capsules were generally rejected by patients suffering from painful menstruation, even if red was one of the favored colors. Red also met with very little approval among patients suffering from intestinal complaints, whereas red was welcomed by those suffering from anginal complaints (possibly because Nitroglyn, a long-acting red tablet containing nitroglycerine, is a frequently prescribed drug)'] (Schindel 1967: 912).

Whether these processes of association and recognition are subject to a mechanism which, as Eco (1976: 17) demands for semiotic processes, is "culturally recognized and systematically coded" cannot be decided for the time being because of the sparse material available. The already quoted recommendation by Kissel and Barrucand (1964) that laxative placebos should be brown and taste salty but that soporific placebos should be bitter is a cautious implicit assumption – though without empirical substantiation – of the validity of a pharmacological color and taste code.[59] If such codes exist and the model developing from them should prove adequate, then their existence can be assumed to be closely linked with a mechanism that Koch has described within the framework of his theory of "socio-semiotic structuralism": "Der biophysische Mechanismus, der es auf irgendeiner Stufe erlaubt, Unendlichkeiten bzw. relativ größere Mengen von Diskreta bzw. Verhältnissen in übersichtlichere ökonomische Verhältnisse zu überführen, soll Strukturator bzw. Struktur genannt werden" ['The biophysical mechanism that permits infinities or relatively larger amounts of discrete quantities or proportions to be converted at some stage into clear economic proportions shall be designated structurator or structure'] (Koch 1971: 4).

If the principle of Koch's "structurator" is applied to the efficacy of the three factors summarised in Figure 12, then the following definition results:

Sensorily perceptible qualities of drugs can influence their effects to the extent to which they are suitable for structuring the complexity of the pathological process:

(1) by establishing a fixed, affirmative relationship between the current event and that knowledge of the confrontation between suffering and healing that has already accumulated and is also largely sensorily perceived and structured by sensory qualities (factor 1);

(2) by placing on the same footing as the threateningly new, deranging aspects of the illness something complementary or similar which, together with them, inaugurates a new, surprising and thus powerful order (factor 2);

(3) by compensating in a comforting way for unpleasant, distasteful sensations with acceptable, pleasant sensations (factor 3).

These definitions might be anchored in operational terms by designating factor 1 as /affirmation/, factor 2 as /simulation/ and factor 3 as /gratification/.

The anticipatory references of //placebos// transmitted by consciously or unconsciously executed structuring processes of this kind can best be described as signposts to the location or the provisional vectorial direction of their possible effects. Sebeok therefore refers to the placebo as an "attenuated symbol" or – quoting a usage by Peirce – as a "sign which has a symbol for its indirect interpretant" (Sebeok 1979a: 132).

But to return to the chronology of placebo research. As indicated above, its real beginnings are generally dated back to 1945 with the publication of Pepper's article "A note on the placebo". This article gives a precise specification of a research desideratum and makes a terminological proposal founded primarily on historical factors: /placebo/. There was an overwhelming response to Pepper's Note, and within a few years a completely new branch of research had been established, one in which the essential fundamentals were developed methodologically for what was to be referred to – from the late 1950s onwards, after the invention of neuroleptics – as /psychopharmacology/. In 1947 one of the notable symposia of the "Cornell Conferences on Therapy" was devoted exclusively to the placebo problem. The early 1950s saw the beginning of systematic empirical and experimental research into everything that was to be achieved pharmacologically without active pharmacological substances. In 1946, Jelinek performed the very first experimental investigations into the pain-relieving effect of placebos. His results were replicated and described in closer detail in the 1950s by numerous authors, first in the USA but soon afterwards in Europe. In 1950, Cleghorn observed that the quantitative increase in adrenocortical hormone secretion induced in patients with anxiety neuroses by injecting nothing more than physiological saline solution was the same as that induced in healthy probands by injecting the pituitary hormone ACTH, which is specific to this effect. (For bibliographic data on the stated authors, cf. Kissel – Barrucand 1964: 213–234). Lasagna and coworkers (1958) showed that the effects of placebos could be described in part with dose:effect ratios and time:effect ratios, which had previously been interpreted as a mere consequence of the intake, metabolisation and excretion of active pharmacological substances. It was also found, however, that patients could become psychologically and physically addicted to placebos, responding to discontinuation of the non-specific preparations with specific withdrawal symptoms (Vinar 1979). Kissel and Barrucand (1964: 42–43) published a summarised report of a number of cases in which the administration of placebos had even led to severe toxic side-effects with cardiac decompensation and those dermatological symptoms typical of allergic reactions.

Another prematurely thematised drawback of placebo therapy concerned the ethical issues relating to its application: Was it still possible in the age of the enlightened, emancipatory doctor-patient relationship to treat people without or even against their knowledge of the content of the therapy, even if this was done in the context of clinical therapy for their own benefit or in the context of clinical research for the benefit of third parties?[60] 1961 saw the publication in the USA of the first two detailed research bibliographies on the placebo problem, edited by Mooney and by the National Institute of Health (bibliographic references in Schindel 1967: 915). In 1961 (Rinkel 1963) and 1966 (Rickels 1968), two successive psychiatric world congresses each held a symposium on non-specific factors in drug therapy.

One of the few authors to thematise the semiotic dimension of the phenomenon in the direct context of placebo research, at least in elementary terms, is the American psychiatrist Whitehorn. In an article published in the *American Journal of Psychiatry* and declared as a personal comment on the problem of placebo therapy, he comes up with a definition of his own, one that differs from those quoted above in the very aspect of specificity, an aspect of special interest at this juncture:

> For purposes of abstract discussion, it is convenient to designate as "placebo" effects all those psychological and psychophysiological benefits or detriments which quite directly involve the patient's expectations and depend directly upon the diminuition or augmentation of the patient's apprehension by the symbolism of medication or the symbolic implications of the physician's behavior and attitudes." (Whitehorn 1958: 663).

By interpreting the placebo effect as an elementary correlation between the patient's apprehension and semiotically relevant factors, which he describes in very general terms as "symbolic", Whitehorn assimilates into his definition the trail of a specificity whose further analysis eludes a pharmacological but not a semiotic approach. With respect to Peirce's trichotomy (to which Whitehorn makes no reference whatsoever), this correlation does, however, conceal indexical (cf. Sebeok 1979a: 132) and – as is shown at a later point – iconic elements.

Whitehorn describes elsewhere a prerequisite for this correlation, whose formulation conforms impressively with Eco's already quoted criterion for the semioticity of inferences: "... a 'placebo effect' should not bring discredit on the patient. It does not mean that illness is absent or feigned... Instead it indicates a preparedness to be helped, a willingness to trust a help-giver, and a responsiveness to the physician as a person as well as to him as a culturally established symbol of healing." (Whitehorn 1958: 663).

If this trail continues to be followed, then it is not irrelevant whether a specific placebo is round or angular, red or white, solid or liquid. Its application thus demands a very specific selection from the armamentarium of professional routines generated by the application of medical therapies in the course of time. In each concrete case, this selection is the outcome of an individual service tailored to the expressed symptoms and needs of the patient and adapted to the context and the situation. Another practical example, to which Kleinsorge (in: Hippius – Überla – Laakmann – Hasford 1986: 19–20) has referred in a different context, illustrates quite clearly that placebo therapy is relatively ineffective without this service and the doctor-patient interaction involved in it: An attempt was made in the Netherlands to introduce officially into therapy a placebo that can be prescribed without further explanation by any doctor and produced – in accordance with standardised specifications – by any pharmacist. These standard placebos proved, however, relatively ineffective. Kleinsorge associates their ineffectiveness with news of this practice having spread among patients within a short time. The fact may rather be, however, that these standard placebos were completely non-specific, hollow significants, as it were, not only from the pharmacological but also from the semiotic aspect. Placebos cannot be prescribed in the Federal Republic of Germany. Prescription practice has, however, found a way round this – one recommended explicitly by Kuschinsky (1975: 666), for example – which appears to be far more effective than the Dutch model and does indeed permit provision of that service referred to here that is needed to make the application of placebos specific from the semiotic aspect: The German armamentarium stocks a large number of preparations whose pharmacological inefficacy is either considered proven or whose pharmacological efficacy has remained unproven in controlled double-blind trials. As these preparations are available in every conceivable color, mode of application and taste under a wide range of names and indications, it is easy to select and prescribe the appropriate preparation for a large number of different contexts, situations and symptoms. Preparations containing pharmacologically defined substances but prescribed or applied by doctors in full awareness of their inefficacy are referred to in the placebo literature as "pseudoplacebos".[61] In a survey among practising doctors in the Federal Republic of Germany, Classen and Feingold (1985) found that 54% of them prescribe //pseudoplacebos// regularly (without detailed frequency data). Another result of their study at least indicates the qualities of the respective individual preparations by which the doctors are guided. The authors asked the same doctors what qualities might influence the efficacy of drugs, apart from the active substances contained in them. (In line with standard placebo research practice, the authors refer to these properties as "nonspecific characteristics" (Classen – Feingold 1985: 131)). According to these authors,

> Almost all the physicians are of the opinion that nonspecific characteristics do influence the efficacy of medicines: as the most powerful one the instruction sheet attached to drugs was mentioned by 75% , followed by the colour (60%), the price (47%) and the form (40%) of the drugs. Furthermore, mode of application (39%) and taste (32%) are supposed to influence their efficacy. (Classen – Feingold 1985: 131).

Although the question of //pseudoplacebo// application was not necessarily linked in substance with the question of efficacy rating in that study, these qualities may be assumed to be the essential orientation characteristics for those doctors when prescribing //pseudoplacebos//. A reliable decision on whether this orientation depended on a system that might adequately be described in terms of a code model can admittedly not be based on these data.

Further research into the placebo phenomenon was influenced methodologically in essential features by the development of constructs and instruments based on social and personalistic psychology. This influence resulted in the traditional pharmacological hypothesis of the non-specificity of placebos being viewed in more relative terms. Even in the first decade of placebo research the interesting observation was thematised that distinct //placebo effects// – depending on experimental or clinical conditions – were by no means to be observed in all patients or probands treated with //placebos// but in only about one-third of them. In subsequent decades, a great deal of energy and scrupulous methodological exactitude was applied to the question – one that has yet to be answered – of whether so-called placebo responders can be distinguished consistently from non-responders with variables determined sociodemographically or by personalistic psychology.[62] The placebo phenomenon was thus linked for the first time in a working hypothesis with a certain specificity, at least with respect to those persons involved, acting and interacting.

Lasagna, Mosteller et al. (1954: 774), for instance, discovered in a study on placebo therapy for postoperative pain that regular churchgoers were represented in the "responder group" significantly more often than in the "non-responder" group. In a study by Rickels (1968: 11) on the pharmacological placebo therapy of anxiety neuroses, patients with a low "vocabulary verbal intelligence" benefited significantly more from this therapy than a parallelised control group of above-average intelligence.

In the Sixties and Seventies, attempts were made in numerous studies to determine the correlation between various constructs of personalistic psychology and placebo responsiveness, to lend empirical support to forming the theory of possible determinants of the placebo phenonemon.

Two constructs investigated with outstanding frequency, though by no means with conforming results, are "acquiescence" or "acquiescent response set" (Pichot – Perse 1968) and "suggestibility". Both constructs play an important role in psychological artefact research too (cf. Bungard 1980), and it is not surprising that they intrude into the investigation of a phenomenon that is reputed in the tradition of the pharmacological perspective, in which it remains initially inexplicable, to be an artefact. Despite the extent of statistical correlation having indeed been significant in individual studies, the overall picture emerging from this research approach was rather of a contradictory nature. With respect to the relevance of the "suggestibility" construct to placebo research, Gallimore and Turner come to the following evaluating conclusion: "The cumulative evidence however is persuasive that neither primary nor secondary suggestibility is a reliable or effective predictor of placebo response." (Gallimore – Turner 1977: 51).

The hypothesis that expectations placed on a specific therapy and preliminary experience gained with it by all those involved must have a crucial influence on its measurable effects has, however, been reliably founded within the framework of these endeavours (e.g. Wheatley 1968). The very contradictions in placebo research based on personalistic psychology resulted in the formulation of a fundamental contradiction whose theoretical proximity to Eco's dialectics between codes and messages may at least be of interest for the semiotic significance of the placebo problem. This fundamental contradiction between a "situationstheoretische(n)" ['situation-theoretical'] and an "eigenschaftstheoretische(n)" ['quality-theoretical'] explanatory model of the placebo effect is described by Janke (1986). The validity of such quality-theoretical models – and thus the feasibility of forming systematically codified interrelational structures – is linked by Janke to two fundamental questions: "1.) Handelt es sich bei der Reaktivität auf Placebo um ein Merkmal im Sinne einer Eigenschaft, das in hinreichendem Maße zeit- und situationsinvariant ist? 2.) Hängt Placebo-Reaktivität mit anderen Persönlichkeitsmerkmalen zusammen, etwa allgemeiner Art wie Neurotizismus, Extraversion, Suggestibilität, Jasagetendenz oder spezifischer Art wie Einstellungen gegenüber Psychopharmaka?" ['1.) Is reactivity to placebo a quality in the sense of a sufficiently invariant feature with respect to time and situation? 2.) Is placebo reactivity connected with other personality characteristics of a general kind such a neuroticism, extraversion, suggestibility, acquiescence, or of a specific kind such as attitudes towards psychopharmaceuticals?'] (Janke 1986: 152).

With respect to the context of special interest at this juncture, these two questions would have to be supplemented for an analogous semiotic model of qualities by two others: Is there a time-constant correlation between placebo effects and sensorily perceptible qualities of those objects used as //placebos//? And: Is the systematisation and cultural codification of this correlation sufficient (in Eco's sense) for it to be described adequately in terms of a code model?

If, on the other hand, the placebo effect were to be regarded as a "situation-theoretical" event, then neither constructs based on personalistic psychology nor sensorily perceptible qualities of //placebos// would really be suited to theoretical interpretation of the fundamental mechanisms of this effect in terms of a code model. The secret of the surprising effects of placebos within the framework of association between the sufferer and the healer would continue to be a rewarding object of psychological and semiotic consideration, but from a completely different perspective, one characterised by the dominating influences of the individual case, of the subjects involved, of the concrete situations, and by a relative lack of intersubjectivity and horizontal comparability. The possible connection between semiotically relevant characteristics of a drug and its effect would then be, as it were, the "rezeptionsästhetische" ['reception-esthetical'] (Warning 1975) realisation of an intersubjectively valid code of colors, shapes, tastes and application rituals, an expression of "personal constructs" (Kelly 1955) or "idiolectal concretions" (Eco 1976: 137) that could not be comprehended without reference to the subject and the situation.

2.3. Experimental aspects: structural gain through arousal

In an experimental study, Schachter and Singer (1962) examined the influence of the concrete situation in which a drug is administered on its possible effects and their subjective perception and interpretation by the probands. Besides a pharmacologically specific and potent substance, //adrenalin//, they also used pharmacologically non-specific //placebos// in two parallelised proband groups. The results of their study – though not performed in the direct context of placebo research – are, however, of great interest to the context being dealt with here, for a different reason. From the methodological viewpoint, their study seems quite remarkable because it not only compares the application effects of a pharmacologically active substance with those of a pharmacologically inert substance, as is perfectly normal within the scope of placebo research, but because it goes one step further: Numerous situational details of this application are altered systematically – but imperceptibly for the probands – and can thus be included in this comparison as independent variables.

Schachter and Singer examined the effect of subcutaneous injection of a single dose of adrenalin or physiological saline solution (= placebo) on 184 healthy male college students in a total of 7 different treatment stages each comprising 23 to 27 probands. All probands were informed that they were participating in a study designed to examine the effect of a vitamin preparation by the name of /Suproxin/ on vision. The probands were informed in different ways at the individual treatment stages of possible side-effects of the administered /Suproxin/, which was, in fact, either //adrenalin// or a //physiological saline solution//: One group of probands, who were given an adrenalin solution without their knowledge, was given adequate information on the side-effects to be expected, such as palpitations, trembling hands and flushing (= initiation stage: "informed"). Another group of these probands, on the other hand, was informed of possible side-effects, such as itching or headache, that were by no means to be expected in view of the known specific effects of //adrenalin// (= initiation stage: "misinformed"). A further group of probands treated with //adrenalin// and all those treated with the //placebo// injection were given no information at all on possible side-effects (= initiation stage: "ignorant").

Special attention was paid at the planning stage to systematic changing of the situation in which the probands believed, after administration of the substance, that they were awaiting the announced experiment, namely a vision test. (The entire study had been announced to them, after all, as an investigation into the effect of a /vitamin preparation/ on vision).

Each proband in turn was led into a waiting-room in which another person besides himself, also introduced to him as a "proband", was awaiting the announced vision test. This other person was, however, in actual fact a member of the research team, whose task consisted in filling in the alleged waiting-time with preset, standardised actions and remarks as drastically as possible through the production of "emotion-inducing cognitions" (Schachter – Singer 1962: 383). This stooge either produced a euphoric atmosphere with imaginative slapstick activities of comic effect in that specific situation, using properties located in the waiting-room, or he expressed distinct anger at the pointlessness of and the unreasonable demands made by the alleged experiment. During the period in which the administered substances were taking effect – which was declared as a "waiting-time" – the extent to which the respective genuine proband was influenced by the situational set-up staged by the stooge and the extent to which he participated in the actions of euphoria or anger or even initiated such actions himself were watched by unseen observers. In addition, each proband made a self-rating of his physical and emotional well-being during this phase by filling in a questionnaire with a four-stage scale.

This highly complex experimental design by Schachter and Singer thus incorporated a total of three independent, systematically modified variables:

(1) the subcutaneously injected substance (adrenalin/saline solution); (2) the initiation stage ("informed", "misinformed", "ignorant"); (3) the cognitive-emotional design of the reaction time, which was declared as a waiting-time (euphoria/anger).

Of those dependent variables taken into account and determined within the framework of this study, two appear to be of special importance:

(4) the occurrence of announced or – depending on degree of initiation – unannounced side-effects, determined quantitatively by proband self-rating (at a rational scale level) and (5) the cognitive-emotional adaptation of the probands to the – environment-orientated – waiting situation, determined quantitatively by self-rating (at rational scale level) and by observations of behaviour (at interval scale level).

The outcome showed that the occurrence of side-effects was relatively independent both of the degree of initiation and of the design of the waiting situation, and varied almost exclusively with the injected substance. Significant differences were thus determined here only when the placebo-treated and the adrenalin-treated groups were compared. This outcome is initially contradictory to what would have been expected on the basis of empirical evidence provided by placebo research – that similar therapeutic results can be observed with similar therapeutic conditions even if these therapeutic conditions differ distinctly with respect to their pharmacological efficacy. Whilst this contradiction is by no means to be ignored at this juncture, it is not to be the subject of further discussion either.[63]

The emotional adaptation of the probands to the waiting situation provided a far more differentiated picture. The degree and the direction of this adaptation are found to have varied both with the degree of initiation and with the situational characteristics of the waiting situation but – contrary to the working hypothesis expounded by Schachter and Singer – hardly at all with the pharmacology of the injected substance. Those adrenalin probands who had been adequately informed of possible side-effects reacted significantly

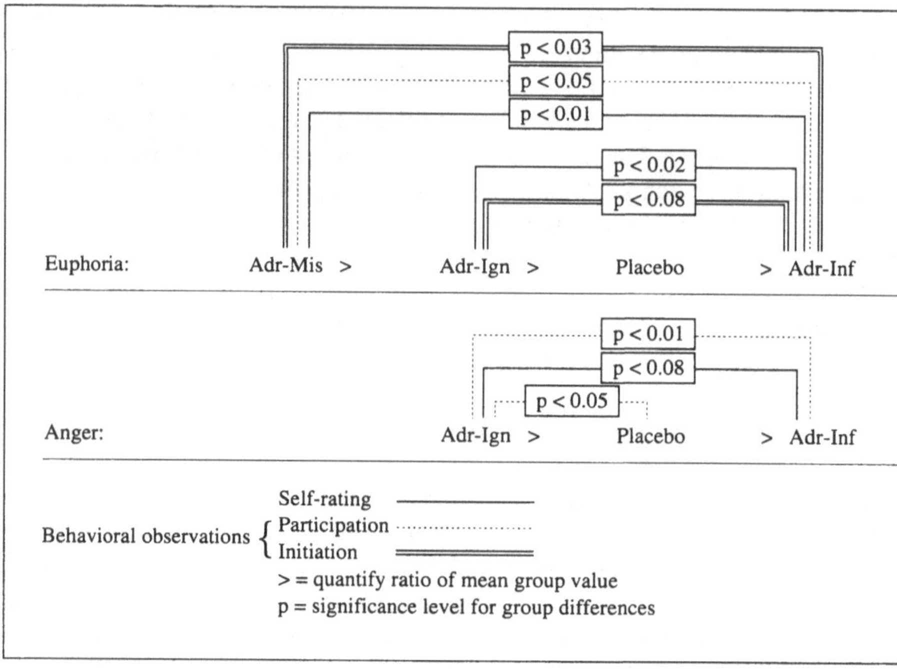

Figure 13: Inter-group comparisons of Schachter and Singer's experiment.

less frequently with anger or euphoria on their own part, both in the /angry/ and in the /euphoric/ waiting situation, than those who were misinformed or left in ignorance. The emotional reactivity of the placebo probands was quantitatively between that of the "informed" and that of the "ignorant" adrenalin probands. This quantitative difference was not significant, however, except in comparison with one control group and in one waiting situation. Figure 13 gives a survey of these quantitative ratios, the significance levels of the direct comparisons, and the different sources of rating data.

Schachter and Singer interpret the consistently different degrees of manipulability in the various proband groups roughly as follows: They argue that, at least in the adrenalin probands, the injection of a pharmacologically highly effective substance – one that moreover acts as a stimulant specific to the sympathetic nervous system – triggers off a distinct rise in the general level of arousal and attentiveness, thus provoking a state commonly referred to in the context of psychophysiological research as "arousal" or "sympathetic activation". If distinct physical, emotional or cognitive changes were to take place in such a state of generally increased attentiveness or if such changes were to be induced by situational changes in the environment, continue Schachter and Singer, then the probability of these changes becoming effective factors determining behavior and experience would depend directly on whether or not the change can be explained by the experience and information available to the proband or – in more general terms – whether the change rather questions or rather confirms his previous hypothesis or his previous world knowledge (a term not used by Schachter and Singer). In other words: The /degree of innovation/ of a change (which for its part behaves in direct proportion to the amount of information measured by the Shannon/Weaver method) behaves in direct proportion to the emotional "Plastizität" ['plasticity'] (Schultz-Gambard 1983) of the person affected by it.

Jospe (1978) has given special emphasis to the explanatory and integrative potency of this hypothesis for the heterogeneous field of placebo research. Summing up, he writes:

> When people are in a state of arousal, they may experience very disparate emotional states or no emotional states at all, depending on the concurrent cognitions. This emotional plasticity leads people to search for cognitive sources that could be causally associated with their experienced physiological state and that could provide a label for it. A person taking a tablet, for example, is in a state of arousal ... and has learned to associate pill taking with relief of some sort ... As a result of complex conditioning processes, visceral changes are initiated. These changes may be relatively undifferentiated physiologically and almost always take place contiguously with some set of cognitions (e.g., "This will make you feel better" or whatever the instructions, expectations of other communications or perceptions, tacit or not, in the schema are). The placebo effect can then, according to such a view, be interpretated as having three components: physiological arousal, emotionally relevant cognitive or situational factors, and a perceived causal link between these factors. A person who is not aware that he or she is being treated cannot exhibit the placebo effect; this is surely axiomatic. (Jospe 1978: 144).

Under both waiting-time conditions, the emotional manipulability of the (ignorant) placebo probands in Schachter and Singer's study was quantitatively between that of the informed (= Adr.-Inf. in Figure 13) and of the misinformed or even ignorant adrenalin probands (= Adr.Mis. or Adr.Ign. in Figure 13). This sequence is fundamentally compatible with Schachter and Singer's hypothesis: They had not been informed of possible effects of the injection and also noticed significantly fewer such effects. Consequently it was less possible for them than for the informed adrenalin probands to explain any changes occurring (= Adr.-Inf. in Figure 13) but also less necessary than for the misinformed or ignorant adrenalin probands (= Adr.Mis. of Adr.Ign. in Figure 13). Schachter and Singer nonetheless expressed surprise at this result, since they had actually assumed that the level of attentiveness could not be raised distinctly, i. e. no arousal provoked, by an injection of pharmacologically non-specific //saline solution//. And indeed, the placebo probands in Schachter and Singer's study failed to meet any of the criteria set by the authors for attainment of this state. On the other hand, it has been demonstrated and replicated within the framework of placebo research that state-of-the-art application of medical preparations – regardless of whether or not they contain pharmacologically effective components – is quite capable of provoking an increase in attentiveness and arousal in the sense of sympathetic activation.[64] This conclusion is also drawn by Jospe in the passage quoted above from his placebo monograph. The production of arousal may even be one of the main functions of many of the rituals developed within the framework of confrontation between sufferer and healer and involving a high degree of cultural codification: Adjurations by medicine men and shamans, drawing up a fluid into a hypodermic syringe (whose subsequent de-aerating has even advanced to a stock theme in movies), all preliminaries for the injection process, including dabbing alcoholic solution onto the injection site – a measure of virtually no antibacteriological significance, the prescription rituals detailed more closely in Chapter 1, rubbing in liniments, /therapeutic/ tonometry, the diagnostically futile stethoscopic auscultation in what is referred to in Germany as the "Kassendreieck" [panel triangle][65], and most especially the phenolic, bitter, clinical smells, tastes, colors and names of the prescribed medications. All these are highly significant, culturally traditional, but constantly renewed significates, all of which flow into one common message, roughly:

"Watch out – something important is happening now; a gestalt of healing is being formed here, one that is spatiotemporally visible and limited, yet esoterically mystic and analogous in many respects to the structure of suffering."

Or, in more analytical terms: "Strukturgewinn bedeutet Ordnungsgewinn, Ordnungsgewinn 'rettet die Welt'." ['Structural gain implies enhancement of order, and it is enhancement of order that "saves the world".'] (Koch 1971: 7)

The view proposed by Schachter and Singer has a number of advantages for methodological integration of the heterogeneous findings of placebo research into the context being dealt with in this chapter:

(1) It permits exact definition of the concepts of semiotic "inference" and sociopsychological "attribution" already mentioned in conjunction with Netter's "causal factors" of the placebo effect, and thus a more precise answer to the question: Through what associations do sick or suffering individuals attain "structural gains" (in Koch's sense)? Namely through the passive experiencing of arousal, through the unconscious reception of messages such

as "Something special and of significance with respect to the gestalt of suffering is happening here", and through the contingent re-interpretation of the "Erfahrungswelt" ['world as experienced '] (Six 1983: 122) in which the threateningly new that is associated with the illness finds a safer and less threatening place for the time being. Those associations whose starting material is represented by sensorily perceptible qualities of pharmaceutics can be adequately described as semiotic "inferences", provided that they conform with a culturally widespread pattern. Those associations motivated by social interactions between the sufferer and the healer are, in contrast, rather to be described as "attributions".

(2) It is neutral with respect to the dialectics between codes and messages (cf.Eco 1976). Within the framework of their theory of emotions, Schachter and Singer take into account both the validity of intersubjectively communicable codes and standards and the special significance of mastering them. Their theory thus offers room for the next contradictory observation: that the interchange of signs has of necessity to be controlled by rules but repeatedly infringes the rules – or frequently attains its special significance only by infringing the rules – in actual implementation. The genuine probands in their study were able to interpret the unusual behaviour of the stooges as angry or euphoric only by applying behavioral standards. The behavior of these stooges was, however, exceptionally influential on their own behavior with respect to their own emotional "plasticity" (Schultz-Gambard 1983: 465) for another reason too: because of its total failure to conform with the acquiescent behavior that has come to be expected of those taking part in psychological tests.

(3) As a model, it helps clarify possible interferences and contradictions between the three factors summarised in Figure 12, factors playing a crucial role in determining the influences of sensorily perceptible qualities of pharmaceutics on their effects. According to the differentiation proposed in Figure 12, these qualities are exceptionally influential (within the terms of the desired therapeutic effect) when they confirm the individual apprehension and the related associations of the sufferer in dealing with pharmaceutics (= factor 1). On the other hand, they may be influential and valuable when they admittedly contradict this apprehension but instead put the familiar old and the unexpected new into a surprisingly conclusive relationship of similarity or complementarity to each other (= factor 2). Such a process might have led to the misinformed adrenalin probands interpreting their inward tension with exceptional consistency as an outcome of their great euphoria or of their anger, whereas objective observation suggests that the tension resulted at least in part from the injection, and the emotion at least in part from the manipula-

tion by the stooge. Sensorily perceptible qualities of drugs can, after all, also exert a crucial influence on their effect if they have outstanding esthetic appeal, are impressive, and generate sensory pleasure in some way regardless of the individual apprehension in contact with drugs (= factor 3). Within the framework of Schachter and Singer's theory and in the context of the passage quoted from Jospe (1978: 144), this factor, probably the most negligible of the three differentiated here, is connected with the fact that esthetically conspicuous and pleasantly stimulating objects are far more inclined to generate what the authors refer to as arousal than neutral or repulsive objects.

This model – though theoretically integrative, nonetheless highly abstract in other respects – can be brought down to earth in a clinical context with one practical example. This particular example does have a certain amount of practical significance for the social reality of drugs in contemporary medical science because it occurs with great frequency, possibly even more frequently than the application of //pseudoplacebos// discussed above. What is meant is the application of so-called "impure" placebos.[66] According to Müller-Oerlinghausen (1986: 89), these are drugs containing pharmacologically defined substances which (in contrast to "pseudoplacebos") may well develop effects of a proven pharmacological nature. These effects have, however, nothing to do with the desired therapeutic effect forming the rationale for application. One vivid example of this is the rubbing-in of ointments with a warming and hyperemisating[67] effect to treat degenerative or inflammatory joint trouble. This rubbing-in has no effect whatsoever on the objectively measurable perception of pain; in other words, it has neither "curative" nor "symptomatic" action. In cases of inflammatory joint disease, it is even likely to make matters worse. The popularity of these ointments is nonetheless undiminished among both doctors and patients. That popularity depends, however, on the ointments' being effective. The efficacy of this therapy can be interpreted and clarified in very precise terms with the three-factor model presented in this chapter:

In the first place, the generation of external warmth and the stimulation of the cutaneous circulation ("hyperemia") in one locally confined region is a distinct, unusual and decidedly pleasant stimulation that can confidently be expected to raise the level of attentiveness (= factor 3). In addition, the region where this stimulation is taking place is that very region at which the inwardly felt morphological disorder is projected outwards. (It is for this reason that so-called //nitro-patches// for angina pectoris therapy are generally worn direct over the heart, although the active substance contained in them cannot diffuse direct into this organ nor develop its pharmacological effect there.) There is thus a significant – in this case indexical – similarity relationship between the illness and the remedy (factor 2). The assumption that the selected therapy might be helpful in treating joint trouble furthermore complies with an association that is widespread and confirmed autoreflexively for its part by this new empirical experience: Warmth has healing properties (= factor 1).

This is admittedly an impressive but not necessarily representative special case, in which all three factors outlined in Figure 12 may take effect without disturbing one another. This special-case character may, on the other hand, also be an empirical cause of this form of ointment-based therapy being so effective against joint trouble and therefore so popular. One of the leading brands on the German market, whose proprietary name /Rheumon/ conceals distinctly prepropríal elements that may also be associated with factor 2 (cf. Figure 12), was prescribed 2.5 million times in the Federal Republic of Germany in the 1984 calendar year and was thus 16th on the list of those medical preparations most frequently prescribed (Schwabe – Paffrath 1985: 177). Müller-Oerlinghausen (1986: 89) suspected that "impure" placebos might well be more effective on principle than pure – in other words, pharmacologically totally inert – placebos. This finding, which has virtually no empirical substantiation, might be explained within the framework of our model by the fact that "impure" placebos can indeed develop pharmacological effects. Whilst initially of no relevance whatsoever to the desired physiological-therapeutic effect, they are ideally suited to generating arousal. They thus offer the patient – as a special service in comparison with "genuine" placebos and "pseudoplacebos" – the opportunity to venture physiologically into that process that we have endeavoured to formulate in this chapter: structural gain.

2.4. Placebo effects and Peirce's trichotomy

We have considered sensorily perceptible qualities of drugs as "structurators" of outstanding relevance to semiotics and have discussed some quantitative and qualitative aspects of their semiotically specific efficacy, based on examples taken from placebo research. The sometimes astounding effects of pharmacologically non-specific medical preparations have proved to be essentially of a "symbolic" nature with respect to Peirce's trichotomy and with the definition formulated by Whitehorn (1958: 663) taken into account. At times, however, the signs that can be reconstructed with these effects also fulfil "indexical" functions, especially when they give anticipatory indications of the direction or location in which the preparation takes effect. It is mainly to round off this system that the question of whether contact with pharmaceuticals also opens up indications of the efficacy of "iconic" signs is discussed here. The use of masks, amulets and figurative properties in a large number of Red Indian and schamanist healing rituals shows that iconic signs in particular may occasionally have important therapeutic functions, at least from an ethnomedical perspective. In today's enlightened pharmacological therapy, such elements will seldom be expected, and even then only in a very rudimentary form. One such rudiment is given closer consideration in this chapter with a comparison between two headache remedies. The conspicuous under-representation of iconic signs among the semiotically specific factors of drug effects might be connected with the fact that similarity experiences mediated by iconic signs are extremely obvious and hardly unconsciously perceptible. The largely unconscious and unreflected reception of sensory qualities that may well be effective is apparently, as suggested by some findings of placebo research, a preliminary condition which, whilst not essential, is conducive to their effectiveness.[68] A modern-day patient with expectations of pharmacologically specific therapy may possibly be capable of embarking on treatment with signs (instead of with active substances) only if intake is an unconscious process. This constellation possibly reflects in the patient the ambivalent attitude, characterised by a sense of threat and by interest, of modern pharmacology at the outset of placebo research.

Today, iconic signs are most likely to be effective in the clinical context when they get through to the recipient via the back door, as it were. This may be the case with one of the two headache remedies reproduced in Figure 14.

Figure 14.1 shows an Old English remedy for treating headaches, reproduced by Nöth (1977: 34) from Cockayne (1865: 20).

Figure 14.2 reproduces an advertisement from a contemporary German pictorial with an enlargement of a detail taken from it. This advertisement can also be interpreted in the broader sense as a remedy or at least as a recommended therapy against headache, despite its being embedded in a mass-communication framework. As a syntagmatic composition, it is identical with the series of advertisements analysed in Chapter I as a /recipe for success for aspirants/ (cf. Figures 4 to 8), apart from the protagonist figure and the offered product being clearly outside the structural framework outlined in Chapter 1. The comparison drawn below concentrates essentially on the //product// itself rather than on its figurative representation:

Nöth (1977: 34) himself recognizes in the use of the Old English remedy a "Gebrauch von Zeichen anstelle eines physiologisch-medizinischen Vorgangs" ['use of signs instead of a medico-physiological process'] and a theory based "primär nicht auf einer medizinischen sondern vielmehr auf einer semiotischen Grundlage" ['primarily not on medical but rather on semiotic prin-

> Wiδ heafod ece hundes heafod ȝebærn to ahsan & sinδ pe heafod Leȝe on.
> (Against headache = Burn a dog's head to ashes and apply the ground head.)

Figure 14.1

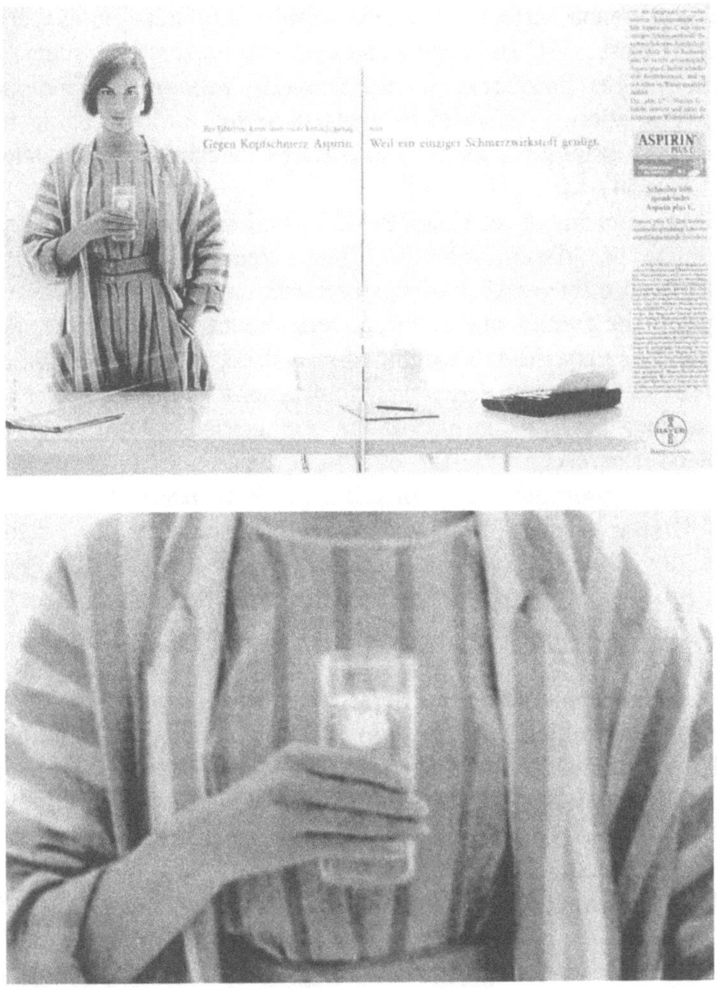

Figure 14.2

Figure 14: Traditional and modern therapies of headache.
(14.2 Reproduced by permission of Bayer AG, Leverkusen.)

ciples'] (Nöth 1977: 34). Obviously the "semiotic principles" in this concrete case are largely identical with what was identified above (cf. Figure 12) as the second factor in the influence of sensorily perceptible qualities on the effect of medication. Nöth summarises these principles as follows: "Der Heilungsprozeß wird in der magischen Therapie in Form von Zeichen dargestellt, und zwar ikonisch (durch die Similaritätsrelation) und indexikalisch (durch die Kontiguitätsrelation...). Statt durch die Therapie einen physiologischen Prozeß einzuleiten, erfolgt eine semiotische Abbildung eines erwünschten Heilungsprozesses." ['The healing process is represented in magic therapy in the form of signs, both iconic (in the similarity relation) and indexical (in the contiguity relation...). Instead of a physiological process being induced by the therapy, a semiotic depiction of a desired healing process takes place.'] (Nöth 1977: 34).

Analogous elements can also be identified in the example of the recommended use of //Aspirin plus C//. These elements are connected with a sensorily perceptible quality of this preparation, one that was given prominence within the framework of the advertisement but is visible, audible and even tangible every time the preparation is used, even without this advertisement, provided the user remains within a certain distance of it (a distance that is indicated by the gesture of the protagonist in Figure 14.2): //Aspirin plus C// is effervescent. On the one hand, this sensorily perceptible quality – being both prominent and pleasant – lends itself to the induction of arousal. On the other hand, it also depicts the desired healing process semiotically as an autoreflective demonstration model, as it were. This depicted healing process is for its part complementary in many ways to the experienced symptom //headache//. We can image it as a tingling vitalisation of the pain-stricken head, discharging the existing tension into numerous small quantums. Now designating this depictive relationship as "iconic" is certainly not without its problems, as the significate represents a totally fictitious process. This relationship does, however, offer a feasible (though not the only conceivable) theoretical explanation for the claim peddled in the advertising slogan – and one that may well be empirically verifiable – that /effervescent/ //Aspirin plus C// gives relief faster than other conventional headache remedies. A pharmacological explanation is in all events lacking.[69]

What cannot be left unchallenged in some respects, however, is the interpretation put forward by Nöth that semiotic depiction is a substitute for the initiation of a physiological process. For this depiction does not replace this physiological process but induces it – whilst using another mechanism, yet no less effectively than would be the case with a pharmacologically effective substance. A biochemical /code/ or /end piece/ to a semiotic induction process was presented and discussed in another context in Chapter I: the secretion of //endorphins//, those endogenous, pain-relieving substances that develop their effect at the same receptors in the central nervous system as externally applied analgesics of the opiate type.

In a study of postoperative pain tolerance, Levine, Gordon and Fields (1978) examined the secretion of //endorphins// as the central mechanism of placebo analgesia. They treated the traumatic pain of freshly operated patients with pharmacologically non-specific placebos – in other words, placebos that had no active substances (and were thus "genuine" or "pure"). The placebo effect was found to be reversible by supplementary administration of //opiate antagonists//, i. e. exogenously applied substances that inhibit the effect of //opiates// and thus of //endorphins// on the central nervous system.

They thus succeeded in antagonising a purely semiotic – and thus, in pharmacological terms, non-specific – medication effect by means of active pharmacological substances.

If this mechanism is assumed to function with respect to the effect of /effervescent/ //Aspirin plus C// as well, this preparation could be described in the narrower pharmacological sense too as a "compound preparation", with the effects of exogenously administered //acetylsalicylic acid// and endogenously "effervescently" secreted //endorphins// supplementing each other. In this model, the effect of the //acetylsalicylic acid// would be pharmacologically, and that of the endorphins purely semiotically, induced. Both effects, on the other hand, would undoubtedly be specific in a general analytical sense. In his critical review of the way in which the terms /specific/ and /non-specific/ are used in the context of placebo research, Grünbaum comes to the conclusion that these terms are "tantalizing words" (Grünbaum 1985: 11), doing little towards providing a well-defined description of the placebo phenomenon. He suggests discriminating between various /specificities/ to assist terminological clarification. Although the discriminating criteria put forward by Grünbaum are totally different, the attempt made in this chapter to place a semiotic "specificity" alongside the pharmacological one might be seen as one possible way of implementing Grünbaum's proposal.

3. De attractionibus electivis: the modelling of /similarity/ in the history of pharmacy and chemistry

> The mind has learned that beauty can make things good, bad, stupid or enchanting. The mind dissects and analyses a sheep and a penitent sinner and finds humility and patience in both. It investigates a substance and observes that in large quantities it is a poison, in smaller quantities a stimulant. It knows that the mucous membrane of the lips is related to the mucous membrane of the intestine, but knows too that the humility of those lips is related to the humility of all that is saintly. It mixes things up, unravels them again and forms new combinations (...) For the spirit of man is the great opportunist, but cannot itself be seized hold of anywhere; and one might almost believe that nothing is brought about by its influence but decay.
>
> Robert Musil

3.1. Terminological case studies of /similarity/: Mnemosyne, anthropomorphia, and Maxwell's daemons.

In Spring 1949 the first post-war German congress for internal medicine was held in Heidelberg. It took place amidst the rubble of social Darwinism, and one of its focal concerns was the endeavour to find a new anthropological approach to the relationship between disease and cure. The endeavour was pursued in a spirit of cautious enquiry by those who had retained the capacity to mourn the immediate German past. Alexander Mitscherlich[70], who had been a reporter at the Nuremburg trials together with Fred Mielke, gave one of two introductory papers on "Psychosomatic Medicine", the main programmatic theme of the congress. The choice of this particular theme focused attention – possibly quite by chance – on an increasing awareness of the presence of signs in the process of disease. And this new awareness merged in productive combination with the prevailing spirit of cautious enquiry. In one of the concluding discussion papers Josef Meinertz spoke, among other things, on the subject of similarity:

> Die ursprünglich starke Neigung des Menschen, alles und jedes miteinander in Beziehung zu setzen und eins als Bild des anderen zu behandeln, diese Ähnlichfindung, wenn man so sagen darf, ist nicht durchweg willkürlich verfahren, sondern hat von Urzeiten her die im Leben am stärksten verwurzelten Vorgänge mit einer gewissen Typik in den Kreis ihrer symbolischen Identifizierung gezogen. [The original and pronounced inclination of mankind to build relationships between anything and everything, and to treat one thing as the image of another, this detection of similarity, if I may put it like that, does not proceed altogether arbitrarily. From earliest times it has displayed a kind of pattern in the way it has drawn those occurrences most deeply rooted in human life into an area where they can be identified by means of symbolic interpretation.] (Meinertz 1949:59)

What is most important in this contribution is the rhetorically inconspicuous phrase: "If I may put it like that." The "detection of similarity" calls for caution; it can quickly arouse suspicion, especially of procuration. It establishes relationship between things previously unconnected, it is seductive, tempting comparisons which change, rescue or even endanger the things compared. The practices hiding behind this apparently cumbersome idea are powerful, dangerous, confusing, stimulating, and comforting. In the "fight between l'ordre et l'aventure" (Appollinaire, quoted from Eco 1984b: 188) it constantly changes sides, if I may put it like that.

It is impossible to imagine ordinary proto-scientific dealings with disease which do not include such "detection of similarity". Actual disease can only be conceived of through comparison with previously experienced, observed, or imagined disease. Such comparison is conditioned by motives of fear, grief, pain, and the need for consolation, and thus becomes aggressive, fraught and speculative. The presence of disease confuses; the detection of similarity lends structure.

The everyday concept of /similarity/ is imprecise. As "equivalence" it indicates logical relation, as "analogy", logical operation; as "metaphor" it is a rhetorical figure, as "isomorph" the result of analytical observation; and as "icon" it becomes a sign with complex indications.[71] /Similarity/ is present whenever signs – even arbitrary, unmotivated signs – are produced or perceived. It is even possible that a substantial body of general semiotic theory is involved in the attempt to outline its meanings. Nevertheless, the concept /similarity/ is avoided, not without reason, by semiotic terminology. It does not appear as an entry in relevant lexicographical works on semiotics (Bense – Walther 1973; Nöth 1985, 1990; Sebeok et al. 1986), although it is listed by Greimas and Courtès (1979: 316). Now and again, in conjunction with one of the above terms, it serves as an auxiliary concept used to define others. For example, in the framework of a general theory of metaphors (Nöth

1985: 514) or along Peirce's attempt to develop it as a criterion for "iconicity" (reviewed and criticised by Eco 1975: 260). However, the lack of terminological precision peculiar to /similarity/ leaves these attempts at definition and explanation open to dispute and minimises the value of their contribution to research. According to Eco, geometric "similarity" ("similitudine" or "similitude") is the only concept of similarity which has found adequate definition.

In this chapter /similarity/ will assume a vital role as an orientating concept. Lack of terminological precision will have to be accepted, especially as it is rooted in the very nature of the process described as "detection of similarity" and cannot be overcome by means of pure definition. /Similarity/ is nebulous, rhizomatic, multiform. For these very reasons it needs to be modelled so that it can eventually take part in a proto-scientific structure of relationships where hardly anything of it will remain "but decay" (Musil 1953–60, 1: 179). Yet this decay is significant. It is a constitutive process in the cultural function of medication as the medium between suffering and a return to health. When a means to health, in Latin *remedium* (or *medicamentum*), emerges from herbs, drugs, elixirs and chemical compounds, then such decay is playing a vital supporting role.

In the midst of the disjunctive clarity which stretches between /sameness/ and /difference/, /similarity/ establishes a twilight zone where the Order of Things (cf. Foucault 1970, 1983a, b) is neglected in favor of an order of the inner representation of "things". When two //things// are similar to each other, or, more precisely, are held to be similar to each other, then they are not completely different, but neither are they entirely the same. Magritte frequently refers to the vital distinction between /similarity/ and /sameness/ in his letters to Foucault:

> The words Resemblance and Similitude permit you forcefully to suggest the presence – utterly foreign – of the world and ourselves. Yet, I believe these two words are scarcely ever differentiated, dictionaries are hardly enlightening as to what distinguishes them. It seems to me that, for example, green peas have between them relations of similitude, at once visible (their colour, form, size) and invisible (their nature, taste, weight). It is the same for the fake and the real, etc. Things do not have resemblances, they do or do not have similitudes. Only thought resembles. It resembles by being what it sees, hears, or knows; it becomes what the world offers it. (Magritte 1983b: 57–58)

Orientation by means of the concept /similar/ makes it possible for this chapter to pursue what is of interest and relevance to semiotic theory through certain stages of the history of remedies, whether these stages are determined by mythological or by rational principles. Myth and Logos are bound together by similarity.[72] It is true that in both diachronous and synchronous situations close contact with pain and death can hardly be borne without the dialectic intervention of mythical "*bricolage*" (Levi-Strauss 1966) and sharp rational analysis. /Similarity/ will become especially interesting when it can be established, threatened, rescued, and above all modelled by the use of signs, both iconic and otherwise, and when the use of signs is accompanied by the use of remedies. Examples of such modelling of /similarity/ have been examined in the previous chapters, some in detail, some in survey. At this point the question of their historical contingency must be raised and resolved. Whenever someone displays "[den] Aufweis angetroffener Ähnlichkeiten" ['indications of encountered similarities'] (Benjamin 1984: 125) in connection with remedies, whether in a theoretical essay, during a clinical wardround, in a papal encyclical, on a doctor's prescription, or on the "Directions for use" leaflet enclosed with some medicament,[73] then we should be prompted to examine the role played in this context by semiotics. Orientation by means of a criterion that is neither necessary nor sufficient but indicates – indexically – empirical directions is an established tradition among medical "thought styles" (Fleck 1979 125–126). Within this tradition the detection of similarity will be regarded here as a symptom of semioticity.

Brief consideration of the relativity of /similarity/ in certain individual languages suggests that two perhaps fundamentally different emphases of meaning can be derived from the undifferentiated lexeme in German, Latin, Ancient Greek and Italian.

Firstly, synchronous /similarity/, which draws comparison in a historical and more or less sudden relationship, uniting what was previously disunited by means of comparison but without including /before/ or /after/ in the act of comparing. This emphasis of meaning clusters around the Indoeuropean root *sem*, which approximates the English 'one': Latin *similis*, Ancient Greek *homoios*, Italian *simile*, French *similaire*, English 'similar'. Its nominal derivatives are: Latin *similitudo*, Italian *similitudine*, *similarità* or *somiglianza*, French *similarité* and English 'similarity'. A prime function of this /similarity/ is the reduction of complexity in the surrounding world through a structuring of experience. Synchronous /similarity/ engenders hypotheses, whether in everyday "personal constructs" (Kelly 1955) or in scientific discourse. "Geometry" and "comparative anatomy" are its oldest and most productive fields of operation. In as far as it can be quantified, the scope of this "similarity" correlates less with the accuracy of the hypotheses it engenders than it does with their outcome. The person whose argument depends extensively upon similarity may not necessarily be right, but he will make an impression.

Secondly, diachronous or anamnestic[74] /similarity/ extends around the Latin particle *re*, and thus assumes a historical orientation in the broadest sense of the word. Anamnestic /similarity/ connects what is present to what is past by indicating that the here and now is reminiscent of the past and gone. In English and French '*resemblance*' is the corresponding lexical homograph. A function of this /similarity/ which is not immediately apparent but highly relevant to present discussion is its capacity more or less to cancel separations that have already taken place. In certain extreme instances it can even, for a few hallucinatory moments, reconstitute a lost paradise.

When man was driven out of the Old Testament paradise, he brought with him into a finite existence not only the inconquerable barriers of suffering and death but also a resemblance to the divine that is a transcendental reminder of primordial bliss and, moreover, a "... similitudine cosmica di tutte le cose uscite dalle mani creatrici di dio" ['... cosmic similitude of all things that came out of God's creative hands'] (Giardini 1959: 48).

What could be closer to our hearts than the need to combat the ever-present threat of suffering and death – or to make it bearable, at least – by re-calling this resemblance to our minds? And it is indeed this aspect of /similarity/ which occidental pharmacy sought to make applicable to and in the use of remedies through the doctrine of signatures – although it did not do so with conscious intention, and was therefore all the more successful.[75]

The doctrine of signatures has its classical roots in Pliny's *Historia naturalis*. It was cultivated in the humanistic garden by Paracelsus, highly fertilised in a baroque hothouse by Croll, Glauber, Dalla Porta and some of their contemporaries, and has – growing apace as ill weed during enlightment – retained a remarkable portion of its impact on theory-formation until the twentieth century. Remedies and their natural by-products are related to each other, as well as to the sick person's body and to the *natura naturata* from which they all emerge, by comparisons embedded in a hierarchical system of similarities that provides both theoretical basis and cosmological legitimation for their therapeutic use.

Metaphorologically the doctrine of signatures introduces to pharmacy a trope which stands for "das Ganze der Erfahrbarkeit" ['the whole sum of human experience'] (Blumenberg 1986: 9–10) and which Blumenberg has reanimated as the *legibility of the world*.

> Die Kunst, nemlich der Signatur, ist das Buch, daraus man die Kräfte der Gewächse lernen soll, denn gleichwie ein Apotheker auf seine Büchsen schreibt, was in einer jeden zu finden sei, also braucht die Natur ihre hieroglyphischen Buchstaben und schreibt damit auf ihre Gewächs, was für Kräfte in ihnen liegen. Welche Zeichen nichts anders sein als ihr Geruch, Geschmack, Angriff, Farben und ander Formen und Gestalten. [The doctrine of signatures is the book where we can learn the properties of plants, for just as an apothecary writes upon his boxes what can be found in each of them, so Nature uses

> her own hieroglyphic symbols and writes with them upon her plants to tell what properties they contain. And these signs are none other than their smell, taste, texture, color and other characteristics and qualities.][76]

These words were written in 1659 by the court apothecary in Stuttgart, Johann Gudrius von Tours, in his *Anatomia et Physiognomia Simplicium* (quoted by Schlegel 1933: 95). The metaphor of the world as book refers to:

> … Sinnverlangen an die Realität, gerichtet auf ihre vollkommenste und nicht mehr gewaltsame Verfügbarkeit … nur dem einen anderen Wunsch nach unmittelbarer Intimität [zu] vergleichen, der Gott selbst möge sich als eßbar erweisen, so daß zugleich von ihm nichts bliebe und er doch ganz einverleibt würde: die Inkarnation als Ritual. [… a craving to extract sense and meaning from reality which aims at establishing a non-threatening availability of that reality … comparable only with one other desire for unbroken intimacy. Namely, that God should render himself edible, so that at one and the same moment there should be nothing of him left, although he has been wholly assimilated. This is, of course, the ritual of incarnation.] (Blumenberg 1986: 10)

Right up to the present day, oral ingestion is the most widespread and important means of taking remedies. There are sound biological reasons for this, for the gastro-intestinal tract is in its entirety the most efficient conversion system at man's disposal. It forms that "internal surface" (Foucault 1976b: xviii) which decides on behalf of the organism what part of any ingested substances should continue to belong to it, and what part should not. In ontogenetic terms, though, this apparatus functions less as a conversion system, more as an organ for the consumption of nourishment. As such it is the site of a desire which uniquely reveals the suffering caused by expulsion from paradise: hunger. The psychoanalytical concept of /orality/ can absorb this notion and give it further differentiation. Every instance of oral ingestion is perceived both physically and mentally – and, usually, subliminally – by the recipient as in some degree the ingestion of nourishment. Thus it is action against hunger, and takes place on a primordial level as part of the battle to regain access to paradise and to that ['unbroken intimacy'] (Blumenberg 1986: 10) which returns to the memory so insistently in the desire to render God incarnate. A satisfied infant at the breast may believe for one hallucinatory split second that he or she has won the battle. That is, until the ontogenetic moment when the demands of a limiting reality present him or her with the first and – not only because it is the first – most difficult task in life, the task of individuation. In this difficult situation the infant – facing a threatening and disharmonious reality – searches for some object that will recall a lost and orally symbiotic paradise through similarity; for something that is warm, soft, and, above all, offers a gratification both instant and constant. Winnicott (1974: 2) has identified the "transitional object", which makes its appearance in an "intermediate area of experience between the thumb and the teddy bear", as belonging to a phase when the subject deals with a reality in the form of confrontation with separation by seeking security. The detection of similarity is one possible strategy for the stabilisation of such security. It creates situations between the subject and his or her paradise which Musil (1978: 1337) has characterised as "ungetrennt und nicht vereint" ['unseparated and yet not united']. As far as the psychodynamics of adult life are concerned, Winnicott himself hoped to see his pychoanalytical paradigm applied above all to the phenomena of "addiction" and "fetishism",[77] which he interpreted as the regressive search for secondary transitional objects, and thus as an attempt to re-enter the area of experience associated with them. Rauchfleisch (1981: 57) has suggested that a generalisation of Winnicott's concept could be used in a wider sense to characterise one aspect of the relationship between patient and medicament. It would also appear appropriate and productive in the present discussion to regard medicaments in some respects as "transitional objects" in Winnicott's sense, since this would aid the present process of modelling and of building hypotheses. For the observer with an interest in the theory of signs, such transitional objects are of particular importance, because the establishment of relationship through the detection of similarity which they induce must necessarily be orientated by their appeal to the senses. A structural law that would comprehend their effectiveness would have to conform to the *aliquid stat pro aliquo* type. Transitional objects model similarity within the meaning of the two factors isolated in the previous chapter as taking part in the effects of placebo: factors 2 (= "simulation") and 3 (= "gratification") (see Figure 12). They possess "elektiven Wert" ['elective value'] (Laplanche – Pontalis 1986: 584)[78] for those who make use of them. Thus they lend themselves to a specifically semiotic function according to how far they facilitate "*modelage*" in the sense implied by Kristeva (1969: 29–30):

> Ayant défini la semiotique comme une production de modèles, nous avons désigné son objet, mais en même temps nous touchons à la particularité qui la distingue parmi les autres "sciences". Les modèles des sciences exactes, sont des représentations et comme telles, se réalisent dans des coordonnées spatio-temporelles. Or – et voici surgit la distinction d'avec les sciences exactes –, la sémiotique est aussi la production de la théorie du modelage qu'elle est: une théorie qui, en principe, peut aborder ce qui n'est pas l'ordre de la représentation. [Having defined semiotics as production of models we have designed its object. But doing so we come very close to the peculiarity which distinguishes it among the other "sciences". The models of the exact sciences are representations and as such they materialize within the scope of spatiotemporal coordinates. In other words – and here surges the distinction from the other exact

sciences – semiotics is also the production of the theory of modelling as such: a theory that, on principle, can afford to neglect anything out of the order of representation.]

If we try to find something approximating a philological paradigm for the diachronous detection of similarity or, more precisely, for the strategy of coming to terms with reality which it lends to the comparisons made by memory, then we might well choose an "Urbild geschichtlicher Erfahrung" ['archetype of historical experience'] (Kany 1987: 217) whose objective criteria of truth lag far behind those of "exact" scientific methods, but outstrip them by a long way in terms of illuminating potential for the construction of a modelling theory. The archetype is *mnemosyne*, "die Mutter der Musen und personifizierte Erinnerung" ['the mother of the muses and the personification of memory'] (Kany 1987: 1).

In a detailed monograph, Kany has isolated the methodological and programmatic significance of the concept of *mnemosyne* in the work of three scholars, Hermann Usener, Aby Warburg, and Walter Benjamin. All spent much of their lives in obsessive preoccupation with the phenomenon of «culture». Kany writes:

> 'Andacht zum Unbedeutenden', diese von Benjamin den Brüdern Grimm zugeschriebene Devise hätte das Motto aller drei Gelehrten abgeben können. Denn wo es um Vergessenes und Verlorenes geht, können eine verwitterte Inschrift in einer sonst nirgends belegten Form eines Götternamens, ein Flugblatt der Renaissance oder ein mißglücktes Barockdrama dem philologischen Blick mehr verraten als die großen Werke der Kultur. ['Homage to the insignificant and unimportant' – this maxim, attributed by Benjamin to the Brothers Grimm, could have served as a motto for all three scholars. For when it is a question of the lost and forgotten, then an otherwise unsubstantiated form of the divine name in a weathered inscription, a Renaissance broadsheet, or an unsuccessful baroque drama can reveal more to the searching gaze of a philologist than any of culture's greatest works.] (Kany 1987: 241–242)

But according to Kany's research the phrase re-discovered by Benjamin does not come down to us from the Brothers Grimm but from Sulpice Boisserée, who in 1815 comments in a letter to Goethe on A. W. Schlegel's review of *Altdeutsche Wälder* by the Brothers Grimm "Schlegel lobt an ihnen [den Brüdern Grimm; K. S.] was zu loben ist, aber das nichtige, kleinliche Sinnbildeln und Wortdeuteln, ihre ganze Andacht zum Unbedeutenden, verspottet er mit grimmigem Witz." ['Schlegel grants them [the Brothers Grimm, K. S.] praise where praise is due, but with a furious wit he ridicules their trivial and petty attention to symbolisation and subtilisation, their whole attitude of homage to the insignificant and unimportant'] (Boisserée [1970]: 72, cf. Kany 1987: 234).

Now the strategy for coming to terms with reality outlined in the above discussion, the strategy set in train by the use of medicaments – in that they are accompanied by colors, shapes, aromas, memories of tastes, in short a wealth of sensuous data for the detection of similarity – fits very well into this general pattern. Remedies encourage anyone who turns to their use to work on this data by symbolising and subtilising in such a way. For the person undertaking it, this work will to a large extent be quite "unconscious" (in the psychoanalytical sense, but also in the sense of Proust's "*memoire involontaire*"; cf. Kany 1987: 217) and will emerge as a fundamental component in that emotive work which precedes the successful effect of placebos.

The increasing conformity of medicine and pharmacy with accepted methodologies of the more precise natural sciences, brought to a historical conclusion by the empirical successes of carbon chemistry at the end of the nineteenth century, deprived the concept of *mnemosyne* of a large part of its heuristic significance in the discovery of remedies (without, however, damaging its pragmatic importance in their application and use). While in the pre-industrial era the mystery of disease still demanded an "... Antwort auf ein Unbehagen oder Übel, dessen Ursprünge unbekannt sind oder kaum geahnt werden und dem man gleichzeitig durch Linderung, Anteilnahme, Exorzismus, Ritus und Magie beizukommen sucht." ['a response to discomforts or maladies whose causes were unknown or barely suspected, and could only be dealt with through a mixture of alleviation of symptoms, sympathetic participation, exorcism, ritual and magic...'] (Ongaro-Basaglia 1985: 102), in the twentieth century such responses are increasingly replaced by deliberate battle against the causes of disease, as determined by precise metabolical and biochemical research. Herbs, drugs and elixirs are no longer attributed with healing power because their shapes, colors, aromas or names resemble the forms of a disease, or because they are reminiscent of a saviour figure, of favourable astrological constellations, or of a lost paradise; but because substances they contain have successfully passed through a long series of exclusively synchronous comparisons of similarity. The first chapter examined this process in detail, using the /Aspirin/ paradigm. The cosmological legitimation of extract of willow as *febrifugum*, by means of the precept *ubi morbus ibi remedium*, was a matter of complete indifference to Felix Hoffman when he discovered /Aspirin/. As a chemist his sole concern was to improve //salicylic acid// by "decocting" its unpalatable taste and its corrosive effect on the lining of the stomach. Acetylation was effected by means of a detection of similarity purely synchronous in nature, which had however been cleansed of all tendencies towards the cosmological: "Die Aufklärungsfunktion des Begriffs erfordert unerbittlich das Vergessen seiner metaphorischen

Vorgeschichte." ['The pragmatic and rational function of the concept inexorably demands that we should forget its metaphorical history.'] (Blumenberg 1986: 166)

But the subsequent chronology of //acetylsalicylic acid// definitely shows that there were recurring phases during which empirical investigation was enriched by the entrance of cosmologically motivated elements through the back door, as it were. The interpretation of its analgesic effect as the "inhibition of prostaglandin synthesis" (cf. Chapter 1.3) is perhaps the most vivid example so far of this countermovement, interpreted in Chapter 1 as a realisation of Blumenberg's precept (Blumenberg 1986: 199): "Das Sinnverlangen, rational des Feldes verwiesen, schafft sich Zugänge, ist listiger als die sich selbst zur List ernennende Vernunft." ['Ordered off the field for rational motives, the craving for sense insists on gaining access and is even more artful than Reason assuming the self-appointed title of artfulness.']

In the present context of pharmaceutical history two forms of a predominently synchronous detection of similarity have particular significance. Both have often contributed to a "cunning" opening of back-doors into the course of that history; they are anthropomorphism and – a specific instance of anthropomorphism – Maxwell's daemon.

According to Lacan (1977), /anthropomorphism/, at least in an ontogenetical sense, forms an important chapter in the "past metaphorical history" of /speculation/. As a psychoanalytical semiologist Lacan has focused especial attention on that moment when an infant begins to recognise his own image in a mirror (Latin: *speculum*) as such, and reacts to this dawning of recognition with "affairement jubilatoire" (Lacan 1966: 94):

> This event can take place … from the age of six months, and its repetition has often made me reflect upon the startling spectacle of the infant in front of the mirror. Unable as yet to walk, or even to stand up, and held tightly as he is by some support, human or artificial (what, in France, we call a "trotte-bébé"), he nevertheless overcomes, in a flutter of jubilant activity, the obstructions of his support and, fixing his attitude in a slightly leaning-forward position, in order to hold it in his gaze, brings back an instantaneous aspect of the image. (Lacan 1977: 1–2)

Lacan sees the "mirror stage" as accompanied by especial celebration for the infant because it bestows a gift in the early empirical affirmation of bodily control, thereby revealing an end to passive subjection and inaugurating an "order of homeomorphic identification" (Lacan 1977: 3). The mirror image defined in Lacan's paradigm – which is unrepeatable ontogenetically – is the only one to which Eco grants symbolic character in the narrower sense, because it represents far more than simple mechanical reflection.[79] The "flutter of jubilant activity" which marks this particular distinction has a possible counterpart in anthropomorphism, a counterpart drawn from a collective history of ideas which can contribute to present attempts at the modelling of /similarity/. Eight hundred years before Lacan – although also in Paris – Hugo de St. Victoire wrote in his *Didascalicon*: "Anima ... ad se ipsam rerum similitudines trahens aggregrat." ['Collecting the similarities of things, the soul returns to herself.'] (Hugo de St. Victoire, quoted by Grassi 1984: 79). Grassi characterises the function of the detection of similarity as a cognitive tool for coming to terms with reality in the following way: "Im Geist (mens) entsteht die Einsicht in die "similitudo" als die Voraussetzung für die Übertragung (durch das metaphérein) von Bedeutungen auf das, was die Sinne zeigen: Erst so tritt der Mensch in Verbindung zur Realität." ['Insight into the "similitudo" arises in the mind as a necessary preliminary to the transfer (by means of metaphor) of meanings onto what is grasped by the senses: and this is how man first connects with reality.'] (Grassi 1984: 80).

Anthropomorphism presents itself as a particularly protective, comforting and finely-tuned form of a similarity detection which has something to bestow, something urgently needed by a sick person whose reality is necessarily endangered, or at the very least thrown into disarray. It bestows an opportunity of sensory apprehension which affords far more security than the mere exercise of faith. Wishes for recovery, formulas for exorcism, and healing rituals will be especially efficacious if the sensuous materials accompanying them facilitate what Lacan has called "homeomorphic identification".

The mandrake-root is "... der Prototyp der Gift- und Zauberwurzel schlechthin. Seit undenklichen Zeiten ist der Alraun von Geheimnis und Zauber, von Angst und Furcht, Hoffnung und Glückserwartung umwittert ..." ['...the prototype of roots with toxic and magic properties. Since time immemorial the mandrake-root has been surrounded by an aura of mystery and magic, anxiety and fear, hope and the promise of good fortune'] (Hunnius 1962: 224). It is a particularly vivid example of "homeomorphic identification" which is accessible to different cultural milieus and yet displays a stable cultural identity valid from neolithic times to the silent-movie era (when the subject is treated yet again in Henrik Galeen's film *Alraune* 'Mandrake'). It cannot be cultivated, is rare and therefore costly, and contains, as we know today, properties of considerable pharmaceutical value, besides the alkaloids //hyoscyamine//, //scopolamine//, and //atropine//. The latter two can, in moderate doses, cause alteration in the regulation of vegetative functions such as pupil dilation, glandular secretion, heart-beat, and the tone of blood vessels, while higher doses have a toxic or even lethal effect. Hyascomine, moreover, can produce euphoria and hallucination. Such knowledge allows the use of mandrake-root as *velenosum* and aphrodisiac to be explained in retrospect as to some extent "specific" pharmacological practice. But how did mandrake-root attain its immense importance as a miracle-worker, as talisman, as, next to theriac, probably the most important panacea of the western world? The mandrake-root owes its cultural status less to its comparatively unimportant chemical components than to its shape, and for the purposes of present discussion that means to its semiotic specificity. The mandrake plant puts forth a root of human shape in which a minimum of imagination can recognise arms, legs, hair, facial features, even sexual characteristics. There were male and female mandrake-roots. Some mandrake-roots may resemble a human embryo (cf. Hunnius 1962: 224). Its anthropomorphic shape determines the rituals of its use fairly close to the function of transitional objects as Hunnius reveals, not without a trace of irony:

> Der Alraun mußte ein Mäntelchen bekommen aus Samt oder Seide, mußte in einem kleinen "Särglein" aufbewahrt werden, mußte von jeder Speise etwas zu essen bekommen und vor allem pünktlich jeden Freitag in Rotwein gebadet werden. ... Bei der Verwendung der Alraunwurzel als Amulett oder Talismann, die ja lediglich wegen der menschenähnlichen Gestalt erfolgte, kamen die starkwirkenden Inhaltsstoffe der Wurzel nicht zutage. Der Alraun wurde ja nicht gegessen, sondern nur sorgfältig aufbewahrt. Lediglich Hildegard von Bingen läßt die einzelnen 'Körper'teile entsprechend der Signatur verwenden: den Kopf gegen Kopfschmerzen, den Hals gegen Halsschmerzen, die Beine gegen Podagra usw. Wenn aber jemand so mißgestimmt ist, daß er vor Herzenskummer und Trübsal keine Ruhe findet, so lege er einen Alraun in sein Bett, damit von seinem Schweiße die Wurzel warm werde. [The mandrake-root needed a little jacket made of velvet or silk, had to be kept in a special little casket, was to be given something to eat at every meal-time, and, most importantly, had to be bathed in red wine every Friday without fail. ... When the mandrake-root served as an amulet or talisman, and did so quite simply as a consequence of its resemblance to the human form, the powerful effects of the root's chemical properties were not in evidence. The root was not eaten, it was simply very carefully looked after. Only Hildegard von Bingen recommends use of individual parts of the 'body' according to the signature: the head for headaches, the throat for sore throats, the legs for gout, etc. But if anyone should become so disturbed by a troubled heart or other affliction that rest is impossible, then he should lay a mandrake-root in his bed, so that the root is warmed by his sweat.] (Hunnius 1962: 226-227)

The use of drugs of animal origin was also fundamentally determined by comparable anthropomorphic indications.[80]

The anthropomorphism typified by the mandrake-root is macroscopic, palpable, and directly transmitted by the senses. Even more important for the history of pharmacy up to the present day is a further instance of anthropomorphism, this time microscopic, which can also be used as a reference point in the present modelling discussion. It appears in a vivid intellectual experiment put forward by Maxwell – though admittedly in a completely different context. He proposes two chambers filled with gas, which are to be joined by a single tube. If a condition existed in this connecting tube whereby all slow-moving gas molecules were to pass through it in only one direction and all fast-moving gas molecules in the other, an energy potential would be set up between the two chambers, and this condition – Maxwell's daemon – would "choose", would generate energy solely through the "exercise of [its] cognitive function". (Monod 1972: 63–64)[81]

As a paradigm Maxwell's daemon introduces a whole new genre of microscopic anthropomorphisms, some of which have proved to be more than helpful in the systematisation of attitudes to Nature in the history of pharmacy and chemistry. Above all, Maxwell's achievement brought the speculative element in the construction of theories – which was, of course, in existence before his work – to the fore, and thus stimulated systematic criticism of it.[82] The assumption that chemical reagents have at their disposal characteristics and abilities resembling human characteristics and abilities is a hermeneutic maneuver which has had the most lasting influence, among the natural applied sciences, on pharmacy and on medicine. There are two reasons for paying closer attention to some chapters from the history of this influence, especially in an investigation concerned with semiotic theory:

(1) Because the detection of similarity between macrocosms and microcosms, which is the hermeneutical basis of this influence, can be described as a semiotic procedure or, more precisely, as the correlation of two previously unconnected "S-Codes" (Eco 1984b: 169–172).

(2) Because perhaps the most important and productive ability assigned to "solutions", "substances", "molecules", "receptors", "enzymes", "transmitters" and "metabolisms" is that assigned to Maxwell's daemon – the ability to make distinctions.

Both nitric acid, which in alchemy "is capable of" (Cf. Lämmert 1986: 20) freeing gold from its connections in almost any compound, and the monoclonal antibody, which in modern immunology can "recognise" the cell-membrane of one single population among a thousand, owe their "strong potential for practical results"(Fleck 1982: 122) to this assumed ability. The capacity to "choose" (Monod 1972: 63) attributed to Maxwell's daemon, implies, though, a number of relational similarities between the objects of comparison, objects which in many respects are similar to one another, but in one crucial respect are not. Differentiation presupposes the segmentation of a continuum of similarities. And signs fuctioning on the organisational level of "S-Codes" play a constitutive part in this process of segmentation. When executing its task, Maxwell's daemon compares //gas molecules// exclusively with //gas molecules//, the monoclonal antibody compares //membrane proteins// only with //membrane proteins//: ['The idea of the plurality of things implies their insertion into certain more general connections.']

Some enzymes that are catalysts in "prostaglandin synthesis" mistake //acetosalicylic acid// for one of its natural substrates. They cannot be blamed for this, since the two resemble each other like peas in a pod. For the subject in whose organism it occurs, the mistake happily produces the effect of "analgesia".

It would be possible to describe the biochemical changes in an organism brought about by medicaments as semiotic processes, using Sebeok's (1976: 73) concept of "endosemiotic connotation". On the other hand this would scarcely be compatible with the "cultural" and "anthropocentric" perspective of semiotics deriving from Peirce and Eco which forms the basis of present discussion. This study sets out to examine the semiotic content of those models which clarify the effects of widely-used medicaments and heuristically stimulate the search for new substances. These biochemical, pharmacological or physiological models have a far greater freedom from contradiction and a closer approximation to truth than the proto-scientific "personal constructs" (Kelly 1955) which underlie everyday dealings with medicaments. Like these, though, they are often codified projections of invisible microcosms onto a medium accessible to sensory perception, and we are often inspired by an approach that is both empirical and speculative. And like these also, they are particularly accessible to the opening of back-doors to a "craving for sense" ['Sinnverlangen'] (Blumenberg 1986: 199), because their object – that is, medicaments – has "conquered" more "ubiquity" (Valéry 1957–75, XII: 225) than radio telescopes, slipper animalcules, or electron microscopes. It is highly probable that such interpretations of the reality of medicaments, of their development, distribution and use, may have a significant influence on their usefulness for the propagation of ideologies. And furthermore, it is also possible that such semiotic contribution on the part of medicaments as "cultural units" may itself have an important reciprocal influence on the microscopic biochemical process. Some findings in placebo research, for example the "endorphin" hypothesis on placebo-induced analgesia, lend themselves to convincing combination with such a proposition.

The sensuous feelings which may accompany the ingestion or use of medicaments seldom bear a direct relationship to the intended biological effect that is the reason for ingestion. A patient seldom feels, in any sensuous or palpable fashion, how the medicaments he or she has ingested actually work in his or her organism. In many cases the patient simply feels, with the passage of time and the lessening of symptoms, that some effect has taken place. This experience, however, does not provide him or her with an explanation of the effect. Therapeutic pharmacological effects occur in dimensions of the microcosm which are inaccessible to human sensory perception. Prescribers and users of drugs therefore have to rely upon, and are practised in, working upon the sensory material presented to them in the consumption of medicaments through "Sinnbildeln und Wortdeuteln" ['symbolising and subtilising'] (Boisserée [1970]: 72) and through the detection of similarity, processes which help satisfy a craving for sense and meaning. An anthropomorphic use of metaphor in the naming of active substances does not render the effect of medicaments accessible to the senses in this narrower meaning of the phrase. Nevertheless, it does create the possibility of reproducing the mechanism of a proposed effect by means of some model, and on a level that is virtually actual. A //mucoregulant// loosens a /deep-seated/ cough, because it /regulates/ the production of mucous in the respiratory passages. An //ataractic// is calming because body and soul are inundated with /ataraxia/, and a //liver protective// is helpful because it almost tautologically /protects/ the liver.

Within the relaxation training programme developed by Simonton et al. (1980) the metaphorical reproduction of a microcosm in macroscopic dimensions is introduced in an extremely concrete and vivid manner when, for example, tumor patients are challenged by suggestive formulas to visualise the attack, reduction and final destruction of the tumor by thousands of defensive body-cells circulating in the blood. This suggestion is carried out by most participants with full cognisance of its purely symbolic nature, but nevertheless with the expectation of achieving some definite result. The popularity gained by this procedure in recent years can serve as an indication that in dealing with disease – especially with life-threatening disease – a strong desire for this form of similarity-detection continues to play a part, and does so even when there is a conscious or even rational disregard of its lack of empirical truth. An exercise suggested in the authors' handbook runs as follows:

> If you are receiving chemotherapy, picture that drug coming into your body and entering the bloodstream. Picture the drug acting like a poison. The normal cells are intelligent and strong and don't take up the poison so readily. But the cancer cell is a weak cell so it takes very little to kill it. It absorbs the poison, dies, and is flushed out of your body. ... Picture your body's own white blood cells coming into the area where the cancer is, recognising the abnormal cells, and destroying them. There is a vast army of white blood cells. They are very strong and aggressive. (Simonton et al. 1980: 121)

3.2. Paracelsian signatures

In its earlier stages, the history of pharmacy produced an autochthonous semiotic concept which has hitherto received no attention in semiotic historiography, and which histories of medicine and general science have granted only brief handbook entries (Winkler 1926, Tschirch 1933) or mere general and unsystematic discussion in the form of articles (Schneider 1950, Quecke 1955, Erhardt 1956). The concept is the /signature/ of remedies. In 1915 Schlegel ([1933]) published a monograph with the subtitle: "The theory of signatures as a science". The monograph sets out to propagate the theory of signatures as a method of healing rather than reflecting upon it systematically, but nevertheless the work represents a valuable collection of material, especially through its bibliography and through extensive and comprehensive quotation from rare printed sources. It must be obvious that the pharmaceutical concept of signatures, and its history, have a particular part to play within the framework of this present study.

Indications of similarities between objects of the natural world on the one hand and specific symptoms of disease on the other have, in various cultures and philosophical traditions, led to the conclusion that these same objects are appropriate or even designed for the cure of the diseases which resemble them. Arrival at this conclusion seems to be less culturally specific than the teleological interpretation of the context in which it occurs or the choice of sensory characteristics modelling the similarities at issue.[83]

In the medical systems of Western tradition the forming of such conclusions was modelled very early on by a "Kraftbegriff des antiken Okkultismus" ['raw but powerful concept from the occult of classical times'] (Stemplinger 1925: 40):

> Verschiedene Wahrnehmungen führten frühzeitig zu dem Begriff der Sympathie: also erklärte man sich das Mitklingen einer Saite, wenn eine andere angeschlagen wird; so das zwangsmäßige Mitgähnen beim Anblick eines Gähnenden; so die wechselseitige Beeinflussung von Leib und Seele; so das seelische Mitleiden. Auch ärztlicherseits beobachtete man frühzeitig Spuren der Sympathie; man sah bei gewissen Krankheiten scheinbar gar nicht erkrankte Teile ebenfalls Krankheitssymptome annehmen, und beobachtete seltsame Zusammenhänge zwischen einzelnen Körperteilen; so schon Hippokrates. Nach Galenus schied man später idiopathische und sympathetische Krankheiten ... Diese Sympathie der Teile unter sich beim menschlichen Körper übertrugen nun die Stoiker und Neuplatoniker auf den Weltkörper, der ihnen ebenfalls ein einziges belebtes Wesen ist. Wenn bei Heraklit das Weltganze sich spaltet in Streit und Friede, bei Empedokles in Liebe und Haß, bei den Pythegoreern in gerade und ungerade Zahlen, bei Platon in den verbindenden und trennenden Eros, so spricht man seit die Stoa maßgebend wurde, von Sympathie und Anti-

> pathie. [Various insights led quite early on to the concept of sympathy; it was used to explain the simultaneous resonance of one string when another was struck, the compulsive yawning that happens at the sight of another person yawning, the reciprocal influences of body and soul, and spiritual compassion. It was quite early on that physicians, too, were able to observe signs of sympathy. In cases of certain illnesses it was seen that apparently unaffected parts of the body would also develop symptoms of disease, and it could be observed that strange relationships existed between individual parts of the anatomy – this was Hippocrates. Later, according to Galen, distinctions were made between idiopathic and sympathetic illnesses ... The idea that sympathy existed between parts of the human body was then applied by Stoics and Neo-Platonists to the terrestial body as a whole, which, like man, is a single living being. When the cosmos is divided, for Heraclitus into strife and peace, for Empedocles into love and hate, for the Pythagoreans into even and uneven numbers, for Plato into love that divides or unites, then the terms used since Stoicism came to the fore are antipathy and sympathy.] (Stemplinger 1925: 40–41)

In Plato's *Symposium* the physician Eryximachos has the opportunity[84] to point out the close relationship between the dual aspects of love and his own professional practice:

> ... a healthy body is admittedly different from a diseased body and unlike it. Now the objects of the desire and love felt by unlike things are themselves unlike; so the love which exists in a healthy body is different from the love which exists in a diseased body ... hostile elements are the opposites hot and cold, wet and dry, and the like ... (Plato 1951: 54–55 [§186])

Approximately 400 years later Gaius Plinius Secundus Maior (23–79 A. D.) recorded the science and culture of his times. According to Stemplinger (1925: 41), his *Naturalis historia* is: "Eine Fundgrube für die ganze antike Sympathielehre ... zumal er wiederholt erklärt, sein ganzes Werk sei der Darlegung dieses Weltgesetzes gewidmet." ['A treasury of information on the classical theory of sympathy particularly because he repeatedly declares that his entire work is dedicated to explanation of this universal law.']

In the literature of pharmaceutical history Pliny is often described as the father of the Western theory of signatures, although he does not use that term. But there is no doubt that he compiled a wealth of examples which would lend themselves to the modelling of similarity for medical purposes, and which could be referred to by more modern physicians alert to the healing significance of signatures. In 1469 the *Naturalis historia* appeared in print for the first time, only a few years after Gutenberg's first publication of a medical work (Kaiser 1969: 138).

His examples are remarkable above all for their explanations of plant-names, which are drawn from folk-etymology:

> So behauptet Plinius, daß Ochsen, welche nicht zusammen an einem Joche ziehen wollen, durch Auflegung der Lysimachia (Gilbweiderich) sanft und

verträglich gemacht werden können; denn lyei machén, d. h. sie stillt den Streit. Von der Reseda behauptet Plinius, in der Gegend von Rimini, wo die Pflanze noch häufig vorkommt, riefen die an Geschwüren und Entzündungen leidenden dreimal aus: Reseda, heile die Krankheiten ... (reseda, morbis reseda; von resedare = beschwichtigen, heilen). [Pliny maintains that oxen who are unwilling to pull under the same yoke can be made docile and tolerant through the application of Lysimachia [*Lysimachia vulgaris* 'yellow loosestrife'; K. S.], which quells strife. As for reseda, Pliny maintains that in the Rimini area, where the plant is still prolific, persons suffering from sores and infections used to say three times: reseda, heal the sickness ... (reseda, mortis reseda; from resedare = to assuage, allay).] (Stemplinger 1925: 82)

Thus a modelling relationship arises between *nomen proprium* and myth, completely in accordance with findings ascertained by Lotman and Ouspensky (1976: 23): "On peut dire que la signification générale de nom propre a son niveau d'abstraction le plus haut ramène au mythe. C'est précisément dans la sphère des noms propres que se produit cette identification du mot et du dénotat qui est charactéristique des conceptions mythologiques et se marque, d'une part, par les tabous de toute sorte, de l'autre par une modification rituelle de ces noms." ['We could say that at its highest abstractive level the meaning of proper names leads to the myth. It is precisely in the sphere of proper names that this identification between word and denotatum comes into being, one that is characteristic of mythological concepts and ranges from all kinds of taboos to the ritual modification of these names.']

The execution of such ritual modifications makes an important contribution to the appearance of the metaphor of the world as book. Its legibility presupposes that at least some proportion of the information which finds meaning in the metaphor must be linguistically structured. It would be virtually impossible to imagine the /book of books/ as a *herbarium* without words or any other kind of comment. Even if there is a "tiefe Rivalität zwischen der Orientierung der Theorie am Ideal der Abbildung und der am Ideal des Namens " ['deep rivalry between a theoretical approach determined by the ideal of reproduction, and one determined by the ideal of naming'] (Blumenberg 1986: 88), it is nevertheless true that both ideals play a part in the genesis of this particular book, although their contributions are differently weighted. The bridge to the mythological which is built in ritual by the culturally formative *nomen proprium* may help to mediate this rivalry. At the beginning of the sixteenth century, when Paracelsus set out to use the *kunst signatum* 'art of signatures' to facilitate the search for remedies and improve their effectiveness, this step had already been taken: the "legibility of the world" (cf.Blumenberg 1986) had long been accepted, disseminated and safeguarded by a number of "stabilisierte ikonische Institutionen" ['stabilised iconic institutions'] (Blumenberg 1986: 32). The herbaria and bestiaries emerging from the tradition of the old Physiologus (1960) preserved this system through to the Renaissance, and largely consisted of synchronous and – in so far as they dealt with the problem of /creation/ – diachronous findings of similarity. During the Middle Ages, then, they fulfilled both functions of the process of /detection of similarity/ indicated in this study: the structuring of knowledge of the outside world, and the revocation of separation, or the virtual reconstruction of paradise. The relationship with nature which nourished these institutions could, with reference to Eco (1984b: 151), be characterised as follows: "Since every visible entity has an allegorical meaning, the world creatures are not described according to their empirical properties, but according to those properties that display some analogy with the content they are supposed to represent."

Paracelsus made this system empirical in that he was not only fascinated by analogical relationships, but also deliberated upon them systematically. In terms of scientific history his contribution is far less important than that of Linnaeus, for example. But it does have relevance to present discussion, firstly because it was developed in connection with remedies, and secondly because one of the concepts emerging from his theoretical deliberations is a semiotic concept:

> Die natur zeichnet ein jeglichs gewechs so von ir ausget zu dem, darzu es gut ist. darumb wan man erfaren wil, was die natur bezeichnet hat, so sol man an dem zeichen erkenen, was tugent im selbigen sind. wan das sol ein ieglicher arzt wissen, das alle kreft so in den natürlichen Dingen sind, durch die zeichen erkant werden ... wo das nit ist, do wird kein secret in der natur erfunden mit gewisser prob und rechtem wesen. [Nature marks every plant that originates from her with signs indicating for what purpose it is good. So if one is desirous of learning what Nature has marked, one shall recognize from the signs what virtue is to be found therein. And this is what every physician has to know: that all powers which are found inside natural things can be recognised by these signs... Where this is not the case, none of Nature's secrets shall be revealed with certain proof and a righteous character.] (Paracelsus 1930: 86)

Philippus Aureolus Theophrastus Bombastus von Hohenheim – after 1529 he used the name /Paracelsus/ as a literary pseudonym – was born in 1493 or 1494 in Switzerland, the son of a Swabian physician and Swiss mother. After the outbreak of the Swabian war at the end of the century, the family left Switzerland and in 1502 settled in the Austrian town of Villach. Theophrastus, as he was first called, attended the monastic school in nearby St. Paul, and gained some experience of mineralogy and metallurgy in the metal works and mines of the area. From 1510 to 1512 he studied the seven liberal arts at Vienna university, from 1512 he studied medicine in Ferrara, where in 1516 he became *doctor beyder arzneyen* 'doctor of both medicines'. His later literary work contains only the slightest indications of interest in previous models or traditions. If he mentions names, then it is those of earlier opponents whose systems he wishes to demolish. Goldammer (1971) attributes the greatest discernible influence on Hohenheim's theories of cosmology and matter to the Neo-Platonists, Pico and Ficino. The Paracelsian relationship which has perhaps the most importance for the modelling of similarity, the anthropomorphic (or "astromorphic"?) analogy between the "macrocosm" //universe// and the "microcosm" //man// (he generally uses the latter pair of concepts synonymously), is granted a good deal of space in the works of Pico della Mirandola, but also in those of Hermes Trismegistos, which were very widely known by Paracelsus' contemporaries.

Immediately on completion of his studies, Paracelsus began the restless travels through Central and Eastern Europe which continued throughout his life, ending 22 years later with a return to Austria three years before his death. Paracelsus cultivated restlessness "als ein konstitutives Prinzip des Erkennens" ['as a constitutive principle in the gaining of knowledge'] (Goldammer 1966: 76). He was not content with experience gained from reading, he liked to absorb it through the soles of his feet: "Dan das wil ich bezeugen mit der natur: wer sie durchforschen wil, der muss mit den füßen ire bücher treten." ['This is what I have to testify about Nature: he who will research her must tread her books with his feet".][85]

Apart from Paracelsus' predilection for book metaphors (also noted by Blumenberg 1986: 69), a further characteristic of his thought becomes apparent here: a rejection of belief in progress via the traditional textbook. The suggestion that one should gather experience by walking on books is not exactly a sign of bibliophilia. Paracelsus followed a course of medical study which consisted almost exclusively of the dogmatic exegesis of textbooks. Direct confrontation with patients was not part of the curriculum (cf. Lejeune 1941: 1005). This meant that Paracelsus regarded books in many respects as an obstacle erected between the seeker for knowledge and his experience, instead of something that would bring about a productive meeting of the two. He expressed this rejection not only through metaphor, he also took the opportunity of the Midsummer's Eve bonfire of 1527 in Basle to arrange a public burning of books.[86]

His turning to the book of Nature represents primarily a radical criticism directed at traditional exegesis of the natural world, together with denial of the dogmatic authority it exercised. Thus a process was set in motion which after circulation through several organisational systems can emerge in the following codified form:

> Not only in the Middle Ages does every community (be it a church, a country, a political regime, a scientific school) in which the symbolic mode holds need an auctoritas (the Pope, the Big Brother, the Master). The auctoritas is indispensable when there is not a code; where there is a code – as a system of preestablished rules – there is no need for a central auctoritas, and the power is distributed through the nodes of organized competence. (Eco 1984b: 152–153)

What Paracelsus put in place of the exegetic rules he rejected goes one step further than the charismatic laws which introduced the symbolic mode into alchemy,[87] and one step further than rules for the detection of similarity put forward in the Physiologus tradition. This step, quite a trivial one in terms of general scientific history, is of especial interest here, particularly since it involves the application and systematisation of a semiotic concept which is a fundamental determinant of the Paracelsian relationship to the book of Nature – namely the /signature/.

Although Paracelsus' earlier writings are often concerned with signs – albeit collectively and only in passing – he later developed a comprehensive systematology, mainly during the time coinciding with his return to his childhood home in Austria.

The Paracelsian *zeichen* 'sign' is a widely comprehensive concept, playing a constitutive part in the relationship of man to the universe and, as will be seen, very closely connected with Paracelsus' notion of what nowadays would be called "culture". Likewise, */signatum/* is a general concept, no more clearly differentiated than /sign/ and often used synonymously; it does tend, however, to be used as a technical term. Use of the Latin participle construction (in contrast with Augustine's */signum/*) leads one to suspect the existence of a triadic concept, but there is no further evidence for this. */ars signatum/* or */ars signata/* is the intentional, deliberate – that is, the non-intuitive – traffic with signs which can be productive as well as receptive. For Paracelsus, though, rooted as he is in the diagnostic tradition of medieval semiotics, the receptive aspect of sign interpretation bears far greater weight in everything that constitutes this *ars*. In Paracelsian cosmology there are three *signatores*, producers of signs, which are more or less the originators of all the material processed by the *ars signatum*: *mensch* 'man', *archaeus* 'creator' and *astra* 'stars'.

Finally, */signatur/* (plural = */signatura/*) is a special kind of *signata* systematically differentiated by Paracelsus. At the same time it is also the semiotic concept which his entire theory of signs aims to unfold. It is possible to distinguish two functions of this concept which are still present in the modern notion of signatures:

Firstly, the function of topographic organisation, where a large number of objects are placed in a closed, systematic relationship with one another, making it possible to identify and, when necessary, retrieve any individual object or determine its location, from among an otherwise indistinguishable mass of information – as library books, for example, are classified by their signatures or shelf-marks.

Secondly, the function of indicating origin, which, given a large number of objects bearing "signatures", makes it possible to infer who produced, modelled, painted or made them.

Although Paracelsus does not explicitly draw these distinctions, their unconscious presence in his thought is nevertheless made clear by the fact that he assigns to those *signatura* whose *signator* is man functions which are related to organisation and the forming of hypotheses, while those *signatura* whose *signatores* are *archaeus* or *astra* are used in constructing bridges to natural mysticism and the metaphysics of creation. Within the referential framework at present being developed for /similarity/, this would mean that human *signatura* may be connected with the synchronous detection of similarity, while celestial *signatura* may be connected with the diachronous.

Paracelsus treats the problems of a theory of signs most systematically and comprehensively in the ninth book of his treatise *De natura rerum*, which, according to the first edition of 1572, was written during 1537.[88] This ninth book, entitled "De signatura rerum naturalium", has the following introduction:

> In this Booke it is convenient for us speaking of the Signature of things in the first place, to declare by whom things are signed, and who the Signator is, and how many things there be that are signed. You must therefore know, that things that are signed are of 3 sorts. The first sort of them Man signs: the second, the Archeius: the third, the stars of supernaturall things. Therefore upon this account there are three Signators: Man, the Archeius, and Stars. Moreover, you must note, that impressions signed by man do bring with them a perfect knowledge, and judgement of hid things, and import the knowledge of their hid vertues, and faculties. (Paracelsus 1650: 100–101)

For Paracelsus, reading the book of Nature unites two often quite distinctly different cognitive activities: pansophism and botany, brooding and collecting. With regard to both methodology and content he shuns no contradictions, marks, in fact, a point of intersection in the history of science: "Das, was in ihm zusammengeflossen war an Traditionen, teils empirisch-rationaler und spekulativer, teils geheimwissenschaftlicher Art, wurde in der Folgezeit in zwei Richtungen entwickelt, die sich beide auf ihn beriefen: einmal eine stärker rational-wissenschaftliche der ärztlichen Paracelsisten und Chemiker, dann in eine stärker geheimwissenshaftliche alchemistisch-theosophische." ['The traditions which flowed together in his work, those of a rational, empirical nature, and those belonging to mystical doctrine, were subsequently developed in two directions, both referring back to him. Firstly, by Paracelsians and chemists, in a more markedly rational and scientific pursuit of medicine; and secondly, by alchemists and theosophists, in a body of more markedly mystical teachings.'] (Goldammer 1971: 22).

The division persists in present-day Paracelsian scholarship, where on the one hand he is gently ridiculed as "der magische Waldesel aus Einsiedeln" ['the magic ass from Einsiedeln[89]], and on the other, in accordance with his motto "wissen und nit wähnen" ['seek to know, not vainly suppose'], is honoured as the "Vorläufer der Chemie und Pionier der Pharmakologie" ['forefather of chemistry and pioneer of pharmacology'] (Schipperges 1976: 76). Paracelsus remained equally fascinated by the speculative and empirical aspects of alchemy. He took great pleasure in being both amazed and admired. At the same time, however, he did not linger in a state of magical fascination; he did not attempt a hermetic appropriation of it, or seek to make capital out of it, unlike many of his contemporaries. He was not a mystery-monger but a man eager for experience, who made his knowledge available to all.

Through the appearance of man as *signator*, both the topographical, organisational aspect of the concept of signatures and the indexical and inferential potential of signs for the generation of hypotheses were rendered productive for the art of medicine. In the *Labyrinthus medicorum errantium* of 1537 something like a programmatic statement may be found: "dan signatum zeigt an das locum, das locum zeigt an sein noturft, und die noturft wird ersettigt durch inventricem." ['because the signature indicates the locus, the locus indicates its necessity, and the necessity is gratified with invention.'] (Paracelsus 1928b: 212).

Schipperges comments: "Der Hinweis auf den organhaft verankerten 'locus' mit seiner pragmatischen Eingebundenheit in den therapeutischen Eingriff deutet darauf hin, daß mit der Signatur weniger ein naiv aufgebautes statisches Entsprechungssystem gemeint ist als vielmehr ein – sicherlich entscheidendes – Glied in der dynamisch bewegten Kette eines kompletten Indikationsprozesses." ['Reference to the position of the "locus" in the organism, with its pragmatic integration in the process of therapeutic intervention, is an indication that the signature is not so much part of a naively structured static system of correspondances, but rather forms an undoubtedly crucial link in the dynamically articulated chain[90] of an entire diagnostic process.']

In so far as the art of medicine is an *ars signatum*, it enables the practitioner, independent of any interpretative authority but guided by the transmission of a codified body of knowledge, to search Nature for similarities and to organise them. The following passage is taken from the treatise *Von den natürlichen Dingen*, written around 1525:

> darumb ich solchs hie anzeig, ist alein die ursachen, dass vil [viele Autoren; K. S.] von kreutern schreiben und nichts aus dem brunnen der arznei, als nur alein vom hören sagen, und alle arzt wollen gleich auf solch hören sagen bauen, und ist ein sant. der do wil ein arzt sein, der muss vom grunt reden und sein grunt nemen aus dem liecht der natur, nit von den hören sagern, von wegen des, das sich niemands mög bekümern und beschweren in den verborgnen heimlikeiten der natur. darumb hats die natur verzeichnet und befilcht alein, das ihr die zeichen lernen kennen. dan ihr mochten sprechen, wer kan in das kraut sehen was in im ist? der rot bart ist ein zeichen, der schwarz auch, die kleidung und anderst; von den allen muss der mann erkent werden. [The only reason why I state this here is that so many authors write what they have learned about plants from hearsay and not from the fount of the physic. All medical men want to build upon such hearsay, yet it is nothing but sand. He who will be a physician must talk of the foundations and develop his foundations from Nature's light, not from those hearsayers, for the very reason that no one should give thought or concern to Nature's hidden mysteries. That is why Nature has endowed all things with a sign, and you have to do no more than learn to read these signs. Now you may raise the objection: Can one look into a plant to see what is inside? No, its signs alone show what is inside. The red beard is a sign, the black one too, and clothing and other things; it is from all these that the man must be recognised.] (Paracelsus 1930: 87)

Paracelsus most certainly does not shy away from contact with the practical magical knowledge coming, for example, from the doctrine of sympathy, from the Cabbale, or from alchemy. In many instances he adopts the "symbolic mode" (Eco 1984b: 143–156) cultivated by these philosophies. As a "phänomenologischer Forschungsansatz" ['phenomenological research approach'] (Schipperges 1976: 77), however, his doctrine on the signatures of natural science takes one important step further than what Eco, in another context (1977a: 111), has called "pansemiotische Metaphysik" ['pansemiotic metaphysics']. The importance of this step was very early recognised within the framework of a general theory of medicine. Bartolomeo Castelli, for example, in his *Lexikon medicum Graeco-Latinum*, first published in 1598, writes that Paracelsus introduced the theory of signs into medicine chiefly because he wanted to shed the suspicion of magic from himself and his doctrines: "Signata ars Paracelso dicitur Caballa, estque ex illius mente, pars Astronomiae, & introitus ad Medicinam; verum ob Magiae suspicionem vitanda." ['Cabbale is called the art of signata by Paracelsus, and it is coming from this mind a part of astronomy and introduced to medicine; in reality to avoid the suspicion of magic.'] (Castelli 1713: 669)

This becomes particularly apparent in his development of the alchemistic *ars spagyrica*, the art of separating substances. According to Scholastic dogma on the 'hylomorphic' nature of chemical combinations, the matter (Greek *hyle*) and form (Greek *morphe*) of a substance are inextricably bound together and determine its incidence in nature as well as its possible chemical reaction with other substances. The idea deriving from corpuscular theory – still "heretical" in the sixteenth-century – that any given chemical element could equally well appear in solid, fluid, crystalline, colored or colorless combinations was not compatible with this dogma or with its assumption of the "absolute unity of substance, guaranteed by its substantial form" (Hooykaas 1939: 166). The dogma was resolutely contradicted by Paracelsus in his assumption that minerals have life in the same sense as fluids or aggregrates of natural matter and are therefore capable of combination with these. Hooykas, in his thorough investigation of the Paracelsian theory of chemical combination, regards Paracelsus' "hylozoistic" system as a connecting link between Scholasticism and the corpuscular theory of natural science (Hooykaas 1939: 167), and concludes: "Die paracelsische Theorie der chemi schen Verbindung ist ein Versuch, mit Hilfe der chemischen Erfahrung die feste Mauer der mittelalterlichen Spekulation zu zertrümmern." ['The Paracelsian theory of chemical combination is an attempt to shatter the protective wall of medieval speculation with the aid of practical chemical knowledge.'] (Hooykaas 1939: 175)

A theory of the primacy of external form perceptible to the senses – as opposed to a theory dealing with internal and invisible microscopic characteristics that could only be deduced logically by means of a long series of laboratory experiments that might remain inconclusive – would lend itself more readily to compatibility with "pansemiotische[r] Metaphysik" ['pansemiotic metaphysics'] (Eco 1977a: 111). But it is precisely this which Paracelsus, working within alchemistic tradition, was able to achieve. The motivation for this venture was not, however, the alchemist's desire for the transmutation of baser metals into gold, or the search for the philosopher's stone, but the search for the active principle concealed within a remedy, the /*arcanum*/. In the context of the development of organic chemistry outlined in the first two chapters in this book, Paracelsus' "chemiatrics" lay an early foundation stone for pharmaceutical "specificity". His "spagyrical" theory of combination, which accords to the internal /*virtutes*/ of chemical combinations the capability of making distinctions and entering into selective bonds, is also an early precursor of Maxwell's daemons.

Quecke (1955) summarises the development of the doctrine of signatures throughout the course of Paracelsus' work. Within a general theory of signatures there are four distinct branches or disciplines that are referred to by Paracelsus with a fair degree of terminological consistency:

Chiromantia, the first of these branches "...geht bei Hohenheim weit über die Handlesekunst hinaus. Er versteht darunter eine Wissenschaft, die aus

Linien, Runzeln und Furchen von Händen und Füßen und aus dem Geäder Folgerungen der Eigenschaften eines Menschen, einer Pflanze oder irgendeines anderen Naturproduktes zieht." ['... involves far more than mere palmistry. According to Paracelsus, it is a science which can draw conclusions about the characteristics of a human being, a plant, or any other product of the natural world, from the lines, creases, or folds in hands and feet, and from veins.'] (Quecke 1955: 44)

The second of these branches, *physionomia*, tends to support the topographic and organisational aspects of the traditions of */signatur/* and medical semiotics: "Jede Krankheit hat ihre physionomia, die sich meistens in Form und Farbe ausdrückt. Beispiel für das letztere ist die Gelbsucht, für das erstere die Elephantiasis. Die Krankheit ist in der Lage, die angeborene Form des Körpers zu ändern." ['Every disease has its own physionomia, usually expressed by means of form or color. An example of the latter is jaundice, of the former, elephantiasis. Disease is in the position of being able to change the congenital shape of the body.'] (Quecke 1955: 45).

The third branch of Paracelsian doctrine on signatures is designated by different terms in different sections of the works: *proportio*, *substantia*, and *habitus*. Here, the search for a "Konstruktionsprinzip und der Architektonik des menschlichen Körpers" ['constructional principle and the architectonics of the human body'] (Quecke 1955: 47) becomes thematic, while a "psychologische Gestaltdeutung beim Menschen" ['psychological interpretation of human form'], in the sense of nineteenth-century physiognomy, is also hinted at.

Finally, the fourth branch is perhaps of most importance for the topographical and organisational aspect of the concept of signatures. It falls slightly outside a general framework, and was not allowed for in the original tripartite structure of the signatures doctrine (Quecke 1955: 48). Paracelsus introduced this fourth branch in the final version of his *Astronomia magna*, where, following a discussion of *chiromantia*, *physionomia*, and *substantia* as the most important branches in the doctrine of signatures, he continues: "und zum vierten ist mos und usus, das ist, weis und geberd, wie sich der mensch erzeigt und stelt." ['and fourthly there is custom and usage, this is manner and gesture, how man appears and behaves'] (Paracelsus 1929: 176). Quecke comments: "Die Deutung dieses Teils der Signaturenlehre bereitet dem Verständnis einige Schwierigkeiten, bricht sie doch scheinbar mit dem Grundaxiom der "kunst signatum", der Anzeigung einer Eigenschaft durch den äußeren Eindruck, dem Rückschluß von der Gestalt auf den Gehalt." ['Explanation of this section of the doctrine of signatures presents some difficulties to the understanding, since it appears to depart from the fundamental axiom of the "ars signatum", from indication of a characteristic through external impressions, from an arrival at content through form.'] (Quecke 1955: 48)

This infringement does show some degree of consistency as a continuation of implications inherent in the theory of chemical bonding. The "arrival at content through form" which is grounded in sensory perception and therefore open to confirmation, is joined by a new and fundamentally less finely tuned alternative, namely the arrival at content through usage ("*mos et usus*").

This observation is by no means revolutionary, and played no great part in the history of pharmacy for a long time after Paracelsus. It contains, however, what is in essence an almost "structuralist" idea quite in keeping with Barthes' programmatic precept (1965: 106): "Dès qu'il y a société, toute usage est converti en signe de cet usage."

As a result of Paracelsus' thematisation and systematisation of the problem of signs during his search for new organisational principles, his thirst for knowledge led to an astonishingly analytic interest in the phenomenon of «culture», and consequently in "semiotic specificity". Again, this idea is developed most fully in the introduction to the ninth book of his treatise *De natura rerum*, from which a long passage is now quoted:[91]

> But that wee may explain briefly, and truly all the signes, or markes, it wil be necessary in the first place, that wee speak of those signes of which Man is the Signer. Those being understood, you may the more rightly understand the rest, whether naturall, or Supernaturall. It is therefore known, that the Iews carry about them, upon their cloak, or coat a yellow sign.[92] And this is nothing else but that mark by which they would have you, when you meet them, to know that they are Iews. So a Serjeant is known by his divers coloured coat, or sleeve. So every Magistrate apparells his servants with his own colours, and liveries.
>
> Every Mechanick marks his work with a certain sign, that every one may know whose work it is.
>
> For which end Carriers wear the liverie of their master or city, that it may be known whom they serve and from whence they travell, that thereby they may goe the safer.
>
> So every Souldier wears a marke, or badge, as colours, black, white, yellow, green, blew, or red, & c. that he may be distinguished from the enemie. Hence it may bee known that this is Cesars souldier, that the Kings, this an Italian, this a French souldier, & c.
>
> These are signs which belong to order, or office, of which many more may be reckoned up. But yet because wee have intended to describe the signes of naturall, and supernaturall things, wee shal not fill up this book with other signes.
>
> As concerning those signes, which Man makes, which do not only respect order, office, or name, but conduce to the knowing of his knowledge, age,

> dignity, degree & c. You must know concerning Money, that every kind thereof hath its peculiar triall, and marke, by which it is known how much it is valued at, who is the Master of it, and in what place it is usually currant. Hence is that German proverb, money is no where more in request than where it was coined.
> The same is also to be understood of things that are looked upon and examined by men sworn and appointed for that purpose, before they bee signed: as Cloth which is marked with peculiar marks, by which it may be known, that in examining they were found good, and proved. Why is a seal put upon Letters but that there is a certain bond, which it is lawfull for no man to violate? For a seal is a confirmation of Letters, whence they are of all men accounted ratified. Without a seale an Acquitance is void, and of no force.
> After the same manner many things are marked with few letters, names, or words, as works, which being writ upon the outside but with one word, doe presently shew what is contained within.
> The same rule also there is for glasses and boxes in Apothecaries shops, all which are discerned by peculier names, or papers put upon them. Unlesse that were done, who could discern as many Waters, Liquors, Syrups, Oyles, Powders, Seeds, Unguents, & c. and all simples? After the same manner doth the Alchymist in his Elabatorie mark with names, and papers all Waters, Liquors, Spirits, Oyles, Flegms, Crocus, Alcali, and all species, that thereby hee may when there is occasion make use of any of them, and know them: without the help of which his memory could never bear them.
> So also may all houses and buildings bee marked with numbers or figures, that the age of evry one of them by the first sight of the number may presently be known.
> These and other things that are marked I was willing to shew to you, that these being comprehended, I might bee the better understood by you in the rest, and so the signification of every thing might bee the more plain, and clear. (Paracelsus 1650: 101–103)

In so far as it is conveyed by signs, /similarity/ here moves further and further in the direction of what Cassirer (1955: 67) has called "a mere concept of relation and reflection." The /similarity/ of logical thought thus becomes differentiated from the /similarity/ peculiar to mythological modes of thought. (Cassirer's criterion would also serve as a rough guide in the delineation of previously discussed distinctions between "synchronous" and "diachronous" detection of similarity, and between the topographic/organisational and origin-indicating functions of the signature). In the passage quoted above, Paracelsus may be seen as giving a comparative list of different S-codes current in contemporary culture, where he finds a system of attributes operating through clothing to be of particular interest.[93]

In pharmacy, however, relational and organisational concepts are especially effective on "glasses and boxes in Apothecaries shops". The labelling of such relations will slightly later act as a starting-point for the systematisation of information on the effects of herbal remedies. /Signatur/ thus becomes an important point of orientation for "pharmacognoscenti" (Tschirch 1932: 1702ff). Valentin (1950: 30) has called Paracelsus the last great physician-apothecary. The professional differentiation of gathering, organising, preparing and preserving medicines grew ever more distinct during the sixteenth century. The establishment and maintenance of an organised system has been from its very beginnings an essential part of the apothecary's calling. The architecture of his dispensary is determined by capacious, compartmented storage shelves, usually of symmetrical design and filled with jars and phials which are themselves an invitation to finely differentiated classification. A "Porphyrian" system (cf. Eco 1984b: 464) arose, anticipating the analytic precision of the Linnaean system, but retaining a secularised concept of /use/ and /usability/ in the sense of the Paracelsian *mos et usus*. The modelling of similarity granted by the doctrine of signatures thus goes one step further than the "gnostic myths emerging from doctrines on sympathy" (Melandri 1968: 749). In so far as this modelling activity is under obligation to the ideal of "botanising", it institutes an "order of things" (Foucault 1970) which falls into alignment with the accumulation of information:

> The system of signatures reverses the relation of the visible to the invisible. Resemblance was the invisible form of that which, from the depths of the world, made things visible; but in order that this form may be brought out into the light in its turn, there must be a visible figure that will draw it out from its profound invisibility, ... the space inhabited by immediate resemblances becomes like a vast open book; it bristles with written signs. (Foucault 1970: 26–27f)

In the next century, however, it was the "pansophic" aspect of the concept of signatures which had a fundamentally greater impact on the history of ideas. This was set out speculatively fifty years after Paracelsus in the work of Jakob Boehme (1575–1624),[94] and in the *Magia naturalis* by Giovanni Battista Dalla Porta (1545–1615), first published in 1569. In 1608 a physician, Paracelsian and Rosicrucian from Anhalt, Oswald Croll (1560–1609), published a *Tractatus de signaturis internis rerum* in the appendix to his *Basilica chymica*. His systematic use of signatures in the recommendation of remedies is of interest to the semiotic theoretician. According to Winkler (1926: 950), he distinguishes between "I. Pflanzenteile, welche in ihrer Form einem menschlichen Körperteil ähnlich sind, daher für irgendein Gebrechen dieser Teile verwendet werden. II. Mittel welche in irgendetwas mit einer Krankheitserscheinung Ähnlichkeit haben. III. Mittel (hauptsächlich tierische), welche durch ihre Gleichheit oder gleiche Eigenschaften helfen. IV. Gifte, welche häufig durch gleiche Gifte erfolgte Vergiftungen beheben."

['I. Elements of plant-life which are similar in form to some part of the human body and therefore applied to any kind of affliction in those parts. II. Preparations which in some respect or other bear similarity to a symptom of disease. III. Preparations (mostly of animal origin) beneficial because of their similarity or the similarity of certain of their properties. IV. Toxins which frequently remedy poisoning caused by similar toxins.']

The doctrine of signatures exerted a particularly formative influence on the theory of Western medicine during the seventeenth century and the first sixty years of the eighteenth century, without, however, fundamentally increasing the body of analytic information on the effectiveness of remedies. The search for an /arcanum/ that had been initiated by Paracelsus, and may be seen as an early antecedent to pharmacological "specificity", made hardly any progress for several hundred years. Chemistry's more extensive incorporation of aspects of corpuscular theory, an important precondition for the analytic competence finally achieved by chemistry in the nineteenth century, did not happen for a long time, and found its first powerful opponent in the eighteenth-century *phlogiston* theory evolved by Georg Ernst Stahl (1659–1734).[95] The chemist Johann Rudolf Glauber (1604–1670), though, did form the hypothesis of an affinity between elements, deducing it from his work on inorganic salts and acids, whose derivates he also used as remedies – the //sodium sulfate// (= /Glauber's salts/) which he produced is a laxative still available in the chemist's shop of today. He is responsible, too, for the *Tractatus De Signatura Salium, Metallorum et Planetarum*, published in 1658. There is no evidence of a hidden affinity between his interest in corpuscular theory and his theory of signatures; nevertheless the treatise betrays a well-developed feeling, both descriptive and analytic, for the detection of similarity:

> Erstlich soll und muß man dieses wissen, daß alle Gestalten der Vegetabilien, als Bäumen, Kräuter und Erdgewächsen wie auch der Animalien, als Menschen und Viehes und der Mineralien allein von dem Circul und dem Quadranten herkommen darbey man das runde und auch das langlecht bey allen Gliedern und Leibern sehen kann. Dann des Menschen Leib wie auch der Stamm von einem Baum ist rund und darbey langlecht und ein jedes Glied am Finger oder Zweiglein des Krauts oder Baums also formiret ist also daß sowohl der Cirkul, als Quadrant darbey zu finden. [Firstly we ought and need to know that all vegetable shapes, such as those of trees, plants and roots, as well as all animal shapes, such as those of man and the beasts, and the shapes of all minerals, derive solely from the circle and the quadrant, as both roundness and length can be seen in every limb and every body. For man's body, as well as the trunk of a tree, is round and has length, and every section of a finger or of a sprig from a plant or tree is formed in such a way that both roundness and length can be recognised.] (Glauber 1703: 13–14)

The most productive and, in his time, perhaps also most successful attempt to speed the systematic search for an /arcana/ of remedies was made by Friedrich Christian Hahnemann (1755–1843). In the context of this study, however, Hahnemann is of particular importance because he developed an enormous interest in /similarity/, and thus involuntarily became a member of the Paracelsian tradition outlined here. His relationship to Paracelsus was contradictory. He obviously regarded him primarily as a "magic ass" (Schipperges 1976: 76), and since he had to be careful of his reputation – he was a prominent dissident – he lost almost no opportunity of distancing himself from the Paracelsists. In spite of many methodological differences, some parallels between their work are so conspicuous that Hahnemann was obliged to fight throughout his life against the predecessor he so resented – and, from a modern perspective, unjustly resented.[96]

It is the preoccupation of both Paracelsus and Hahnemann with /similarity/ which has far and away the most significance for the present argument. The concept of similarity is an axiomatic focal point in the therapeutic method founded by Hahnemann. It was not by chance that he incorporated its Ancient Greek root in the method's name. The therapeutic principle of "homeopathy" sets out from the assumption that those substances whose application is linked with the appearance of certain previously identified symptoms of disease in the organism can also, by means of a certain technique consisting primarily of "dosages", be used to cure those symptoms – *similia similibus curentur.* This principle contains two initially unobtrusive methodological implications which Hahnemann, however, examined very thoroughly:

(1) The substances in question, and the symptoms of disease which appear following their incorporation, must first be identified empirically, systematised, and thoroughly checked in a repeatable context before their therapeutic application can be considered. The systems of recognised symptoms of disease and the body of all available substances are initially regarded as relatively independent monoplanary S-codes, in Eco's sense of the term. The compilation of such a pharmacopoeia fundamentally consists in an initial meticulous segmentation of these two S-codes and their subsequent selective correlation. A comprehensive Thesaurus which would reproduce the connections between the two in dictionary form is not provided as part of this programme, its entries would reach encyclopaedic proportions.

(2) Hahnemann deliberately refused to regard the connection between "*simile*" and "symptom of disease" as a causal connection, even when it was capable of reliable reproduction. Occasionally, he even went so far as to describe it (rather provocatively, like Monod (1975)) as "coincidence" (Fräntzki 1976: 21). Remedies developed on the basis of this assembly of

knowledge can favorably influence the course of disease, although there is no guarantee of this which could be derived from a mechanistic model. This factor of self-critical uncertainty finds expression in the motto of the homeopathic method, whose Latin predicate is conjugated in the subjunctive: *similia similibus curentur.*

In complete contrast with this, Paracelsus, in his *Nachschrift aus der Vorlesung über die Tartarischen Krankheiten*, writes: *similia similibus curantur.* His *similia* are considerably easier to find than Hahnemann's. They do not have to be sought after in the laboratory, in clinical experiment or in experiments conducted on the self, but more or less allow themselves to be found as one passes through Nature and reads her with open eyes. But this obviously makes their efficacy all the more certain. Hahnemann never referred to this aspect of Paracelsian doctrine. As his system of references is otherwise very precise, this might suggest that he was not familiar with it (cf. Schadewaldt 1972: 267). For obvious reasons he never used the concept of signatures, but neither did he develop any other semiotic terminology connected with a therapeutic system.[97] /Signature/ was first introduced into homeopathic theory some hundred years later as a methodological orientation concept (e.g. by Madaus 1932 and Schlegel 1933).

Hahnemann concerned himself with chemistry from his early studies onwards, though in his time it was not considered a science fundamental to pharmacy and had no place in the medical curriculum. But it was in the field of pharmacy that his learning excelled the skill of any other contemporary, and this, at a distance of two hundred years from the professional split between physician and apothecary, was more than unusual. When he published his *Organon der Heilkunst* in 1810 (Hahnemann 1978) and the six-volume "Reine Arzneimittellehre" (Hahnemann 1822) during the next ten years, he was claiming to replace the traditional therapeutic *ars conjecturalis* 'art of supposition' with a consistently enlightened and rational system. In making such a claim he was admittedly overestimating to some extent both the stage of development reached by contemporary chemistry and pharmacy, and their capacity for progress:

> Sein ursprüngliches Konzept, mit Hilfe eines, wie er hoffte, chemisch genau definierten und exakt dosierbaren Spezifikums eine Pharmakotherapie, die zu reproduzierbaren Ergebnissen führt, treiben zu können, klingt für uns heute sehr modern und einleuchtend. Gerade dies erschien aber manchen seiner Zeitgenossen noch völlig utopisch, und Hahnemann hat sich im Laufe seines Lebens dieser – offensichtlich aus der Praxis gewonnenen – Erkenntnis gebeugt. [His original idea of the possibility of developing a pharmaceutical therapy with the aid of a specific that could be precisely defined in chemical terms and was capable of exact dosage sounds today extremely modern and plausible.

But to some of his contemporaries this idea still appeared to be a utopian dream, and as time went by Hahnemann himself submitted to this view, one obviously formed through practical experience.] (Henne 1973: 1330)

This disappointment is a possible explanation for the fact that an ascetic mind like Hahnemann's, completely opposed to any craving for mythical meaning, could yet design a system which so strongly invites "Sinnbildeln und Wortdeuteln" ['symbolising and subtilising'] (Boisserée 1970: 70, cf. Kany 1987: 234). Such an invitation was clearly not intentional on Hahnemann's part, but contemporary and posthumous critics of homeopathy, as well as the patients who continue to benefit from it, respond to this invitation with zeal.[98] Chemically defined pharmaceutical specifics that could be given in exact doses were virtually unavailable during the first half of the nineteenth century. Sertürner (1783-1841) laid important foundations with his isolation of morphine (1803), but the first real contribution towards the establishment of pharmaco-chemical theory was still almost a hundred years away. Only in 1828 did Woehler's (1800–1882) urea synthesis identify the first known significant relationship in human intermediary metabolism. If Hahnemann had maintained this initial claim to analytic and elucidatory accuracy, he would probably have been forced to conclude that in his day there was no such thing as a remedy in the narrow sense – in modern terms, no "pharmacologically specific" remedy. As a result he would have had to distance himself from any kind of systematised medical therapy. (Such a step was indeed taken by the "therapeutic nihilists" of the Viennese School (cf. Haas 1948)). As there were hardly any defined substances with dependably curative properties, it may have seemed far more promising to process the somewhat greater body of substances known to be harmful, and arrive at a differential analysis of them. In other words, possible dissatisfaction with contemporary conjectural answers to the question "What will restore health (and how)?" led Hahnemann to return to a question which many of his contemporaries held to be conclusively solved: "What actually causes disease (and how)?". The hope attached to this retreat, that adequate means of treatment would more or less automatically be revealed by the identification of probable causes of disease, proved to be extremely productive in the time of Pasteur and Koch, releasing an almost unbelievable potential for progress. And even today immunology, together with genetics, is a showpiece discipline for the formation of hypotheses which fall in the */similia similibus/* category; at the same time it is a new abode for those metaphors of books and reading (Blumenberg 1986) which help articulate the formation of theories in the natural sciences.

3.3. Chemical affinities

> Nun hatte er seit Jahren das Menschenleben fast vergessen und daß er dereinst auch gelacht und gezürnt, töricht und klug, froh und traurig gewesen. Jetzt lachte er nur, wenn unter seinen chemischen Stoffen allerlei Komödien und unerwartete Entwicklungen spielten.
>
> Gottfried Keller[99]

The notion that the infinite variety of natural material compounds can be reduced to a finite number of indivisible elements is a constant formative factor in the history of natural science, from the pre-Socratists up to the discovery of radioactivity. During the eighteenth century this assumption found solid empirical and methodological support. Karl Friedrich Wenzel (1740–1777)[100] put forward the concept of /stoichiometry/ (cf. Chapter 1.2) in his *Lehre von der Verwandtschaft der Körper*, and thus established a basis for an algebraic use of /similarity/ in chemistry. Both Antoine Laurent Lavoisier (1743–1794), in his *Traité Elémentaire de Chimie* (1789) and Jons Jakob Berzelius (1779–1848), in his *Lehrbuch der Chemie* (1808) provide the beginnings of an organised theory of chemical elements. Theory reached its final form in the nineteenth century – John Dalton's "law of multiple proportions" (1807) marks a vital stage in its development – when a periodic table of the elements was drawn up by Dimitri Mendelejeff (1869) and, quite independently, by Lothar Meyer. This table remains fundamentally unchanged and is valid to the present day.

Nineteenth-century pharmacy was able to draw little benefit from the classificatory system represented by the table – which is easily as comprehensive as the Linnaean system. It is solely designed to give access to accurate information, and is therefore of no assistance in the finding of diachronous similarity, or in a meditative search for the threads of meaning which permeate creation and bind it into an articulate whole. As an empirical system the table is almost flawless, but no-one can draw any kind of comfort from it. Analytic chemistry tends towards exploration of the division of substances rather than towards the reversal of separations that have already taken place. After a length of time that could be called a latent period, twentieth-century pharmacy will again set out, more or less from scratch, on a search for remedies that will use the framework of this massive system as a guide. Traditional knowledge and methods will be almost completely forgotten, modern pharmacy will be extremely successful in its search – but it is this very success which will open new back doors for the finding of diachronous similarity.

The Linnaean system classifies relationships that are visible to the naked eye – the bonding of chemical substances or of their constitutive elements is less accessible to observation. These relationships are essentially dependent upon "unsinnlicher Ähnlichkeit" ['insubstantial similarity'] (Benjamin 1984).[101] Chemical combinations make their first appearance in the analytical laboratory as relational constructs. The formation of systematic hypotheses is preceded by the formulation of problems, for example:

Which substances A and B react or do not react with which substances C and D? And which constituents a_1 to d_n supply an explanation for this reaction or lack of reaction?

Botany, zoology and chemistry – according to Peirce (Walther, in Peirce 1985: 34) – all describe inductive scientific methods. But in chemistry no obvious species offers itself as a paradigm which could be used to establish connections with the productive areas of comparative anatomy or morphology. Circumstances encouraging belief in the possibility of such a connection – a connection which the doctrine of signatures did all it could to sustain – were finally dispersed in the nineteenth century.[102]

For a long time chemistry played only a subsidiary role in culture's confrontation with science. Nevertheless, it is still of importance in the context of present discussion. Argument in the following section will concentrate, in part, on showing that a discipline whose later success depended on its analytic nature was, in its beginnings – even in the heart of the Enlightenment – supported and shaped by anthropomorphic ideas. It is, though, important to emphasise that the theoretical structure of modern chemistry owes no allegiance to these ideas. It had no need of them in the course of its development into an independent member of scientific discourse – indeed, it can even be maintained that these ideas would have hindered the speed of its development. In the context of this study, chemistry's early dependence on anthropomorphism is, however, of considerable importance, since this connection helped make chemistry culturally acceptable, and thus created a climate where the events described by chemistry could later be so widely understood that they achieved what has already, with reference to Valéry, been called the "conquest of ubiquity". It is perhaps an especially happy coincidence that one of the men responsible for chemistry's connection with anthropomorphism – and shortly to be discussed in more detail – maintained a pronounced critical distance from anthropomorphism as an actual cognitive approach.[103] Consequently it will be more difficult to dismiss the anthropomorphisation of analytic chemistry as a symptom of Romantic philosophical fashion, or to confine it historically to a period of reaction against the Enlightenment. We will return to this point.

An important precondition for the development of a theory of chemical combination in the eighteenth-century was the widespread acceptance of the kind of rational analysis practised by Descartes or Newton. If these examples had been missing, the attempt to reduce the reaction or absence of reaction in chemical combinations to a number of invisible elements by conducting a hierarchically structured series of experiments would have been quite unthinkable. Following this change of perspective, /sympathy/ is superseded by two other concepts of similarity which are usually used synonymously, and which precisely determine the terminological focus of the theory of chemical combination: *attractio* 'attraction', and *affinitas* 'affinity'. /Affinity/ was a leading concept in the natural sciences even at the time of Albertus Magnus (1193–1280). Only in the eighteenth-century, however, does it become a working concept in chemical experiment. From then on, the practical laboratory activity which it presided over consisted in the direct confrontation of the simplest possible reagents, reagents whose composition was empirically and reliably established – mostly salts, minerals, inorganic acids and bases. If any changes in color, shape, smell, taste, composition or any other measurable parameter took place during the confrontation, then these changes would permit conclusions to be reached on the affinity or degree of affinity between the reagents used.[104] One outcome of this experimental procedure was the compilation of a "table of affinities", which may be regarded as a predecessor to the later Periodic Table of the elements. Adler (1987) meticulously reconstructs both the function of the concept of affinity in theories of chemical combination and its "metaphorical history" (cf. Blumenberg 1986: 166). He identifies contributions made by E. F. Geoffroy (1672–1731), P. J. Macquer (1718–1784) and the Swedish chemist Torbern Bergman (1735–1784), a colleague and former pupil of Linnaeus. Geoffroy was responsible for the first tables of affinities, while Macquer was the first to develop a compilatory typology for the various kinds of chemical affinity: "Bei dieser Typologie handelt es sich eigentlich um die Einführung der geometrischen, der Cartesianischen Methode in die Chemie, deren Exaktheit der späteren Quantifikation den Weg bereitete." ['This typology in fact introduces geometric, Cartesian method into chemistry, a method whose accuracy prepared the way for later quantification.'] (Adler 1987: 62).

In 1775 Bergman published what was to become a standard work on the theory of chemical combination. His "Disquisitio de attractionibus electivis" (1968) caused a journalistic sensation that was probably quite unintentional on his part. Its readership consisted of the newly emerging "bürgerlichen Öffentlichkeit" ['bourgeois public sphere'] (Habermas 1984), described by Poerksen (1978: 64) as follows:

... die Naturwissenschaften erschließen ein in den verschiedenen Richtungen sich ausweitendes Wissens- und Erfahrungsgebiet und erreichen zunehmend das allgemeine Lesepublikum der Gebildeten; Ende des 18. Jahrhunderts interessieren sich Adel und Bürgertum für naturwissenschaftliche Fragen. Damit wandelt sich die Rolle des Naturwissenschaftlers; im Zuge der Säkularisierung übernimmt er zunehmend Aufgaben, oder läßt sie sich aufdrängen, die vorher im Rahmen von Theologie und Kirche versehen worden waren: die Funktion der allgemeinen Weltinterpretation. Mit dem Aufstieg der Naturwissenschaften beginnt auch die Zeit des naturwissenschaftlichen Schriftstellers. [... the natural sciences opened up areas of knowledge that were broadening in several different directions, and increasingly attracted a general reading public drawn from the educated classes; in the late eighteenth century the nobility and middle classes began to display a distinct interest in scientific matters. The role of the scientist was transformed. The secularisation of society increasingly pressed upon him duties previously fulfilled by theology and the church – he became responsible for interpretation of the world. And the increasing importance of the natural sciences brought increasing importance to the scientific writer.]

Bergman's word-pair /*attractio electiva*/ functioned as a definition. It grew out of the attempt to give greater precision to the terminology of chemical theory, and to free it from metaphorical antecedents.[105] Chemical substances react with other chemical substances by dissolving their old bonds and forming new bonds with them on the basis of a greater elective attraction. Chance plays no part in this; the process demanded systematic description which would enable the determinants of election to be calculated. The Latin lexeme *electio* closely corresponds to the English 'choice' (German = *Wahl*). Almost immediately *attractio electiva* was taken up as an irresistible topic of conversation in German eighteenth-century salons, circulating under the name of *Wahlverwandtschaft* 'elective affinity'.[106] Bergman's attempt to bring the subject into some kind of order obviously did not take the strength of public interest into account. The most hotly debated question was: "Who – or what – makes the choice?". And this is most definitely not what chemists were asking.

Goethe was clearly aware of a discrepancy between the views of scientists and society. He remarks upon it in the third of his *Vorträge über die drei ersten Kapitel des Entwurfs einer allgemeinen Einleitung in die vergleichende Anatomie, ausgehend von der Osteologie*, written in 1796.

Sie [= die Teile der Mineral-Körper; K. S.] haben nach ihrer Grundbestimmung gewisse stärkere oder schwächere Verhältnisse, die, wenn sie sich zeigen, wie eine Art von Neigung aussehen, deswegen die Chemiker auch ihnen die Ehre einer Wahl bei solchen Verwandtschaften zuschreiben, und doch sind es oft nur äußere Determinationen, die sie da oder dort hin stoßen oder reißen, wodurch die Mineral-Körper hervorgebracht werden, ob wir ihnen gleich den zarten Anteil, der ihnen an dem allgemeinen Lebenshauche der Natur gebührt,

> keineswegs absprechen wollen. [Each (= each element in mineral compounds; K. S.) has, according to its nature, certain inherent tendencies that may be more or less pronounced. When these tendencies are actually displayed they seem to be a kind of preference, and this is why chemists attribute the privilege of choice to mineral elements manifesting such affinities. Yet often it is merely external conditions which propel the elements in one direction or draw them in another, thus giving rise to mineral compounds, although at the same time we hardly like to deny them inclinations which are proper to them as a part of nature's universal vitality.] (Goethe 1956: 203)

This same "privilege of choice" was to preoccupy Goethe more fully between the spring of 1808 and the autumn of 1809, and was to call forth a similar tension between the detachment of critical irony and a frank acknowledgement of fascination. Germany's first social novel (cf.Adler 1987: 9) was the result.

At the age of nineteen Goethe personally experienced what both biography and autobiography describe as a striking instance of medical skill. In July 1768, while studying in Leipzig, he was overtaken by a mysterious illness which still resists more modern attempts at diagnosis and was known at that time as *Blutsturz*, 'hemorrhage' (Göres 1981: 26).[107] There is every reason to believe that he may have undergone a serious adolescent crisis at this time. He had attended university in Leipzig for two years without feeling he had accomplished anything of personal value: "Das Bewußtwerden, bei vielfältiger Tätigkeit im Grunde nichts erreicht zu haben, mochte eine als Krankheit erscheinende, psychisch-physische Kapitulation bewirkt haben." ['The realisation that all his varied occupations had, in fact, resulted in very little, may have precipitated a physical and mental collapse that could have been diagnosed as disease.'] (Göres 1981: 27)

He left university in a mood of resignation and immediately returned to the irritating yet secure confinement of the family home in Frankfurt, where he stayed for almost two years. In the following autumn and winter he suffered several relapses, and was cured by a Frankfurt doctor, Johann Friedrich Metz. Goethe writes about him retrospectively in the eighth chapter of *Dichtung und Wahrheit*:

> The physician was an inexplicable, sly-looking, friendly-speaking, and, moreover, abstruse man … Active and attentive, he was consoling to the sick; but, more than by all this, he extended his practice by the gift of showing in the background some mysterious medicines prepared by himself, of which no one could speak, since, with us, the physicians were strictly prohibited from making up their own prescriptions. With certain powders, which may have been some kind of digestive, he was not so reserved; but that powerful salt, which could only be applied in the greatest danger, was only mentioned among believers, although no one had yet seen it or traced its effects. To excite and strengthen

> our faith in the possibility of such an universal remedy, the physician, wherever he found any susceptibility, had recommended certain chemico-alchemical books to his patients ... (Goethe 1848–1849, 1: 291–292).

Following the example of an "ecstatic" (Sudhoff 1932) woman friend, Susanna Katharina Klettenberg (1723–1774), who was a member of Metz's circle and conducted private studies in her own small chemical laboratory, Goethe eagerly began to read the recommended works: "We turned to the works of Theophrastus, Paracelsus and Basilius Valentinus; as well as those of Helmont, Starkey, and others whose doctrines and directions, resting more or less on nature and imagination, we endeavoured to see into and follow out." (Goethe 1848–1849, 1: 293)

This account, written forty or so years after the event, betrays a certain critical distance between the maturity of an experienced natural scientist and the speculative enthusiasms of his youth. Nevertheless it also contains the admission that they were beneficial to him, and at a time when his health was seriously threatened:

> In the meantime a very serious trial was preparing for me; for a disturbed, and one might even say, destroyed digestion, excited such symptoms that, in great tribulation, I thought I should lose my life, and none of the remedies applied would produce any further effect. In this last extremity, my distressed mother constrained the embarrassed physicain with the greatest vehemence to come out with his universal medicine; after a long refusal, he hastened home at the dead of night, and returned with a little glass of crystallised dry salt, which was dissolved in water and swallowed by the patient. It had a decidedly alkaline taste. The salt was scarcely taken than my situation appeared relieved, and from that moment the disease took a turn which, by degrees, led to my recovery. I cannot say how far this strengthened and enhanced our faith in our physician, and our industry to make ourselves partakers of such a treasure. (Goethe 1848–1849, 1: 293)

In 1770 Goethe, now twenty-one, resumed legal studies at Strasbourg university, and successfully completed them less than two years later. While in Strasbourg he pursued the practical and experimental interest in chemical reaction which had been awakened in Frankfurt by regularly attending lectures on chemistry held by J. R. Spielmann (1722–1783). It was probably here that he encountered the chemical concept of affinity for the first time, in any kind of systematic form. (Adler 1987: 34,74)

Goethe's later study of natural science in connection with his *Farbenlehre* 'theory of color' belongs to a period when "bourgeois public's" (cf. Habermas 1984) opinion, like Goethe's own, was beginning to be shaped to some extent by its interest in chemistry. The systematic deliberation on this fashionable topic which took place during the last decade of the eighteenth century and the first ten years of the next – Goethe's novel *Die Wahlverwandtschaften* appeared in 1809 – is summarised by Adler as follows:

> Goethe war nicht einem einzelnen Werk, etwa dem Bergmans für die Chemie seines Romans verpflichtet, er stand innerhalb einer Tradition. Diese beruhte auf der Stoa, und auf Plotin, sowie auf der neuplatonischen Philosophie der Renaissance, beginnt aber als moderne chemische Tradition mit Newton und Geoffroy und erreicht in den Werken Macquers und Bergmans im achtzehnten Jahrhundert ihren Höhepunkt. Diese Tradition wurde nicht zuletzt deswegen bedeutsam, weil sie durch zahlreiche andere Forscher erweitert und in den einflußreichen Lehrbüchern der Goethezeit variiert und verbreitet wurde. Die Wahlverwandtschaften entspringen nicht etwa einer Übertragung der Farbenlehre. Im Gegenteil, Goethe dachte sogar 1793–1797 daran, die Farben nach den Gesetzen der Verwandtschaft zu behandeln. Der Roman beruht nicht auf einer zufälligen Begegnung mit der Chemie, sondern entsprang einer langjährigen Auseinandersetzung, die sich jedoch erst im Roman selbst vollkommen niederschlug. [Goethe's novel was not indebted to any single work, such as Bergman's, for its chemical content. It stands within a tradition which reaches back to the Stoa and Plotinus and includes Renaissance Neo-platonic philosophy; but the modern chemical tradition begins with Newton and Geoffroy, and reaches an eighteenth-century high point with the works of Macquer and Bergman. The tradition gained importance through its development by numerous other scientists, and was variously discussed and disseminated in the many influential handbooks published during the late eighteenth-century. 'Die Wahlverwandtschaften' should not be viewed as a by-product of the 'Farbenlehre', quite the reverse – between 1793 and 1797 Goethe even contemplated an approach to color which was to follow the precepts of <Verwandtschaft> [= affinity; K. S.]. The novel is not based upon a chance encounter with chemistry, but grew out of a long period of analysis which only found its full and complete expression in the novel.] (Adler 1987: 83)

In 1799, when Goethe had been living in Weimar for some years, society salons there were inundated with chemical conversation. Kuhn (1972: 268–269; cf. also Adler 1987: 81) cites an eloquent and wonderfully malicious passage testifying to this. It is taken from Joseph Rückert's "Bemerkungen über Weimar":

> Herr Scherer, der seit mehreren Jahren unter dem Titel eines Bergrats von dem Herzoge einen ansehnlichen Gehalt zog, erhielt bald nach seiner Rückkehr aus England, wohin er vor einigen Jahren eine gelehrte Reise angestellt hatte, den Befehl, wöchentlich, sonnabends von vier bis fünf Uhr, chemische Vorlesungen für alle Stände zu halten. Der Plan war zweckmäßig und ein rühmlicher Beweis von dem Patriotismus des Fürsten. Jedermann, der es bedarf, sollte hier das Brauchbarste und Nötigste aus dieser Wissenschaft zur Aufklärung in seinen Geschäften erlernen. Die Neugierde und das Interesse des ganzen Publikums waren auf die angekündigten Vorlesungen gerichtet. Der Saal füllte sich mit einer großen Menge Zuhörer, worunter sich auch Damen aus beiden Ständen befanden. Der Herzog selbst mit seinem Prinzen erschien öfters in den unterhal-

tenden Stunden. Herr Scherer ließ ein chemisches Handbuch drucken und teilte es bogenweise unter sein Publikum aus. Nah am Parke wurde ihm für seine Präparaten und Experimenten die untere Hälfte eines großen, schönen Gebäudes eingeräumt, und der Herr Bergrat übte sich so stark und belagerungsmäßig, daß die Bewohnerin des obern Teils des Hauses eine Bittschrift für die Erhaltung ihres Lebens bei dem Regenten einzureichen für gut fand, weil sie jeden Moment in die Luft gesprengt zu werden fürchtete. Umsonst! Der patriotische Plan mußte durchgesetzt werden. Man sprach jetzt in Weimar von nichts anderem als von Gas, Oxigna, brennbaren Stoffen, leicht- und strengflüssigen Dingen. Alle Weimarer und Weimaranerinnen schienen Chemiker und Weimar ein großer Schmelzofen werden zu wollen. [Herr Scherer had been drawing a handsome salary from the Duke for several years in return for his services as Minister of Mines. Soon after his return from England, where he had been travelling in connection with scientific interests, he received an order asking him to deliver weekly lectures on chemistry, to be held before the general public every Saturday between the hours of four and five. The proposal was highly expedient and offered resounding proof of the Duke's patriotic care for his subjects. Anyone who wished to could now learn all about the most important and the most practical aspects of this science, and apply them to his own affairs. The entire public awaited the forthcoming lectures with interest and curiosity. The hall was completely filled by a large audience which included women from both upper and lower classes. The Duke himself was often present at these entertaining occasions, accompanied by his son and heir. Herr Scherer published a chemical textbook, and distributed it as it appeared, section by section amongst his audiences. The lower floor of a fine large building near the park was made available to him for his preparations and experiments, and the Minister of Mines in fact set about his work with so war-like a fervour that the lady who lived on the upper floor saw fit to petition the Regent to spare her life, for she was afraid the house might explode beneath her at any moment. But in vain! The patriotic plan had to continue. People in Weimar talked about nothing but gas, oxides, inflammable substances, easily fusible and non-fusible objects. The whole population of Weimar was set on becoming chemists, and turning Weimar itself into one great smelting furnace.][108]

Goethe's social novel was a reflection of erotic experience, its dialectics vividly oscillating between the poles of union and separation. Chemistry and its theories of combination represented far more to him than an ornamental framework of ideas for the novel. *Die Wahlverwandtschaften* is the distillation of a craving for meaning in a solvent of good common sense. "Daß diese Auseinandersetzung mit einer chemischen Theorie in einem klassischen Roman, ja im ersten deutschen Gesellschaftsroman, geführt wird, sollte nicht zu der Ansicht verleiten, daß hier die Naturwissenschaft nur ästhetisch dargestellt und verwertet wird. Selbst im Bereich des Ästhetischen behält die Naturwissenschaft ihre eigene Gültigkeit, ihre Wahrheit." ['The fact that this analysis of chemical theory is conducted in a novel belonging to the period of German classicism, indeed in Germany's very first social novel, should not give rise to the false supposition that the representation and evaluation of natural science are purely esthetic. Even within the realm of esthetics natural science maintains its own validity, its own truth.'] (Adler 1987: 9)

In the autumn of 1809 Goethe himself wrote an advertisement for the newly published *Die Wahlverwandtschaften*, which appeared in the *Morgenblatt für gebildete Stände*. In it, he remarks:

> Es scheint, daß den Verfasser seine fortgesetzten physikalischen Arbeiten zu diesem seltsamen Titel veranlaßten. Er mochte bemerkt haben, daß man in der Naturlehre sich sehr oft ethischer Gleichnisse bedient, um etwas von dem Kreise menschlichen Wissens weit Entferntes näher heranzubringen, und so hat er auch wohl in einem sittlichen Falle eine chemische Gleichnisrede zu ihrem geistigen Ursprunge zurückführen mögen, um so mehr als doch überall nur eine Natur ist und auch durch das Reich der heitern Vernunftfreiheit die Spuren trüber, leidenschaftlicher Notwendigkeit sich unaufhaltsam hindurchziehen, die nur durch eine höhere Hand und vielleicht auch nicht in diesem Leben völlig auszulöschen sind. [It seems that the author's long-standing preoccupation with the study of natural science gave rise to this rather curious title. He could have drawn attention to the fact that similes derived from ethics are often used in natural science in order to bring something far removed from the sphere of human experience somewhat closer to it, since he wanted, through the portrayal of a moral situation, to trace a chemical simile back to its spiritual origins, and is justified in doing this since Nature is everywhere undivided, signs of a dark and passionate necessity penetrate even the realm governed by free and unclouded reason, and only a higher law can extinguish them, in this life, though perhaps never completely.] (Goethe, quoted by Ritzenhoff 1982: 5)

At the beginning of the nineteenth century the concept of *attractio electiva* had proved its worth in analytic deliberation, and the educated reading public did not want to forget its metaphorical antecedents. Goethe took up this refusal with a sure sense of its underlying astuteness. In *Die Wahlverwandtschaften* 'Elective Affinities' (Goethe 1975, 1971), he orchestrates a postlude for the concept whose fictional nature is firmly established from the very beginning. The first words of the novel are: "Eduard – so nennen wir einen reichen Baron im besten Mannesalter" (Goethe 1975: 3). ['Edward – this is the name we will give to a wealthy baron in the prime of life].[109] Adler (1987: 141) comments: "Im Augenblick des Benennens reflektiert der Satz auf das Nennen selbst." ['The sentence deliberates upon the process of naming even as it performs it.']

Edward, whose baptismal name is /Otto/, as we learn in the third chapter, lives with his wife Charlotte and several friends, guests and servants in his own mansion, surrounded by grounds which he lovingly landscapes with the pleasure of a connoisseur. Their relationship is frank and egalitarian, characterised by shared interests and an enviable appreciation of their separate identities. They are shining bright examples of an enlightened aristocracy. Very soon a friend of Edward's youth enters the action of the novel, a Captain by profession and Otto by name. In the sixth chapter Charlotte's niece, Ottilie, comes to complete the quartet of main protagonists, after her proposed arrival has been discussed by the others. From the fourth chapter onwards it is clear not only to the reader but to the fictional characters of the novel as well, that Edward will fall in love with Ottilie, and the Captain with Charlotte. The most interesting aspect of this constellation – one that is certainly not unusual in fiction – for this present study, is that for the four adults involved it becomes an occasion for sincere mutual discussion of what truly binds or separates them. The chaotic feelings of hope and fear that usually hinder such discussion are contained and structured in a model of similarity that was produced and developed for quite different purposes. Edward, Charlotte, the Captain and, in the reader's imagination, Ottilie too – even though she is not actually present at this point in the novel – compare the imminent changes in their relationships with the process of chemical reaction:

> 'Provided it does not seem pedantic', the Captain said, 'I think I can briefly sum up in the language of signs. Imagine an A intimately united with a B, so that no force is able to sunder them; imagine a C likewise related to a D; now bring the two couples into contact: A will throw itself at D, C at B, without our being able to say which first deserted its partner, which first embraced the other's partner.' 'Now then!' Edward interposed: 'until we see all this with our own eyes, let us look on this formula as a metaphor from which we may extract a lesson we can apply immediately to ourselves. You, Charlotte, represent the A, and I represent your B; for in fact I do depend altogether on you and follow you as A follows B. The C is quite obviously the Captain, who for the moment is to some extent drawing me away from you. Now it is only fair that, if you are not to vanish into the limitless air, you must be provided with a D, and this D is unquestionably the charming little lady Ottilie, whose approaching presence you may no longer resist.'
> 'Very well,' Charlotte replied. 'Even if, as I think, this example does not precisely fit our case, I still consider it a good thing that today we are for once fully in agreement, and that these natural and elective affinities should hasten me to tell you something in confidence' (Goethe 1971: 56–57)

While the bodies of the four protagonists experience a powerful natural force which threatens to deprive them of their self-control, their minds combat impending separation by seeking security and orientation:

> Zwischen den Gegensätzen von Geist und Körper liegt aber eine Fülle von Fähigkeiten, Affekten, Erscheinungen, welche die Vermittlung von Ich und Welt erzielen: Fühlen, Einbilden, Denken, Erkennen und Sehen, Verstehen, Verhalten, Beziehen und Lieben. In der Welt der Wahlverwandtschaften beruhen diese auf Ähnlichkeiten, Übereinstimmungen und Korrespondenzen, die zumindest durch Assoziation als <Verwandtschaft> aufzufassen sind und die zum

> Teil auch der Struktur der <Wahlverwandtschaft> folgen. [The opposites of mind and body carry a wealth of abilities, affects and phenomena that mediate between the individual and the external world: feeling, imagination, thought, recognition, seeing, understanding, behaviour, relating, loving. In the world of Goethe's Elective Affinities, all these are based on similarities, agreements and correspondances which, by association at least, are to be interpreted as <affinities>, and which also, to some extent, follow the patterns of <elective affinity>.] (Adler 1987: 187–188)

In the sphere of human relationships Goethe's novel examines /similarity/, its traditionally contrasting opposite, /polarity/, and the accompanying problem of maintaining harmony between mind and body. Thus one of the most important areas of thought conditioning the influence of Schelling's natural philosophy on medicine (cf. Tsouyopoulos 1982), pharmacy (cf. Petersen 1978, Oldenburg 1979) and pharmacology (cf. Heischkel 1958) during the late eighteenth century also comes under consideration in *Die Wahlverwandtschaften.*

The fourth chapter of the novel introduces the chemical simile and is, moreover, rich in allusions to contemporary discussion on scientific method. It begins by describing the preparation of a topographical map of the entire estate, "fixed by trigonometrical measurements the Captain had been making" (Goethe 1971: 46). Then all papers, documents and reports concerning the estate are to be arranged in an archive and "reduced to a satisfying order" (Goethe 1971: 47).

The next step taken involves the remedies available on the estate: "The domestic dispensary, which had consisted of only a few medicines and remedies, was enlarged. Charlotte was industrious and helpful by nature and through discussion and by reading comprehensible textbooks she was enabled to be so more effectively and more often." (Goethe 1971: 47)

The dispensary has hardly been brought up to date when the Captain suggests that a field-surgeon he knows might be sent for to instruct them all in the use of the new remedies: "'… an excellent man in his trade and one who has oftentimes treated me for serious internal troubles too, and better than a specialist might have done; and immediate aid is, after all, what is most seriously missed in the country'" (Goethe 1971: 48).

Almost immediately afterwards Charlotte's concern to "do away with anything that might be harmful or deadly" (Goethe 1971: 48) brings her into conversation with the Captain about the lead-glazing on her crockery and the verdigris on her copper-ware: "… she had him instruct her about this and the instruction had naturally to begin with the fundamental principles of physics and chemistry." (Goethe 1971: 48)

Finally, Edward's "taste for reading aloud" also changes significantly:

> He had a very melodious deep voice and had in earlier days been well-received and well-known for his lively and sensitive recitation of oratory and poetry. Now it was other subjects that engaged him and other books from which he read, and as it happened these had for some time been principally works on physics, chemistry and technical matters. (Goethe 1971: 48)

After these preliminaries, which take up only a few pages, the remainder of the chapter develops the chemical analogy during the course of an evening conversation between the Captain (whose name is Otto), Edward (whose baptismal name is Otto), Edward's wife Charlotte, and her niece Ottilie, who, however, is only present as a topic, not in person. Lämmert (1986: 21) analyses the disarming simplicity of this authorial device by posing a rhetorical question:

> Das Schema ist so einfach, daß pflichtschuldig sensible Literaturwissenschaftler es gar nicht glauben wollten. Wo bleibt in diesem Schema der erotische Konflikt, wo die ganze Seligkeit aus Neigung und Leidenschaft, wo der ganze Jammer aus Entsagung und Edelmut, die der Roman vor uns ausbreitet? [The scheme is so simple that sensitive and responsible critics found themselves unable to believe it. Where was the erotic conflict, all the bliss of passionate attraction, all the agony of generous self-denial which the novel lays before us?]

The conflict of the novel, on the one hand so vividly creative, on the other so chaotically destructive, is resolved – if only for a moment – in an irresistibly simple and therefore extraordinarily consoling "order of homeomorphic identification" (Lacan 1977: 3). This pattern represents an ordering process, previously referred to in this study as "structural gain", which enables participating subjects to maintain an illusory certainty that separation is not painful, that paradise itself can indeed be reconstructed even after it has been lost.

Edward, without of course being aware of Lacan's notion of the "mirror stage" (cf. Chapter 3.1), nevertheless directly refers to it when he turns to Charlotte at the beginning of their evening conversation: "'It is a metaphor which has misled and confused you,' said Edward. 'Here, to be sure, it is only a question of soil and minerals; but man is a true Narcissus: he makes the whole world his mirror.'" (Goethe 1971: 50)

In Plato's "Symposium" (1951, 1957), Aristophanes tells a myth which explains erotic attraction between the sexes as a yearning attempt to re-create the original hermaphroditic state of paradise before the Fall.[110] There was originally a third sex,

> ... with the characteristics of both male and female, but now the name alone remains, and that solely as a term of abuse. Secondly, each human being was a rounded whole, with double back and flanks forming a complete circle; it had four hands and an equal number of legs, and two identically similar faces

upon a circular neck, with one head common to both the faces, which were turned in opposite directions. It had four ears and two organs of generation and everything else to correspond. (Plato 1951: 59 [§189]).

These beings, Aristophanes continues, were so all-powerful that they attempted "to climb up to heaven and set upon the gods" (Plato 1951: 60 [§190]). Zeus then cut each of them in two, to weaken them, and at the same time to make them more numerous and therefore more profitable to the gods. Apollo was entrusted with the cosmetic details of the operation; he smoothed and rounded off the new beings, but left a few wrinkles around the navel, "to remind man of the state from which he had fallen" (Plato 1951: 61 [§191]):

Man's original body having been thus cut in two, each half yearned for the half from which it had been severed. When they met they threw their arms round one another and embraced, in their longing to grow together again, and they perished of hunger and general neglect of their concerns, because they would not do anything apart... So they went on perishing until Zeus took pity on them, and hit upon a second plan. He moved their reproductive organs to the front: hitherto they had been placed on the outer side of their bodies, and the processes of begetting and birth had been carried on not by the physical union of the sexes, but by emission on to the ground, as is the case with grasshoppers. By moving their genitals to the front, as they are now, Zeus made it possible for reproduction to take place by the intercourse of the male with the female. His object in making this change was twofold; if male coupled with female, children might be begotten and the race thus continued, but if male coupled with male, at any rate the desire for intercourse would be satisfied, and men set free from it to turn to other activities and to attend to the rest of the business of life. It is from this distant epoch, then, that we may date the innate love which human beings feel for one another, the love which restores us to our ancient state by attempting to weld two beings into one and to heal the wounds which humanity suffered." (Plato 1951: 61–62 [§191])

Lillyman (1983) puts forward the initially startling hypothesis that the relationship which develops between Edward and Ottilie during the course of Goethe's novel both borrows and elaborates upon the fundamental idea in Aristophanes' myth. He views the "... analogy of chemical affinities as a Goethean update of Plato" (Lillyman 1983: 128). "It is, indeed, repeatedly emphasised throughout Die Wahlverwandtschaften, that when Ottilie and Edward do something together, they become indispensable to one another, become as it were identical and suggest a wholeness or completeness, the ultimate goal in Aristophanes' characterization of love." (Lillyman 1983: 131).

Lillyman supports his hypothesis with argument based on evidence of Goethe's intense preoccupation with Plato's thought before and during his work on *Die Wahlverwandtschaften*, and on the text of the novel. Here he finds Goethe's repeated references to the existence of a synchronous physical harmony between Edward and Ottilie to be of particular significance. For example, their handwritings are so alike that they themselves can hardly tell them apart. They astonish their audience by accompanying each other perfectly on flute and piano without previous rehearsal or arrangement. Perhaps the most impressive support for Lillyman's argument comes, however, from the fact that they frequently and simultaneously suffer quite sudden attacks of a kind of migraine which affects each of them on opposite – and therefore corresponding – sides of the head.

Lillyman's argument makes an important contribution to the present attempt at the modelling of similarity, since it suggests a particularly clear example of one function of "diachronous finding of similarity" that has already been discussed, namely the virtual reconstruction of a lost paradise. Thus in "Die Wahlverwandtschaften" similarity becomes the source not only of structure and topographic order, but also of welcome consolation, and it invites a "Sinnbildeln und Wortdeuteln" ['symbolising and subtilising'] (cf. Boisserée 1970: 72). It offers access to a structuring of experience in the face of threat. When Bergman's *attractio electiva* enters the everyday world of human relationships, it becomes – although this was never his intention – a point of departure for structural gain, and it thus facilitates establishment of "semiotic specificity". A useful description appears in Ottilie's diary:

> There are many kinds of memorial and memento which bring us closer to those who are far away and those who have departed, but none is more meaningful than the portrait. There is something exciting about being with a much-loved portrait, even if it is not a good likeness,[111] just as there is sometimes something exciting about arguing with a friend. You have the pleasant feeling that you are divided, and yet can never be separated. (Goethe 1871: 164)

When he was twelve Charles Sanders Peirce wrote *A History of Chemistry*, but the manuscript has never been found; eight years later, in the 1859 Harvard year-book, came "My Life written for the Class-Book". The following is an extract: "1847. Began to be most seriously and helplessly in love. Sought to drown my care by taking up the subject of Chemistry – an antidote which long experience enables me to recommend as sovereign." (Peirce 1982: 2)

3.4. Pharmacological receptors

> Im Jahr 1932, als ich im Ausland war, begann ich mir klar zu werden, daß ich in Bälde einen längeren, vielleicht einen dauernden Abschied von der Stadt, in der ich geboren bin, würde nehmen müssen. Ich hatte das Verfahren der Impfung mehrmals in meinem inneren Leben als heilsam erfahren; ich hielt mich auch in dieser Lage daran und rief die Bilder, die im Exil das Heimweh am stärksten zu wecken pflegen – die der Kindheit – mit Absicht in mir hervor. Das Gefühl der Sehnsucht durfte dabei über den Geist ebensowenig Herr werden wie der Impfstoff über einen gesunden Körper. Ich suchte es durch die Einsicht, nicht in die zufällige biographische sondern in die notwendige gesellschaftliche Unwiederbringlichkeit des Vergangenen in Schranken zu halten.[112]
>
> Walter Benjamin

By the fourth decade of the nineteenth century, at the very latest, the influence of natural philosophy (of Schelling's in particular) on the theory of medicine had rather abruptly come to an end. The rift between the two disciplines is confirmed by the fact that until well into the twentieth century the historiography of natural science presents a fundamentally distorted picture of natural philosphy's attempt to view mind and matter as one dynamic entity. It tends to reduce this attempt to a set of speculations, and to confine it to a few somewhat peripheral theoretical movements such as "vitalism" and "theurgy"[113]. Any speculative desire was barred from scientific discourse. Justus von Liebig (1803–1873) is typical of a new generation of angry young men whose work in the scientific laboratory was highly promising, but whose rational distance from tradition now and again took the form of something like exorcism. After occasional attendance at Schelling's lectures in Erlangen on natural philosophy he called it "die Pestilenz, der schwarze Tod des Jahrhunderts" ['the Plague, this century's Black Death'] (quoted by Wurster [year of publication not indicated]: 154). But it must be remembered that pharmacists in the medicine of the Romantic period who had taken their general direction from natural philosophy, like Johann Heinrich Wilhelm Grabau (1837) or Ignaz Bertele, a pupil of Schelling's, had also followed a similar pattern in their rejection of the theory of signatures.

Ackerknecht (1977: 149) characterises medicine in the second half of the nineteenth century as 'laboratory medicine', thus distinguishing it through its practical environment from Hippocratic 'bedside medicine', from the 'library medicine' of the Middle Ages, and from the 'hospital medicine' which grew out of the *Birth of the clinic* (Foucault 1976b) in the eighteenth century. The four walls of the laboratory are the orthogonal germ cell of a new 'pharmacological' body of theory whose sober, thorough approach was finally successful in tackling a problem which the first two chapters of this study examine in some detail and present as being already "solved". This is the problem of pharmacological 'specificity'. A few years after Sertürner's isolation of morphine, Francois Magendie (1783–1855), with the extraction of //strychnine// from the seeds of //nux vomica//, isolated another 'alkaloid' possessing a high degree of pharmacological effectiveness. His pupil Claude Bernard (1813–1878) lent vital impetus in both practical and theoretical areas to the acceptance of pharmacology as a discipline fundamental to medicine. Bernard developed experimentation on animals as a basic means to the pursuit of knowledge within the four walls of the new working environment. Bynum (1970: 520) identifies two particular nineteenth-century innovations as contributing to the fact that the question of correlation between the 'structure' of chemical combinations and their physiological effect received increasingly close attention in medical journals of the latter half of the century. Here, of course, the question is dealt with far more successfully than it was by Hahnemann fifty years previously.

(1) The discovery of various 'anaesthetics', such as //ether//, //chloroform//, and //laughing-gas//. From a chemical point of view these were all simple, sub-molecular combinations not occurring naturally. Since they were produced synthetically, chemists had good verified knowledge of their structure. These chemicals also had obvious physiological effects that could be clearly defined: they caused characteristic changes in consciousness and perception which included the particular phenomenon of brief elimination of pain.

(2) The discovery of antagonistic effects limited to certain narrowly defined physiological reactions and to certain distinct physical organs. For example, //physostigmine//, an extract of the Calabar bean, could be seen to stimulate the salivary glands to a measurably greater level of secretion, while the 'alkaloid' //atropine//, an extract of belladonna, caused the level of secretion to fall back.

This amassing of constant correlations drew the attention of laboratory research to a "structure/activity relationship" (Peters 1970) that is still the basis of much new theory in the pharmacology of today. Its first precise definition as an outcome of experimental procedure probably came from James Blake (1814-1893) when he called it the "apparently analogous action of isomorphic substances when introduced directly into the blood" (quoted by Bynum 1970: 522). Further consolidation of a correlative connection between the formerly "monoplanar" (Eco 1984b: 169) systems of physiology on the one hand and analytic chemistry on the other was provided in significant measure by the collaborative work of Thomas Richard Fraser (1841–1920) and Alexander Crum Brown. The influence of 'structural pharmacology' reached a temporary high-point with Thomas Lauder Brunton's *Textbook of Pharmacology, Therapeutics, and Materia Medica*, which was first published in 1885; editions in German, French, Italian and Spanish very soon followed. But in 1895 Oswald Schmiedeberg's (1838–1921) *Grundriss der Arzneimittellehre* found resonance among its specialist readership with the complaint "that all speculation about the structure-function problem [should] be temporarily suspended until more empirical information became available" (Bynum 1970: 538).

In the nineteenth century, however, the "suggestive Kraft praktischer Erfolge" ['implications of practical results'] (Fleck 1982: 122) were unequivocally monopolised by two other disciplines fundamental to medicine – bacteriology and its direct descendant, immunology. Later both were to exert a crucial influence on the direction of pharmacology.

In 1850 Casimir Joseph Davaine (1812–1882) produced a virtual duplicate of *contagium* when he caused anthrax in healthy animals by injecting them with blood from infected victims. He thus supplied powerful empirical evidence for the argument against "anticontagionism" (Ackerknecht 1977: 153), a view which had shaped theory for over fifty years in spite of Edward Jenner's (1749–1823) discovery of inoculation. During the next decades several new causes of disease were discovered in quick succession, and some were verified by use of the microscope. Controversy over the hypothesis put forward by Girolamo Fracastoro (1478–1553) that infectious diseases were transmitted by microcosmic corpuscular //contagia// was finally settled, and almost overnight there came to hand a palpable cause for diseases – a "représentation ontologique du mal" ['ontological representation of the sick and evil'](Canguilhem 1972: 12) – which all together until then had been pathogenetically impenetrable and epidemically destructive. Even more important, however, was the fact that this discovery had clear therapeutic consequences. In 1885 Louis Pasteur (1822–1895) developed a method of inoculation against rabies which, although rather dangerous, was nevertheless a welcome alternative to the otherwise fatal disease. In 1890 Emil von Behring (1854–1917) discovered that blood which was carrying infection contained not only the bacteria causing disease but also, in certain cases, substances which would destroy those very bacteria. He concluded that such //antitoxins// were produced by defense mechanisms in the body which were triggered off by the penetration of disease-bearing bacteria.

A logical next step was the attempt to isolate such substances, to accumulate them in high concentration, and to use the resulting concentrates for therapeutic purposes. In 1893 Behring was encouraged by the successful treatment of diphtheria through the use of serum. This method of treatment was not based on the same principle as Jenner's or Pasteur's method of vaccination, since it was not small quantities of disease-bearing bacteria that were smuggled into the body of the patient to activate immunities, but biologically synthesised substances produced by the immunological systems of other organisms. //Antitoxins// were – as an example of man's conquest of Nature – a powerful complementary answer to the problem of //contagium//. They would have been capable of analogical *représentation ontologique du bien* if they had possessed the same iconic aptness as //contagium// and could have been captured, for example, under the microscope. But science still lacked the necessary basic knowledge of immunology, or any body of verifiable hypotheses on the mechanisms of the effects of //antitoxins// and their chemical constitution. Clarification of this unresolved and ever more urgent problem was the focus of scientific research carried out by Paul Ehrlich (1854–1915). His findings finally led to a model of similarity that even today still determines the organisation of all theoretical knowledge on pharmacological 'specificity'. This model is the receptor model.

Ehrlich was born in a small Silesian town in 1854, and studied medicine in Breslau, Strasbourg, Freiburg, and Leipzig. His doctoral dissertation of 1878 was entitled *Über Theorie und Praxis der histologischem Färbung* 'On theory and practice of histological staining' (Ehrlich 1956). According to several biographers, a passionately curious love for color and coloring accompanied his whole scientific career. Anecdotes tell of a schoolboy prank which involved dyeing white doves blue, and also that he had a huge bouquet of white carnations delivered to his daughter's wedding reception, after previously replacing the water they were kept in with a dye solution, so that they would surprise everyone by turning pink at a certain point in the proceedings (Anonymous [no year of publication indicated]: 9; Marquardt 1951: 80).

Without having any definite therapeutic purpose in mind, Ehrlich's thesis pursues the problem of which chemical characteristics would selectively concentrate certain dyes in certain tissues, cell-clusters or parts of cells, so that these structures could be examined topographically under the microscope as functional entities. His laboratory bench in Breslau university, and later in the Charité hospital in Berlin where from 1878 he was intern under Friedrich Theodor von Frerich (1819–1885), and then senior physician, was permanently and completely covered with splashes of dye.[114] After the death of his clinical mentor, von Frerich, Ehrlich found it hard to work with Gerhardt, his successor, whose research interests were completely opposed to his own. Much later he spoke to his secretary, Martha Marquardt (1951: 25), about the difficulties of this period of his career: "Wie ich damals bei Gerhardt mich so elend fühlte, ging ich immer an meinen Farbenschrank und sagte: 'Das sind meine Freunde, die mich nie im Stich lassen werden.'" ['In those days, whenever I felt really miserable about working with Gerhardt, I would go to my cupboard of dyes and say to myself: "These are my friends, and they will never desert me."']

His work with dye-stuffs first began to have therapeutic consequences in the 1890s, when he used //methyl blue// in chemical experiments directed towards the combat of pain and the treatment of malaria. Around the turn of the century the production of dye-stuffs was one of the most important activities in a rapidly expanding chemical industry, and since an especially detailed knowledge of structural chemistry had been built up in this field, many of the //mother substances// subsequently introduced into pharmacology were originally derivates or intermediate products of synthetic dye-stuffs.

After two years in Egypt spent convalescing from tuberculosis – probably contracted in the laboratory – Ehrlich went to the Berlin Institute for Infectious Disease in 1890 and worked there under Robert Koch (1843–1910). In 1896 he was appointed director of the Steglitz Institute for Serum Research. In 1898 the Institute transferred to Frankfurt with improved staffing conditions and funds, and became the "*Institut für experimentelle Therapie*" which, with the "*Institut Pasteur*" in Paris, became the European centre for all research into immunology.

A fundamental concern in research of the 1890s was investigation of the mechanism and the determinants of the effects of antitoxins. Clinical experience had shown how urgent this problem was, since in many cases Behring's diphtheria serum had had no appreciable therapeutic effect. Ehrlich developed a standardised biological procedure whereby the concentration of antitoxins in various serums could be precisely measured, even though their chemical structures were unknown. By excluding those serums where the level of antitoxin-concentration fell below a certain point, the number of serums with a low rate of therapeutic success could be decreased. Ehrlich assumed that //antitoxins// were biologically synthesised by certain body-cells, and that they must have a complementary and spatial relationship with the toxins of //corynebacterium diphtheriae// which would be similar to the lock and key paradigm.

> It must be assumed that this ability to combine with antitoxin is attributable to the presence in the toxin complex of a specific group of atoms with a maximum specific affinity to another group of atoms in the antitoxin complex, the first

fitting the second easily, as a key does a lock, to quote Emil Fischer's well known simile. (Ehrlich 1957a: 114).

The teleological explosiveness of the 'maximal specific affinity' between bacteriological toxins and antitoxins produced by body-cells made Ehrlich somewhat uneasy. He could not prevent himself from apologising for the hypothesis immediately after its introduction, and distanced himself from the tradition which regarded such affinities with a certain degree of fascination:

> If a chemist were offered the task of finding a physiologically and chemically inert antidote to an alkaloid or some other poison, which antidote must neither destroy the poison nor precipitate it in an insoluble form, but must, nevertheless, render any given quantity of it harmless, he would certainly refuse the task as chimerical. Nevertheless, the living organism can perform this task easily, often within the course of a few days, and with a multiplicity of toxins. To attribute what could be called inventive activity to the body or to its cells, enabling them to produce new groups of atoms as required, would involve a return to the concepts current in the days of [an obsolete] natural philosophy. Our knowledge of cell function and especially of synthetic processes would lead us rather to assume that in the formation of antibodies, we are dealing with the enhancement of a normal cell function, and not with the creation at need of new groups of atoms. Physiological analogues of the group of the specifically combining antibodies must exist beforehand in the organism or in its cells. (Ehrlich 1957a: 114)

But even this "normal" cellular activity follows the Paracelsian program of *signatur-locus-noturft-inventrix* 'signature-locus-necessity-invention' (Paracelsus 1928: 212) with an astonishing closeness. According to Ehrlich's model the cell must choose one specific "physiological analog" from an existing wealth of possibilities, and must then produce a particular and necessary grouping of atoms in sufficient quantity to neutralise a bacteriogenic toxin.

In 1900 an invitation from the Royal Society of Medicine brought Ehrlich to London to give one of the highly prestigious "Croonian Lectures". His lecture presents a model that is speculative yet clearly rooted in laboratory experiment, and offers nothing less than an explanation of the key mechanism which determines a body-cell's chemical reactions with its environment (Ehrlich 1957b).

His analytical study of dyes had revealed that the groups of atoms within a dye-stuff which determine its light absorption properties, and thus its actual color, are not necessarily identical with the groups determining its affinity with certain kinds of tissue or cell-clusters. He transposes this differentiation between the functions of certain groupings (cf. Koch's term /representomorpheme/, introduced in this study in Table 1) to toxin molecules, and here distinguishes between a 'toxophore' group, and a 'haptophore' group responsible for any affinity with cell-clusters or with antibodies. Ehrlich's "side-chain theory", first put forward in its complete form in London, suggests that there are numerous extensions on the surface of the cell and that the surfaces of these extensions themselves have an extremely complex three-dimensional structure. The surfaces of the "side-chains" form the actual heuristic link between the body cell as a complex, living structure in a constant state of change and its potential partner in chemical reaction, which has a comparatively stable structure. According to this model, an organism's //antitoxins// are virtually the result of surplus production, they are side-chains whose surfaces bear a complementary three-dimensional relationship of similarity to the //haptophore groups// of bacteriogenic toxins. This relationship follows the lock and key principle. The theory of side-chains models the "maximal specific affinity" between structures native to an organism and structures foreign to it, and models it, moreover, with a vividness that does not tempt wild teleological speculation. The model gives the processes of theorisation access to the activities of a living cell when it is participating in chemical reaction: *Corpora non agunt nisi fixata*. Ehrlich developed the model within the field of immunology, using the "neutralisation of toxins" as his working example. In the "Croonian Lecture", however, he suggests the possibility that even the very elementary process of cellular energy metabolism can be explained by means of a similar paradigm.

The side-chain theory's special quality of vividness depends not least on the fact that Ehrlich took the risk of illustrating it with imaginative diagrams, even though the structures conveyed by the diagrams are purely hypothetical. The diagrams were first presented to a wide specialist audience in London (cf. Figure 15), and are a vital precondition for the establishment of "lock and key complementarity" as an "iconic institution" in further diagrams produced by natural science during the next decades (cf. Blumenberg 1986: 32). But even more importantly, they are forerunners of the countless doodles drawn by doctors in ordinary clinical practice today when they are explaining the effects of a medicine to their patients.

It was August von Kekulé (1829–1896), a pioneering carbon chemist and the first to discover the ring-like structure of the //benzene atom//, who maintained that "... die Art, wie theoretische Gedanken in Zeichensystemen ausgedrückt werden, sei überhaupt gleichgültig" [the type of sign system used to express theoretical ideas is a matter of little importance'] quoted by Weissbach 1971: 133; cf. Chapter 1.2). Ehrlich followed this dictum ad absurdum in the way he developed his "strong visual imagination" (Mazumdar 1974: 6) into a highly productive cognitive tool. Although he seldom seems

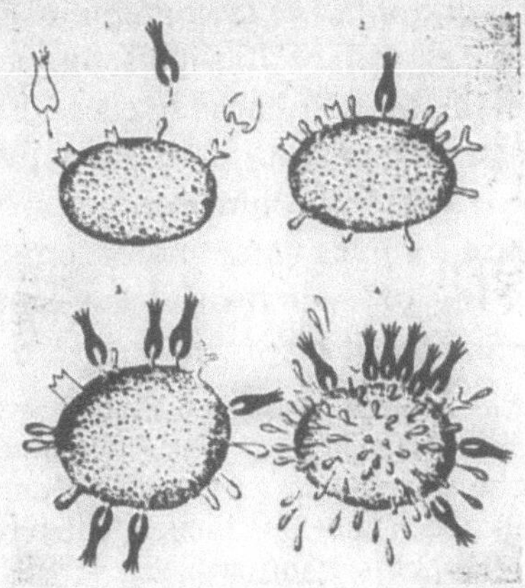

DIAGRAMMATIC REPRESENTATION OF THE SIDE-CHAIN THEORY
(PLATES I AND II)

Fig. 1 "The groups [the haptophore group of the side-chain of the cell and that of the food-stuff or the toxin] must be adapted to one another, *e.g.*, as male and female screw (PASTEUR), or as lock and key (E. FISCHER)."

Fig. 2 ". . . the first stage in the toxic action must be regarded as being the union of the toxin by means of its haptophore group to a special side-chain of the cell protoplasm."

Fig. 3 "The side-chain involved, so long as the union lasts, cannot exercise its normal, physiological, nutritive function . . ."

Fig. 4 "We are therefore now concerned with a defect which, according to the principles so ably worked out by . . . Weigert, is . . . [overcorrected] by regeneration."

Figure 15: A new iconic institution: lock and key complementarity in Paul Ehrlich's 'side chain theory'. Diagram and original captions in Ehrlich 1957b. (The drawings are captioned in the following order: top left, top right, bottom left, bottom right; reproduced by permission of Julius Springer Verlag, Berlin.)

to have reflected on it, he does discuss the method in a letter to his friend C. A. Herter:

> I also, in fact, believe that my real natural endowment lies in the domain of chemistry; and mine is indeed, as you know, a kind of visual, three-dimensional chemistry. The benzene-rings and structural formulae really disport themselves in space before my mind's eye, and I believe that it is just this faculty which has been of supreme value to me in my later studies. (Ehrlich, quoted by Dale 1956: 9).

Martha Marquardt's biography (1951) frequently refers to Ehrlich's almost obsessive habit of recording the problems engaging him by making sketches of them in an idiosyncratic but obviously very vivid visual language. He did this on laboratory pads which he passed to colleagues to look at, but also on the sleeves of his lab-coat, his shirt front or, when he needed more space, with chalk on the floor of his workroom. A photograph of Sir Arthur Conan Doyle (1859–1930) hung on the wall of Ehrlich's room, and his library contained several copies of the Sherlock Holmes novels with personal dedications from the author: "With compliments to my great colleague." Ehrlich's admiration for Doyle's novels – which for him seem to have been a kind of "science fiction" in a truer sense – gives some indication of how semiotics and the semiotic developed a life of their own that assumed a more than marginal importance in the unfolding of his thought:

> Ehrlich las Detektivromane mit Vorliebe, weil er dadurch 'fast vollkommen' von seinen Problemen abgelenkt werden konnte. 'Fast vollkommen', aber doch nicht ganz, denn all diese Hefte und andere 'spannende' Romane, wie überhaupt fast jedes Buch oder Heft tragen außen und innen Farbstiftnotizen, Stichworte, chemische Formeln ... Ehrlich spricht auch, hinsichtlich von Lektüre, von einer 'Affinität', die ihn diejenigen Dinge finden läßt, die zu seinen wissenschaftlichen Problemen oder ihn interessierenden Tagesfragen in Beziehung stehen. [Ehrlich had a preference for detective novels because they provided an 'almost complete' diversion from his problems. 'Almost complete', but still not quite 'complete', for all these volumes as well as other suspense novels, like all his books, are marked both inside and out with notes and chemical formulae written in colored ink... On the subject of his reading Ehrlich also spoke of an 'affinity' which guided him to things that were relevant to his scientific problems or to his daily preoccupations.][115] (Marquardt 1951: 82, 84).

Ehrlich turned towards a new field of enquiry in the first decade of the twentieth century, even before his work in immunology brought him the Nobel Prize for medicine in 1908. As yet no successful means of immunisation had been found, in spite of experiment with both active and passive inoculation against infectious diseases caused by parasites or by bacteria that do not produce toxins. Ehrlich now suggested that it was possible to combat such micro-organisms directly, by means of substances produced synthetically or artificially. Scientists would have "durch chemische Variation zielen lernen" ['to learn to set targets by chemical variation'] (Ehrlich 1957c: 141) in order to attack a selected cause of disease without damaging the affected organism. He saw quite clearly that this presented the medical laboratory with a task of Herculean proportions, for how were such substances to be found: "The exceedingly great difficulty of these studies is evidenced by the fact that hundreds, nay thousands, of substances have to be examined by animal experiments, before a few producing a therapeutic effect can be found." (Ehrlich 1957c: 130).

In 1893 Ehrlich had published a volume entitled *Constitution, Vertheilung und Wirkung Chemischer Körper* (constitution, allocation and effect of chemical bodies), which contained a collection of his papers on topics from the fields of immunology and coloring analysis that had previously appeared in various periodicals. The brief preface to the collection includes the following remark: "Nach meinen Untersuchungen ist die Verteilung d. h. die elektive Verwandtschaft zu bestimmten Organen und Systemen eine Function der chemischen Constitution." ['My researches show that allocation, or, in other words, an elective affinity to certain organs and systems, is a function of chemical constitution.'][116] (Ehrlich 1893: 5).

Fifteen years later he took up this trail again and after long hesitation (cf. Parascandola – Jasensky 1974: 205–206) decided to use the model of similarity embodied in the side-chain theory as a hypothetical basis in the search for effective synthetic medicaments. Ehrlich described the aim of research with conscious reference to the treatise *De sedibus et causis morborum* by Giovanni Battista Morgagni (1682–1771), who revolutionised pathological anatomy, the fundamental medical discipline of his day: "A way is thus shown by which we may enter upon the consideration of the most intricate problems of pharmacodynamics and, so to speak, obtain a fuller knowledge de sedibus et causis pharmacorum." (Ehrlich 1957c: 132) He delivered a paper entitled *Über moderne Chemotherapie* (Ehrlich 1957c) at the annual meeting of the German Dermatological Society in 1908, only one year before he introduced //Salvarsan//, the first specific chemotherapeutic agent in medical history. The introductory paragraphs of the paper present a retrospective survey of the development of his receptor theory. The survey also bears implications for the future – in fact, the basic notion of complementary similarity put forward here in his theory still exerts a heuristic influence on the pharmacology of today:

> Durch die vitalen Färbungen war ich zur Überzeugung gedrängt, daß die übliche Fragestellung zwischen 'Konstitution und Wirkung' eine viel zu enge sei und daß es notwendig wäre, als ein vermittelndes Agens die distributiven Gesetze zu erforschen. Da irgendeine Substanz auf ein bestimmtes Organ, z. B. das Gehirn, oder auf einen Parasiten nur dann wirksam sein kann, wenn sie von ihnen gespeichert wird, ist eine fast selbstverständliche Vorstellung, die sich andeutungsweise bis in die ältesten Vorzeiten der Heilkunde zurückverfolgen läßt. Sprach doch ein mittelalterlicher Forscher direkt davon, daß die Arzneimittel gewisse Spiculae haben müssen, mit denen sie sich an die Organe anheften. Eine praktische Rolle hat aber dieses Axiom in der modernen Pharmakologie nicht gespielt. [Experiment with coloring forced me to conclude that the parameters of previous investigation into the link between 'constitution and effect' were far too narrow, and that it would be necessary to investigate the principles of allocation during the search for a mediating agent. That a given substance can only take effect on a particular organ, e.g. the brain, or on a particular parasite, when it is absorbed by them is an idea that is almost taken

> for granted, an idea which can be traced right back to the very beginnings of medicine. A medieval scientist even said quite explicitly that remedies must have certain little spicules which enable them to fasten onto an organ. But this axiom has had no practical outcome in modern pharmacology.] (Ehrlich 1957c: 140).

This state of affairs was soon to be radically altered. Loewi's "transmitter" theory, Wood and Filde's notion of "anti-metabolites", Watson and Crick's conception of complementary structures in the DNA double-helix and, last but not least, the "endorphine" research discussed in my first chapter, would hardly have been possible without Ehrlich's (or Langley's) model of similarity. A triumphal procession of pharmacological receptor paradigms continues into the present day. The same theoretical concept still gives coherence to our detailed knowledge of the biological effects of synthetic substances, in spite of any apparent inconsistencies or divergencies in method (cf. Table 3).

The model's success is largely due to the fact that it has generated hypotheses which lend themselves to empirical results, and to the fact that it has led to the development of many effective remedies. But its success is in equal measure due to another factor which is of considerably greater interest for the present discussion – the model is extremely accessible and thus has unsurpassable value as an explanatory device, even for the layman, since it satisfies a craving for concrete meaning precisely when critical illness renders this craving acute. The notion that a synthetic substance yields healing power by virtue of a lock-and-key complementarity enabling it to penetrate an organism almost "naturally", and there to conduct a cunning strategy of exchange, is one that is rational but at the same time imbued with mythological significance. It has an empirical basis, and it brings consolation. Both on a heuristic level (in research), and on a practical level for the patient confronted with disease, it brings increased structural clarity through the modelling of similarity. In Ehrlich's receptor model the key metaphor becomes part of a therapeutic rhetoric which assumes "im Milieu gespannter Problemlagen Virulenz annehmen" ['a virulent strength in environments tense with unsolved problems'] (Blumenberg 1986: 405). An extremely vivid example is provided in the fantasy exercises quoted above and offered by Simonton et al. (1980) to tumor patients as a metaphorical weapon in the fight against cancer (cf. Chapter 3.1). It is highly improbable that Paul Ehrlich had such a purpose in mind when evolving the receptor model. But his colorful interest in elective affinity, his "tangential chemistry" (Mazumdar 1974: 10), the unconventionality and even child-like curiosity attached to his "Sherlock Holmes method" (Marquardt 1951: 82) all tend to suggest that his thought was shaped by a semioticity perhaps all the more productive because it was

Table 3: /Receptor/ as a theoretical component of medicinal propadeutics and of popular science.

["Heuristic principles in pharmacology: receptor theory" "Receptor theory starts with the notion that a substance can take effect on a cellular level only when molecules capable of functioning as reacting partners are present. The reacting partner (receptors) must have certain specific characteristics before any given substance (or group of substances) can enter into chemical combination with it. Subsequent physical and chemical change in localised biological conditions at the site of interaction is transformed into a "stimulus" which triggers the "effect" ... A particular receptor can therefore be characterised by describing the properties of substances that react with it. The receptor is then, as it were, the "negative impression" of these substances .... Furthermore the image of a receptor can be used to illustrate competitive antagonism between substances. Agonists are those substances which combine with the receptor and bring about a change in cellular properties (high affinity and "intrinsic activity"); competitive antagonists, on the other hand, enter into reversible combination with the same receptors, but do not trigger change (high affinity without "intrinsic activity"); they thus block the receptor (...). Agonists and antagonists compete for a common receptor. This means that increased concentration of one substance can at "oust" the other from the receptor."] (Kuschinsky & Lüllmann 1978: 3 f.): *Kurzes Lehrbuch der Pharmakologie und Toxikologie.*" ('Short textbook of pharmacology and toxicology')	["How do remedies work?" Investigations into how remedies take effect often refer to what is known as the principle of structure and effect. This implies that certain effects are caused by a certain chemical structure and can be explained by means of it. The principle is grounded in the fact that quite specific sites of effect (receptors) exist for a whole range of natural substances, and these sites must be occupied if the desired effect is to take place. Medication will therefore be effective if, for example, it possesses a chemical structure which enables it to bind to such receptors; the medication may then either take effect itself (by "standing in" for a natural substance), or it may oust a natural substance while remaining without direct effect of its own (so-called competitive inhibition). The receptors too must display certain specific characteristics ... If the chemical characteristics of substances specific to any receptor are known, then their structure will enable conclusions to be drawn about the structure of the receptor. To some extent, then, the receptor can be considered as a negative impression of the natural substances related to it; in other words, receptor and substances belong together like lock and key. Natural substances fit into the lock and open it .... Knowledge about interaction between substance and receptor has even made it possible, among other things, to deliberately produce substances that will not fit a given "lock".] (Ahlheim 1972: 20) *Wie funktioniert das? – Medikamente, Gifte, Drogen.* ('How does it work? – Medicines, poisons, drugs')

spontaneous rather than deliberate. Ebstein (1923: 381) puts forward the idea that the "medieval scientist" referred to by Ehrlich in connection with the side-chain theory is none other than Paracelsus. Unfortunately the idea has not been substantiated. Paracelsus does, however, in that very same chapter of the *Labyrinthus medicorum errantium* which introduces the program *signatum-locus-noturft-inventrix*, describe the effect of a recommended remedy in the following terms: "sein bilt im leib stelt sich an dasselbig ort, dahin sein form gehört." ['its likeness in the body goes to that very place where its shape belongs.'] (Paracelsus 1928b: 210)

4. Reflections on pharmaceutical esthetics

4.1. Drug names as synthetic words: a factor-analytical appraisal

> Dieses Herz- und Nerventonikum könnte heißen: Lavendel-, Rosmarin-, Gänsefingerkraut-, Melisse-, Hopfen-, Baldrian-Tonikum. Das erschien uns zu lang. Deshalb nannten wir es kurz Galama. Zur Stärkung der Nerven, für erholsamen Schlaf und ein ruhiges Herz: GALAMA.[117]
>
> German TV-Spot

In Saussure's (1979) "langue" system, proprietary names are difficult to localise. This problem, exemplified by /aspirin/, was discussed in detail in Chapter 1. Both the "prepropria1" basic forms (cf. Leys 1977: 26) with some rudimentarily denotative semantic components, which are differentiated in the context of onomastic research, and various "postproprial" elements of a more connotative nature that arise only through the repeated use of this name in the "parole" system (Saussure 1979) were found to be involved in its complex linguistic achievement. Proprietary names thus permit at least two functions:

(1) "Individuierung als sozio-psychologisches Korollar zur Identifikationsfunktion von Propria" ['individualisation as a sociopsychological corollary to the identificatory function of propria'] (Kalverkämper 1978: 54) and

(2) the application of rudimentarily denotative yet primarily connotative semantic elements to what has been individualised by (1).

To illustrate the special consequence of this dual function of proprietary names more vividly, it has only to be pointed out that, while there might be still a few German parents naming their children /Adolf/, it is absolutely certain that there will never again be a drug marketed under the proprietary name /Contergan/.[118] This example also illustrates that the concrete implementation of the connotative content of a proprietary name can be controlled only to a limited extent by those who invented it and whose interests are to be represented by it on the market. These persons or institutions nevertheless assert a considerable, certainly often dominating, influence on this process with the instrument "publicity" or, in more precise terms, by their access to the "distributive public". This influence has been dealt with in depth, using the /aspirin/ paradigm, in Chapter 1 and is discussed once again at a more general level and with reference to Haug's (1980) concept of "commodity esthetics" in Section 4.2.

The onset of the actual, often "story-book" (cf. Hangarter 1974a,b) diachrony of the proprietary name occurs only at that moment in which it comes into circulation. Although this diachrony complies with certain conventions, laws and regularities, no clue is found to these when analysis is confined to dual-structured verbal signs alone. This point of view is virtually ignored in the relatively extensive literature[119] on the phenomenon of "proprietary names" from the aspect of linguistic theory. Whilst the name is an important component of the esthetically perceptible armamentarium in the sphere of drugs in particular, this perception is not dominant but has a relationship of constant interdependency with the other, sensorily perceptible qualities of this armamentarium. Yet it is quite feasible that the connotative content of this name is influenced and occasionally given a completely new and unexpected meaning by extralinguistic qualities in their turn. In the case of drugs with very severe side-effects, such as carcinostatics, these side-effects may be triggered by complex conditioning processes acting independently, as it were, sometimes merely due to the perception of sensory stimuli that are normally no more than a concomitant feature of the application of these drugs.

When used as an infusion, for example, some of these cytostatic agents have an intensive red colouring strongly reminiscent of a popular aperitif. Whilst those patients with minimum side-effects tend of make a joke of this association (/Now it's time for my cocktail again/), some patients – those suffering from violent side-effects, especially nausea – often find the mere thought of this aperitif (or of similarly colored liquids) repulsive, and some even go so far as to vomit. If, then, the drug name has a denotative reference to this sensory quality – as in the case of /Dauno*rubi*cin/ – this segment acquires its actual connotative meaning as a reminder of repulsion and nausea only through concrete use of the designated drug.[120]

Ader (1981) has demonstrated the efficacy of complex conditioning phenomena of this kind even in animal experiments. Within an experimental investigation, he combined in various groups of rats administration of the cytostatic agent //cyclophosphamide// with a sensorily perceptible quality by adding simultaneously to their drinking water large quantities of the sweetener //saccharin//, a pharmacologically totally inert substance. The independent target variable of his experiment was the phenomenon of so-called "immunosuppression", a typical pharmacological effect of cyclophosphamide that is reflected quantitatively in the reduced production of endogenous //antibodies// as a reaction to the administration of exogenous //antigens//. In a second test cycle he repeated the application of cyclophosphamide with one group of rats but only added the saccharin to the drinking water in another group. A third experimental group was given totally unchanged treatment. When immunosuppression was measured again, the group treated only with saccharin in the second cycle was found to be exactly halfway in quantitative terms between the other two groups, differing significantly from each of them. Whilst the difference from the group treated twice with cyclophosphamide could be explained conclusively in pharmacological terms, this did not apply to the distinctly higher immunosuppression in comparison with those animals that had undergone exactly the same treatment apart from the second saccharin administration. Ader based his interpretation of the findings on the psychology of learning, pointing out that the repeated addition of saccharin to the drinking water of the middle group must have acted as a "conditioned stimulus", in other words that it had been capable of replacing or imitating – at least in part – the effect of that substance with which it had originally been simultaneously combined. Even in the light of experience based on the psychology of learning, these findings and their interpretation were more than surprising for two reasons:

(1) Because no interdependence with behavior variables had previously been attributed to the phenomenon /immunosuppression/. Unlike phenomena such as /salivation/, /heart rate/ or /galvanic skin resistance/ which have been researched so thoroughly within the psychology of learning, there is virtually no physiological connection between the vegetative nervous system and the immune system.[121]

(2) Because a one-off combination of a conditioned stimulus with an unconditioned stimulus would not as a rule lead to such marked effects as might be explained with the paradigm of classical conditioning.

With respect to the "scale" on which – within the scope of Rossi-Landi's (1978: 56) terminology – the production and reception of sign systems takes place and which extends "dalla piu lucida consapevolezza ... alle soglie del soltanto biologico" ['from the clearest consciousness ... to the threshold of the solely biological'], Ader's findings indicate that the influence of sensorily perceptible qualities on the pharmacological effect of chemical substances does indeed occur, too, at astoundingly low steps on this scale. This interpretation is relatively independent of the scientific paradigm used to interpret Ader's findings.

With the "semantic differential", Osgood, Suci and Tannenbaum (1957) developed in the 1950s an instrument which was to gain some methodological maturity as an important empirical procedure in the context of the psychology of learning and which was attributed in the course of progress-credulous mystification[122] with giving a measurable quality to the "meaning" of lexical elements in terms of linguistic semantics. Osgood and his coworkers contributed to this mystification primarily by giving their monograph the catchy title *The Measurement of Meaning*. In accordance with this perspective, they also developed in their study a learning-theory-orientated model for the signification process ("Meaning as a Representational Mediation Process", Osgood – Suci – Tannenbaum 1957: 5–9) designed to explain the phenomenon "meaning" as an epiphenomenon of the spatiotemporal contiguity of different stimuli, in other words in terms of association theory: "Whenever some stimulus other than the significate is contiguous with the significate, it will acquire an increment of association with some portion of the total behavior elicited by the significate as a representational mediating process." (Osgood et al. 1957: 6).

The vast reductionism of this model becomes obvious the moment it claims to cover the complex phenomenon "meaning" as a superordinate thesaurus (a claim that is reflected in the catchy title *The Measurement of Meaning*). Viewed in this light, the assigning relationship between words and the objects they refer to may be regarded as an important feature of language acquisition; as an analytically explanatory model, however, it certainly fails by far to do justice to the complexity of this process.

Yet the procedure developed by Osgood and his coworkers is well suited to confronting hypotheses that have been framed in the context of semiotics with what is empirically present. In a preliminary approach, that portion of the process "signification" that can be depicted quantitatively with this procedure can be said to be connected rather with that portion of the phenomenon "meaning" that is designated in linguistic terminology as "connotation", whereas it would appear rather to be independent of that portion designated by linguistics as "denotation".[123] The use of this procedure now appears extremely promising for those lexemes to which a "denotative" meaning is generally not attributed within the framework of linguistic semantics: *nomina propria*. Amongst these, interest is centered mainly on those proper nouns that arose only recently in the techno-industrial context but which – as a component of everyday culture – attract public interest and are therefore exposed to a diachronism which, though brief, is often very rich in associations: "proprietary names", meaning specifically in the context of interest at this juncture: drug names.

Osgood, Suci and Tannenbaum (1957: 20) characterise the fundamental methodological concept behind their method as follows: "The semantic differential is essentially a combination of controlled association and scaling procedures." The methodological development of "Osgood differentials" was launched on discovery of the following relation: If specific target words are given a quantitative rating by different probands as to how well or how poorly they suit a series of words and their respective antonyms, and the data obtained in this way are then subjected to factorial principal component analysis, then a large proportion of the variance of these ratings can be explained with just three independent factors. If, for instance, certain nouns as target words are each combined with a number of different adjectives which have to form contrasting pairs but can otherwise be selected completely at random, the quantitative allocations of the pairs of adjectives to the individual nouns are found to correlate with one another in a quite characteristic pattern. If those adjectives in which this correlation is arithmetically exceptionally distinct are grouped together, then each of them can be given a clear-cut allocation to one of the following three "semantic fields":

(1) They belong to the semantic field extending between the two poles /good/ and /bad/, i. e. they denote good or bad characteristics.

(2) Their meaning is related to /strong/ or /weak/.

(3) They belong to that semantic field that might be characterised by the synonyms /active/-/moving/-/fast/ on the one hand and /passive/-/static/-/slow/ on the other.

Such a correlation is also found when adjectives or proper nouns, for example, are selected as target words, and nouns as pairs of comparing words (which must, however, contrast once again in pairs – a feature certainly not without its problems). Taking their bearings from these "semantic fields" – without allowing theoretically for the "semantic field" concept – Osgood and his coworkers designated the three primary dimensions of the "semantic space" (Osgood et al. 1957: 25) postulated by them "evaluation", "potency" and "activity". From the pragmatic standpoint, these dimensions are obviously those properties of greatest value in directing probands confronted with the task of allocating characteristics in an associative way.

Figures 16 and 17 are designed to lend greater plasticity to the principle of Osgood's experimental design, a principle that sounds thoroughly abstract in the description. Figure 16 shows extracts from the instruction text of the questionnaire prepared for data collection within the framework of my own study. Figure 17 reproduces one page from that questionnaire in roughly the form submitted to the probands. The only difference between the different pages of the questionnaire was in the target word printed at the head of each page, i. e. in the concrete drug name. The "Osgood differentials" or "polarity profiles"[124] printed below it were identical on each page of the questionnaire. Closer consideration of the pairs of terms will show that there is nothing random about them but that they were selected with a view to providing as clear a three-factor solution as possible. Each of the three Osgood dimensions is allocated precisely one pair of nouns, one pair of adjectives, one pair of adverbs and one pair of synthetic words (selection of the pairs of synthetic words was based on Ertel's (1969) sampling principle). Sequential effects were minimised by changing the differentials after every three pairs of words, i. e. the /good/, /active-dynamic/ or /potent/ term appears in triples, three times on the left and three times on the right, alternately.

Using this questionnaire, twenty-two different names were rated by forty-four probands with respect to their associative relationships to the twelve differentials presented. A survey of the names used within the scope of the study and the criteria by which they were selected or constructed is given in Table 4.

Thirteen of the investigated names can be allocated unequivocally to one therapeutic indication group. The investigated sample of names contains the proprietary names of five //cytostatic agents//, four //sedatives// and three //analgesics//. Three imaginary names formed by making minimal phonetic changes and intended to be reminiscent of some of the selected proprietary names have been added to the groups of cytostatic agents and sedatives. The individual probands were, however, never confronted simultaneously in their questionnaires with genuine proprietary names plus the imaginary names derived from them, but three "genuine" names were replaced in each questionnaire by three "forged" ones.[125] Finally, all questionnaires contained three further names which were hypothetically assumed to be capable of priming associations that would lead to exceptionally distinct "loadings" on one of the expected three factors resulting from principal component analysis.

One important result of the study by Osgood and his coworkers was the observation already reported in this chapter that the quantitative variance of allocated semantic differentials can frequently be explained to a large extent by three independent factors. By drawing semantic comparisons among the word-pairs correlating with one of these three factors, Osgood formed the hypothesis of a three-dimensional "semantic" "space" whose axes he designated "evaluation", "potency" and "activity".

/Contergan/, the German proprietary name for //thalidomide//, was expected hypothetically for obvious reasons to provoke outstandingly marked negative associations on the evaluation axis. According to the same criterion, the rating of /interferon/ – a non-proprietary name for a group of pharmacological substances on which high therapeutic hopes are placed both by the general public and by specialists – was expected to appear on the same axis in the reverse direction. The choice of /Sagittacin/, the proprietary name of a relatively unknown //bronchial remedy//, was linked to the hypothesis that this name should be rated as extremely moving on the activity axis.[126]

The following questionnaire is part of a scientific study aimed at examining the effect of drug names and its rating. You are given about 40 minutes to fill in the form. The results of the study will not be evaluated for commercial use.

At the top of each page of the questionnaire is a name, written in capital letters and framed. This may be the name of a commercial medical preparation, but it may also be some other proper name or a purely imaginary word. Names protected by copyright are not specially identified.

Below this word there are 12 lines with so-called "polarity profiles". Each of these consists of two terms directly opposite in meaning, between which a 7-step scale is stretched.

For example:

TRANQUILITY o---o---o---o---o---o---o MOTION

You are asked to decide for each of these profiles whether what the name framed in the box above expresses to you fits one end or the other end of the scale better. Three steps are provided on either side of the scale to show whether this tendency in your rating is weakly, moderately or strongly marked. If you find that the name framed in the box above fits both sides of the differential equally well or equally badly, please mark the neutral step in the middle of the scale with a cross. For each differential please mark one of the seven steps identified by circles with a cross. Do not make any crosses between the circles.

This questionnaire is not a test of your knowledge or performance. There is nothing against filling it in in a relaxed atmosphere.

Some of the semantic differentials are not stretched between "real" terms but between meaningless synthetic words. Treat these in exactly the same way as the "real" terms. Imagine the synthetic words to be "genuine" terms from a foreign language of which you have no command but in which you can "find your way". Decide in these cases, too, which synthetic word better fits what the name framed in the box above expresses to you and how strong this tendency is for you.

It is quite clear that your rating will also depend in individual cases on whether or not your are familiar with a drug of the respective name. The name may equally well be reminiscent of another name that has nothing whatever to do with drugs. This would probably influence your decision too. All these influences are unavoidable. Make no attempt to suppress or to reinforce them. What counts is your first, spontaneous impression.

On each of the following pages there is just 1 framed name in the box at the top. Below it on each page are the same 12 semantic differentials. If it makes filling-in easier, do read the framed name aloud. Please keep to just one page of the questionnaire at a time. If you want a short break, it is best to take it at the end of a page.

Figure 16: Instruction text of the questionnaire.

Togal

Tranquility	o---o---o---o---o---o---o	Motion
Dissonance	o---o---o---o---o---o---o	Harmony
Assertion	o---o---o---o---o---o---o	Reserve
Allegro	o---o---o---o---o---o---o	Andante
Light	o---o---o---o---o---o---o	Dark
Delicate	o---o---o---o---o---o---o	Rugged
Hasty	o---o---o---o---o---o---o	Leisurely
Attractive	o---o---o---o---o---o---o	Repulsive
Docile	o---o---o---o---o---o---o	Commanding
Hellillo	o---o---o---o---o---o---o	Sonem
Legem	o---o---o---o---o---o---o	Aafs
Karno	o---o---o---o---o---o---o	Leli

Figure 17: Sample page from questionnaire.

Table 4: Names under investigation. Survey of 22 names each rated by means of the same sematic differentials (cf. Fig. 4.3) [A translation of the German names has been renounced since the important factor was the sound, not the name itself.]

//CYTOSTATIC AGENTS//:	/METHOTREXAT/; /VINCRISTIN; /ENDOXAN/ /DAUNOBLASTIN/; /ALEXAN/.
Names modelled on names of //CYTOSTATIC AGENTS//:	/RETROFLEXAT/; /SINCRISTIN/; ENDOXON/
//SEDATIVES//:	/GALAMA/; /TAVOR/; /VALIUM/; /PLANUM
Names modelled on names of //SEDATIVES//:	/BALAMA/; KAVOR/; /SALIUM/
//ANALGESICS//:	/TOTAL/; /TEMGESIC/; /TALVOSILEN/
Names of various drugs where high factor values were expected:	/CONTERGAN/; /INTERFERON/; /SAGITTACIN/

The mathematical procedure was then as follows: The semantic differentials marked by the proband with a cross were first quantified in such a way that an integer value was allocated to each circle on the seven-step scale – the value /-3/ to that circle closest to the negatively poled term, the value /-2/ to the next circle, the value /0/ to the central circle, and so on up to that

Table 5: Principal component analysis of semantic differentials.
Factor loadings of 12 semantic differentials recorded at interval scale level. Negatively poled terms are on the left. The semantic differentials are arranged in groups, depending on the factor with the highest loading irrespective of positive or negative aspect.

	Factor 1	Factor 2	Factor 3
Tranquility – Motion	+0.78555	+0.17385	−0.20488
Andante – Allegro	+0.80206	+0.15053	−0.18155
Leisurely – Fast	+0.81176	+0.25646	−0.19532
Sonem – Hellillo	+0.68316	−0.37187	+0.14852
Reserve – Assertion	+0.44311	+0.64993	+0.06406
Dark – Light	+0.23226	−0.70071	+0.40057
Delicate – Rugged	+0.30914	+0.76718	−0.15731
Docile – Commanding	+0.28578	+0.78553	−0.04679
Leli – Karno	−0.15235	+0.56900	−0.24603
Dissonance – Harmony	−0.34271	−0.23835	+0.69631
Repulsive – Attractive	−0.15659	−0.38359	+0.72293
Aafs – Legem	−0.01952	+0.02498	+0.76732
	→ /Motion/	→ /Potency/	→ /Evaluation/

circle at the positively poled end of the differential, which was allocated the value /+3/. This yielded twelve interval-scaled variables for which an orthogonal, varimax-rotated principal component analysis was computed for the entire sample.[127] As was only to be expected in view of Osgood's findings and the targeted selection of the semantic differentials used, the result of this procedure was a three-factor solution whose (already rotated) matrix is reproduced in Table 5.

Allocation of each semantic differential to that factor on which it is most heavily weighted irrespective of positive or negative aspect produces – with one exception – the expected picture: The polar terms had been selected in such a way that each of them was to correlate as clearly as possible with one of Osgood's three dimensions. The exception is formed by the semantic differential extending between the terms /light/ and /dark/. As expected, it does correlate positively with factor 3, designated here /evaluation/ with reference to Osgood, but only by a sum far below the amount of negative loading on /potency/ factor 2. This semantic differential, although poled in reverse, must then logically be allocated to this factor. Finally, the first factor is designated here /motion/, a deviation from Osgood et al. (1957) as well as from Ertel (1969). These factor designations should, however, always be used with a certain reserve. The semantic contrasts of all pairs of terms are more or less equally involved, depending on their factorial loadings, in what the factor /means/, and these differences – very subtle in part – simply cannot be embodied in one single term. The factor as such has no meaning at all. It is to some extent a variable introduced synthetically by an arithmetical operation designed merely to illustrate in a structured form the correlative relationships of the empirically present variables.[128]

In a further step, mean values for these three synthetic, independent variables were determined for each single one of the twenty-one names rated by the probands.[129] In this perspective, then, the twenty-one names were recorded as target variables of the investigation, and the probands' ratings as repeat measurements. If the three factors ascertained above are regarded as axes of a three-dimensional system of coordinates, then these mean values as vectorial coordinates yield a plastic image of the rating of the twenty-one names by the forty-four probands. This image is reproduced in Figures 18 and 19, with the factor values of the /evaluation/ and /motion/ axes transferred to a two-dimensional system of coordinates in Figure 18 and the positions on the /potency/ axis shown in Figure 19.

To imagine the position of a specific name in the three-dimensional factor space, the position shown in Figure 18 must always be "pushed back" behind the pictorial plane or (should this amount be negative) "pulled forward" in front of the pictorial plane by the amount shown in Figure 19.

In Figure 18, the drug names are given symbols to indicate to which of the different therapeutic indication groups (cytostatic agents, sedatives, analgesics) they belong. The "forged" names are marked with broken lines. What is striking on initial observation of the two-dimensional system of coordinates is that the representatives of the individual indication groups form relatively homogeneous clusters. The sedatives are without exception on the left-hand half of the /motion/ axis, the cytostatic agents without exception on its right-hand half, and all the analgesics in the direct vicinity of this axis. With regard to the /evaluation/ axis, there is a distinct upward trend among the sedatives and among the analgesics, but a quantitatively somewhat less distinct downward trend among the cytostatic agents. Another conspicuous feature is that the names of those drugs or substances that were included in the investigation on account of their – hypothetically assumed – relatively clear-cut relationships to one of the factors do indeed deviate primarily (/interferon/) or almost exclusively (/Contergan/ and /Sagittacin/) in the predicted direction from the center point of the system of coordinates. If these clusters are then visualised as three-dimensional point clouds, then Figure 19 shows that the sedatives have rather to be "pulled" in front of the pictorial plane of

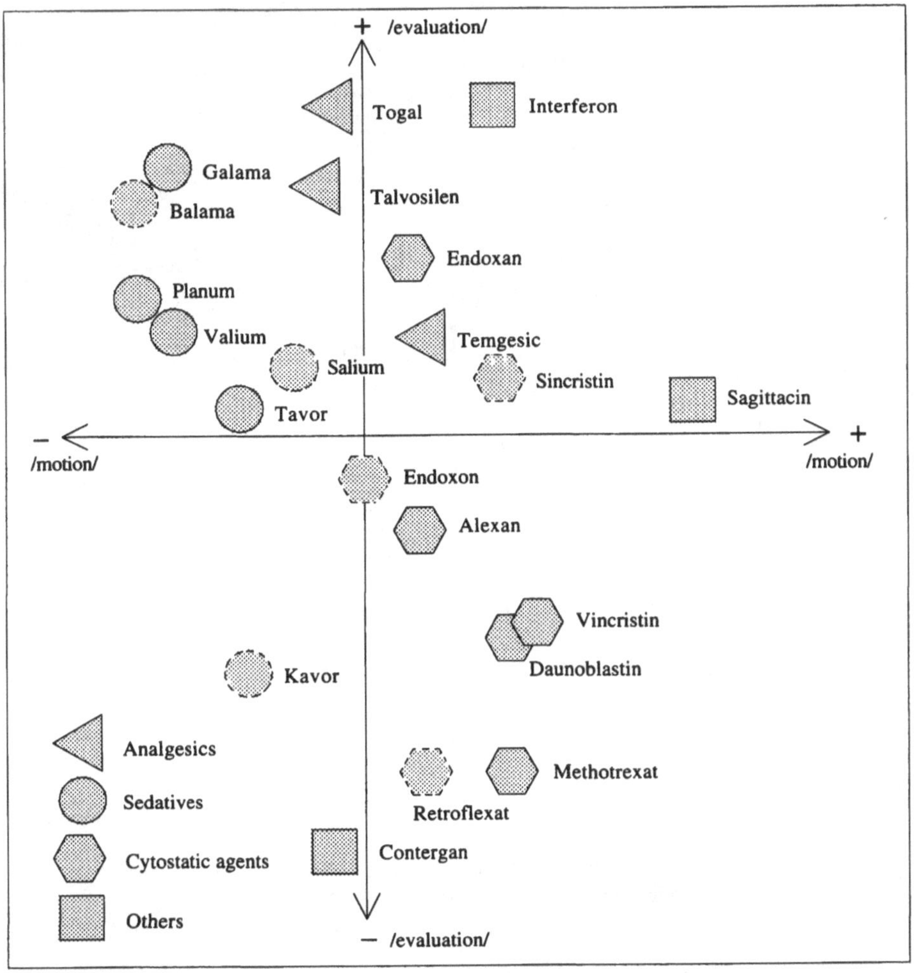

Figure 18: Dimensional mean values of the rating of names in a 2-dimensional space (/evaluation/ and /motion/).

Figure 18 (i. e. towards the viewer), whereas the analgesics show an inclination towards the center point, and the cytostatic agents tend to be located in the positive range of the /potency/ axis behind the pictorial plane of Figure 18 (i. e. away from the viewer). These trends are, however, anything but clear-cut. With /Tavor/, for example, we have a "genuine" sedative farthest away from all names in the positive /potency/ range, whereas /Sincristin/ as a "forged" cytostatic agent is clearly within the negative range, and two

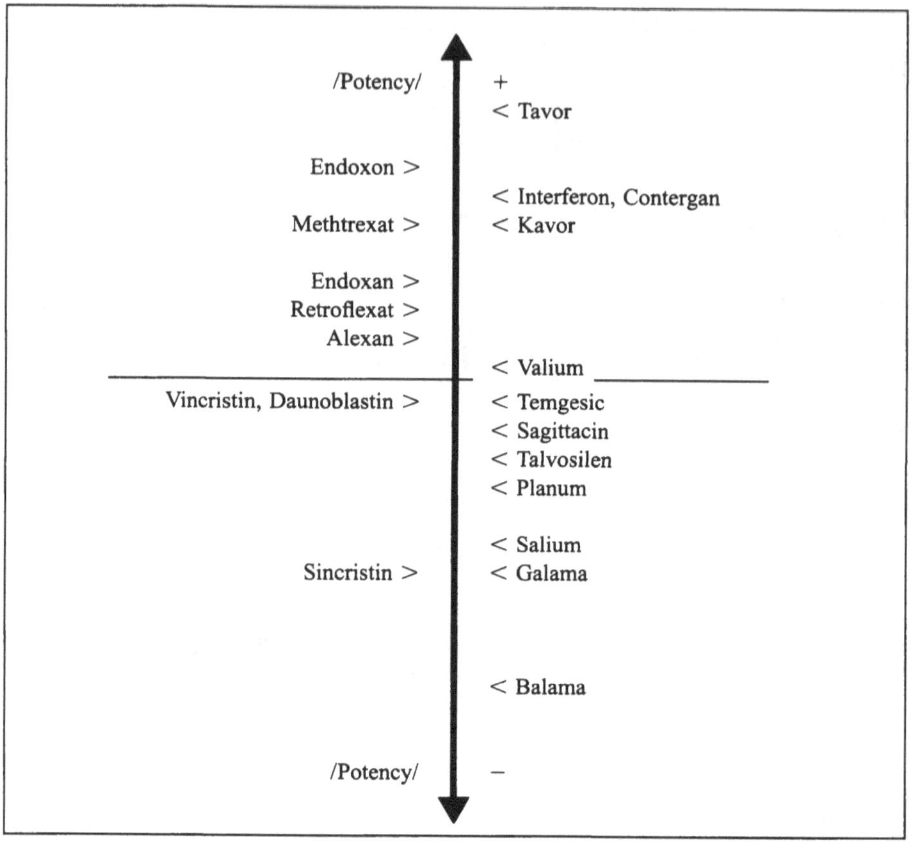

Figure 19: Dimensional mean values of the rating of drug names with reference to the /potency/ axis. (Cytostatic agents to the left of the axis, all other indication groups to the right.)

"genuine" cytostatic agents, /Vincristin/ and /Daunoblastin/ are just within it. Obviously the /motion/ axis makes a greater contribution than the /evaluation/ axis towards discrimination of the investigated names according to therapeutic indication groups, whilst the /evaluation/ axis for its part makes a sharper distinction than the /potency/ axis. But why?

At this juncture it is expedient to recall exactly what the probands were asked to do when filling in the questionnaires. Another point of special importance is the question of who the probands involved in the survey were or, in more exact terms, how their relationship to what they were to rate could be characterised more precisely.

They were all medical students and doctors from the medical school at Cologne University. As a group, they were thus certainly not representative of the general public at large but relatively homogeneous with respect to their familiarity with and their access to drugs. The questionnaires were distributed in the course of the 1985/86 winter semester with a request for voluntary, unpaid participation in the survey. The proportion of questionnaires returned was about 50% among the students and 90% among the doctors (most of whom were known to me personally as colleagues).

The questionnaires asked for the probands' associative rating of various names, some of them recognisable as drug names, others merely imitative of such names. The object being rated in the study, as explained by me, was thus first and foremost only the respective name as an onomato-phonetic object and not its extralingual referent – even if this was recognisable or indeed present. This was emphasised by having the word /name/ occurring fourteen times in the instruction text (cf. Figure 16), but the word /drug/ only four times. The reality of the extralingual referents was nonetheless expected to play a distinct role in influencing the rating of the respective names (a role very much hoped for in view of my specific interest). This effect is exceptionally clear, though certainly not provable within the framework of the chosen test method, in the rating of the names /Contergan/ and /interferon/ which have a selectively high loading on the evaluation axis. It can be claimed that this rating would probably have turned out differently had it not been for the historical forming of the "cultural units" associated with these names. In the case of the name /Sagattacin/, which had been rated as exceptionally /moving/, on the other hand, historical events offer no explanation for this phenomenon. No spectacular properties whatsoever are associated in any way with the drug //Sagittacin//. In pharmacological therapy it is only one relatively obscure //bronchial remedy// among many. The reason for the clear-cut rating is more likely to be found in the denotative reference of the word to the Latin root *sagitta*, meaning 'arrow'. Even so, onomatopoeic characteristics of this dynamically sounding phonetic object may, of course, have contributed to, and possibly added up to, the effect of the denotative reference.

The rating effects shown in Figures 18 and 19 have to be seen as a complex interpreting event in which it is not only the onomatopoeia of the individual names that is involved but also the two "appellative" semantic components of proper nouns described in Chapter 1: On the one hand the denotative references designated as "preproprial" with reference to Leys (1977: 26), and on the other the rather more connotative semantic components characterised analogously as "postproprial" and acquired by a name through what is designated by marking a specific status "all'interno di sistemi semantici" ['inside semantic systems'] of a given culture in the sense specified by Eco (1975: 120). The role of these different components in the rating of the drug names investigated in this study will admittedly have to remain a matter of speculation in the light of the data so far presented. It can, however, be recorded as a provisional working hypothesis that the more clearly what is signified by them generates predictable associations in the community in which it circulates, the more important and influential the appellative functions of the proper nouns become.

In the light of these considerations it first seems quite plausible that it is the /motion/ axis in Figure 18 that makes the greatest contribution towards discriminating the therapeutic indication groups: //Sedatives// are applied in therapy because they develop pharmacological characteristics believed to counteract various forms of //motion// – they tranquillise, counterbalance, harmonise. In contrast, //cytostatic agents// often bring infinite motion, restlessness and dynamics into the situation and the everyday life of patients undergoing treatment with them. This restlessness is, however, never a therapeutic objective but an extremely unpleasant side-effect that has to be taken into the bargain and is rooted in the initial biographic environment in which the patients begin this therapy.

From the pharmacological perspective, the characteristic of //cytostatic agents// is selective destruction of those cell populations with a high reproductive rate, an intensive metabolism and thus a tendency towards rapid proliferation. These biological characteristics are a common feature in a large number of malignant tumors; it is for this reason that //cytostatic agents// are used in these essentially critical diseases. And yet these biological characteristics also affect some natural cell populations, in particular the hematogenic system, the immunological defense mechanism, the mucosa of the gastrointestinal tract, and the gametes. In other words, these substances represent a risk not only to the tumor but also to the person threatened by that tumor.

For many people facing such therapy, this constellation involves the almost brutal requirement of deciding whether it really does offer them more quantity *and* quality of life. With the onset of cytostatic therapy, an almost desperate but clear-cut, menacing situation often gives way to a future-orientated perspective full of new hope yet totally open and uncertain.

If this context played a role in rating the names of the cytostatic agents, then this effect may also be linked with the fact that the questioned medical students and doctors were professionally confronted with this uncertainty, which might well have made demands on them, too. Confrontation with the extremely unpleasant pharmacological side-effects of //cytostatic agents// would also be a possible explanation for the relatively poor placings of the names of cytostatic agents on the /evaluation/ axis.

A comparison of the rating positions of the "forged" drug names in Figure 18 shows all of them to be well within the cluster ranges of their indication groups but at some considerable distance from the positions of those "genuine" drug names from which they are taken and from which they have only a minimal phonetic difference. These distances might result from these "forged" names having, in real terms, no extraverbal referents that might anchor the rating of these names in the everyday working situation of the probands. No doctor, no medical student has ever had any experience with a drug by the name of /Salium/, because there is no such drug. Yet the name /Salium/ is reminiscent of /Valium/, a drug with which such experience has been gained. The fact that the "forged" names, though within the range of the clusters of "genuine" names corresponding with them, are at considerable distances from them might be interpreted as evidence that the rating of the "genuine" names, which was anchored in the everyday working situation, had "colored" the rating of the "forged" names to some extent. The decisive factor in the context under discussion in this study is, however, that "coloring" of this kind has to be conceived as a collective, unconscious process mediated essentially by participation in a cultural circle – for the "forged" names were never rated together with the corresponding "genuine" names by the individual probands. Any one questionnaire contained either one or the other, but never both. Had the probands assessed only the abstract phonetic character of the listed names in their ratings, the considerable distances between these corresponding pairs would have been virtually inexplicable. Within the thematic framework outlined in this study, these distances are something of a quantitatively illustrative reference to that interpretative activity for which Sulpiz Boisserée ([1970]: 72) in the early nineteenth century coined in his ironically sophisticated manner the terms *Sinnbildeln* und *Wortdeuteln* 'petty symbolising and subtilising'. This claim is supported not only by the lengths but also by the vectorial directions of these distances, for the positions of the "forged" names in Figure 18 are – with only one exception[130] – shifted away from the positions of the corresponding "genuine" names towards the center point of the system of coordinates. This finding is outstandingly compatible with the process designated metaphorically in this context as /coloring/ because an object that is partially colored by another – in a washing machine or elsewhere – invariably expresses this quality less intensively than the object from which the coloring originates. This new quality, which it acquires from the associative (or – in the metaphorical image – spatiotemporal) proximity to another object is often little more than a tint or a reflection. However, the object providing the coloring has rarely come into the world with that color. If that object – to keep to the metaphorical image – is an item of clothing, for instance, then its original coloring was influenced with roughly the same intensity but with very different motivations by the manufacturer's product design and the predictable "increment of associations" of the consumer.

There is, of course, no denying the extremely speculative nature of all these interpretative reflections on the data gathered in this context. Nor does the fact that these data were gathered within the framework of an empirical study change this reservation in the slightest. Factor analysis is – at least in the form used in this study – methodologically speaking an exclusively hypothesis-generating procedure. Conclusions drawn on the probability of these hypotheses cannot be derived from it. There are, moreover, some other influences possibly connected with the – prima facie certainly impressive – homogeneity of the clusters in Figure 18. For example, it would also be possible – as a matter of principle – for me to have based selection of drug names for my questionnaire primarily on phonetic combinations that I could intuitively have expected to yield a relatively homogeneous rating response. In this case the same strategy that proved to be hypothesis-compliant in selecting the names /Contergan/, /Interferon/ and /Sagittacin/ might have been used unconsciously to generate this homogeneity through selection of the objects to be rated. Conclusions could then, however, no longer be drawn on specific strategies of "symbolising" and "subtilising" when dealing with specific groups of drugs. A somewhat closer inspection of the names investigated in this study will reveal, in fact, that they have a relatively similar sound within the individual indication groups: The sedative names are shorter and have softer vowels, whilst the analgesic names all begin with the same consonants.

A distinction has to be made, however, between this possible selection effect on my part and another important source that makes some contribution to this impression of purely phonetic homogeneity: The construction of proprietary names in the sphere of pharmaceutical specialities keeps – though in many cases only loosely – to a number of conventions that have developed traditionally in the diachronism of designation. There is, of course, no blueprint for the construction of drug names. On the contrary, a trend to consciously modernistic infringement of traditional rules of this kind has been observed in recent years in the construction of names for new specialities on the market. There is, though, one fundamental, unwritten law still in force in product design, according to which the name of an article has to be compatible with its application and should even back up any indication of the character of this application; this certainly applies to the medical field too. This aspect is taken up once again in section 4.2 in connection with Haug's theory of "commodity esthetics".

The implication of this law for the names subjected in this study to factor analysis is, for example, that those proper names chosen by manufacturers of

//sedatives// for their products can be expected primarily to have "appellative" components denoting and connoting /tranquillity/, /harmony/ and /poise/.[131] This relationship certainly makes a major contribution to the subjective impression of above-random phonetic homogeneity within the individual indication groups. The more unequivocally the therapeutic indication of a drug group correlates with one of the three axes of the "semantic space" (in Osgood's sense), the greater this contribution will presumably be. The hypothesis that this correlation has to be set exceptionally high for the //sedatives// was one of the factors leading to my decision to take special account of the names of this drug group within the framework of this study.

Founded in the product design, this homogeneity of drug names within a therapeutic indication group is present long before the drugs designated by those names become part of the everyday reality of doctors and patients. Now this homogeneity is an ideal means of creating some semblance of order within this reality, a reality that can, as we have seen, be experienced by all those involved as menacingly amorphous and unpredictable. It forms important source material for the construction of structural gain. And the homogeneity of the clusters in Figure 18 may well be something of a portrayal of this structural gain.

Within the framework of his fundamental research into "psychophonetics", Ertel (1969) published some studies involving Osgood differentials that were of a considerably more complex and methodologically more mature experimental nature than the survey presented here. Some of his findings can be used to provide a degree of differentiatiation between the findings processed hypothetically in this chapter.

One special focal point within the framework of Ertel's experiments is the investigation of "synthetic words", sound combinations that can be mastered without difficulty by any competent speaker of a specific individual language but are not present even as proper nouns in the vocabulary of that language. Ertel used such synthetic words both as target terms and as polar pairs of contrasting terms within Osgood differentials. (The meaningless pairs of contrasting terms used in my own questionnaire were taken from one of Ertel's studies; cf. Figure 17). Using factor-analytical operations, he repeatedly reached, within the scope of his studies, three essential dimensions corresponding in content approximately to the dimensions of Osgood's "semantic space" but designated by Ertel with far greater pragmatism as "phonetische Allgemeinqualitäten" ['general phonetic qualities']. In a further study, Ertel asked his probands to rate not only more sound combinations but single sounds, too. He performed this test with all phonemes constituting the German language and was thus able to assign to each individual phoneme three numerical values corresponding to the respective vectorial coordinates of this position in the three-dimensional space of the "general qualities". The obvious step then was to examine to what extent the intensity of the "general qualities" in the synthetic words as a whole could be deduced from the rating of the individual phonemes comprising those synthetic words. For this purpose Ertel reverted to those pairs of synthetic words that had proved in previous studies to be exceptionally useful as polarity pairs because they had exhibited a high degree of factor-analytical correlation with one of the three axes. (In the pairs used in Figure 17 these were the synthetic words /Hellillo/ and /Sonem/ for the "motion" axis, /Legem/ and /Aafs/ for the "evaluation" axis, and /Karno/ and /Leli/ for the "potency" axis.) Ertel then formed the arithmetical mean values from the ratings of the individual phonemes comprising these pairs of synthetic words. With respect to the /potency/ axis and the /motion/ axis (referred to by Ertel with the general quality "agitation"), these mean values for the negatively poled synthetic word then proved to be distinctly lower than those for the corresponding, positively poled synthetic word. With respect to the /evaluation/ axis (referred to by Ertel with the general quality "evaluation"), there was no such correlation. The conclusion drawn by Ertel (1969: 107–115) was that the general qualities of synthetic words can be explained at least in part by the general qualities of their phonetic segments.

If this finding is to be used for differentiation of the hypothesis set up in this chapter, then the validity of this conclusion has to be extended far beyond the framework guardedly formulated by Ertel. Above all it is essential to compare quantitative values that are not known for certain to be comparable. It was from the observation of completely different proband collectives and in part with other semantic differentials that Ertel obtained his data. The pairs of terms used in this study were all used by Ertel too, of course, but within the framework of various studies and never in one single study in the combination of 12 scales selected for my own study. Such comparisons during the course of this chapter are therefore performed with the proviso of their questionable validity.

In Figure 20, those points resulting when the arithmetical average taken from the dimensional values of the individual phonemes comprising each drug name according to Ertel's samples (1969: 94, 101) are entered in addition to the two-dimensional surface points resulting from the drug name ratings obtained in this study.

The phoneme /a:/, which has the highest "evaluation" rating among all vowels in Ertel's sample, occurs three times in the name /Galama/, for example. The phonemes /l/ and /m/, which also occur in this name, are for their

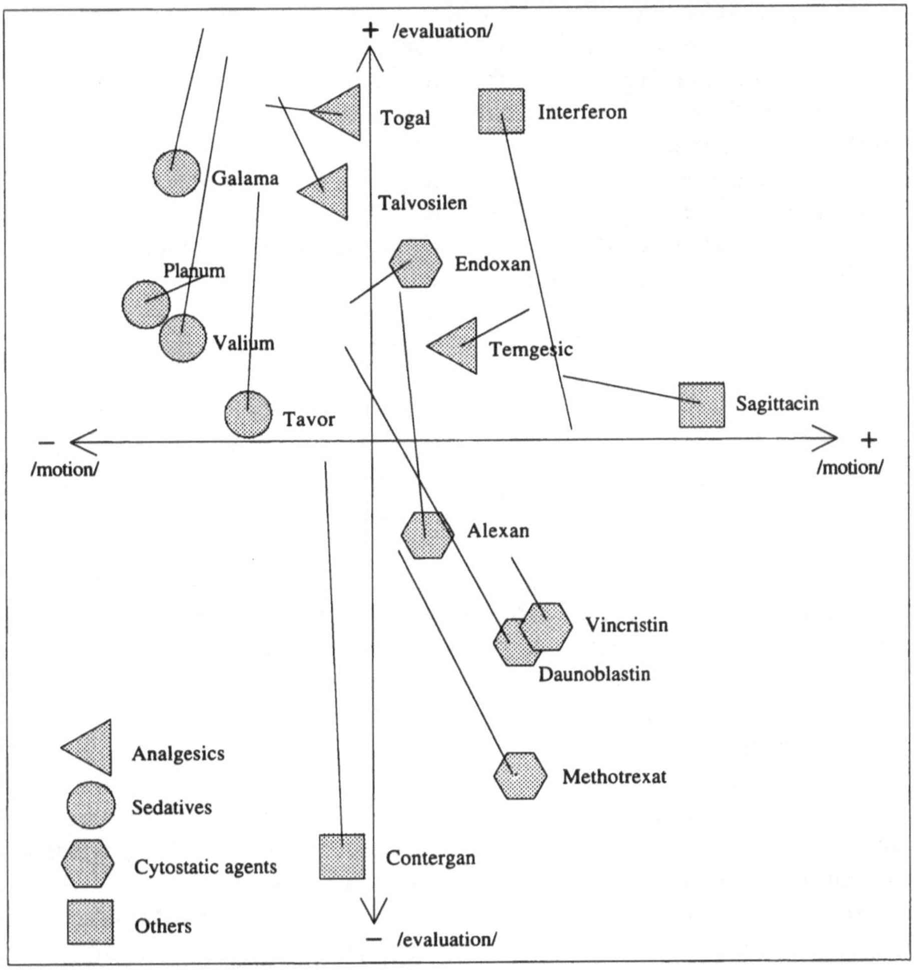

Figure 20: Distances between rated values of drug names and the mean positions of their phonemes following Ertel's sample values.

part those with the highest "evaluation" rating among all consonants in Ertel's sample. This accounts for the arithmetical average of these individual values for the name /Galama/ being exceptionally high on the "evaluation" axis.

If we now turn our attention to the relationships between the rating values of the drug names investigated in this chapter and the mean rating values of the phonemes constituting them in Ertel's sample, we find some conspicuous systematic features:

The names /Contergan/ and /Interferon/, which had been introduced for their expectedly selective axial correlation, and all but one of the sedative names were rated with respect to the "motion" axis almost exactly as might have been predicted in view of Ertel's values. On the other hand, the rating values of these names deviate with respect to the "evaluation" axis by considerable amounts from the positions calculated on the basis of Ertel's sample, with the sedative names and /Contergan/ all having the same direction of deviation. The names of the cytostatic agents deviate from these predictable positions by fairly consistent amounts which, however – with one exception – fall in roughly equal proportions to "evaluation" differences and "motion" differences and which, apart from this one exception, all have the same directions. These relationships can be illustrated geometrically by conceiving as vectors the distances between the spatial points predicted on the basis of Ertel's samples and the spatial points ascertained in this study from the probands' ratings, and entering these vectors into a new system of coordinates related to one joint datum. This has been done in Figure 21. The axes of this new system of coordinates are to be thought of as parallel shifts of the /evaluation/ axis and the /motion/ axis from Figure 20. The distance vectors formed here therefore enclose among one another and with the axis the same angle as would be obtained by ascertaining these vectors in Figure 20. This relationship is marked by giving the axes in Figure 21 only the initial letters /E/ and /M/ as identifiers.

If formation of the mean value from the respective dimensional values of the individual phonemes were a suitable rating procedure for the dimensional allocation of synthetic words in Osgood's "semantic space", then the vectors entered in Figure 20 would represent that effect resulting from the drug names examined here being not only synthetic words or meaningless phonetic combinations but also lexical elements arousing a certain amount of predictable, intersubjective associations. In three of the four //sedatives// examined here (/Tavor/, /Galama/, /Valium/) this effect would then have led to a negative shift on the /evaluation/ axis. An interpretation of this shift, such as the statement that /sedatives have a dubious reputation among the medical students and doctors questioned/, would be a highly speculative matter. What is remarkable, however, is the homogeneity with which this effect can be illustrated.

In four of the five //cytostatic agents// investigated (/Vincristin/, /Endoxan/, /Daunoblastin/, /Alexan/) this shift has roughly equal loadings on the "evaluation" axis (as in the case of the sedatives, in negative direction) and on the "motion" axis (in positive direction). On the other hand, the geometric homogeneity with which this effect occurs within this drug group in the two-dimensional illustration is impressive.

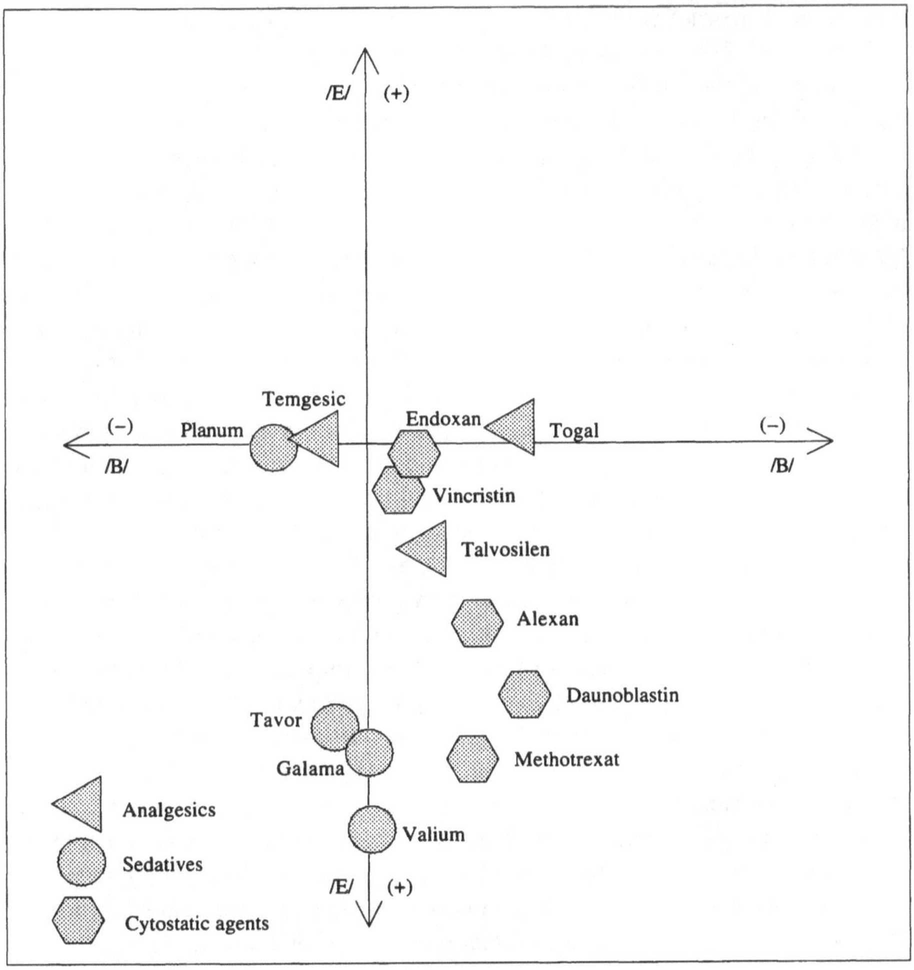

Figure 21: Difference vectors from Figure 20 related to one joint datum.

When we consider the enclosing angles of these seven vectors, the minimum angle between two vectors of different indication groups is found in all cases to be substantially greater than the maximum enclosing angle within these two groups.

The question of the significance of this geometric homogeneity is almost impossible to answer. In the first place it may be totally incidental. It might, on the other hand, be connected with a systematic influence that just cannot be covered by those hypotheses set up to date. It is, above all, questionable whether and in what way this homogeneity correlates with that of the clusters in Figure 18. The vectors of Figure 21 had originated from our comparing the ratings of the probands questioned in this study with set rating values computed on the basis of Ertel's samples. These rating values, we have suggested, may be a guide to how our drug names would have had to be rated as meaningless synthetic words. Ertel (1969:107–115) – to recapitulate – also discussed the value of such rating procedures within the framework of his studies. He came to the conclusion that any such connection is most likely to exist with respect to the "potency" axis, the one not taken into account in this study as it would not have permitted any discrimination to be made between the different indication groups. With respect to the /motion/ axis – the one discriminating best in this study – Ertel still concedes a certain validity to the connection between the dimensionality of synthetic words and the phonemes constituting them, while rejecting this for the /evaluation/ axis. In view of these restrictions, it would seem appropriate to waive any interpretation of this homogeneity with regard to content, for instance with reference to the contents represented by the axes. What has to be recorded, however, is the fact that the impressive intra-group homogeneity of rated drug names obtained by applying Osgood differentials is not totally lost if something varying systematically with the "Allgemeinqualitäten" ['general qualities'] (to quote Ertel's terminology) of its phonetic character is deducted from the dimensional allocation of each of these names. The intersubjective "increments of associations" (Osgood et al. 1957: 6), whose tracks have been followed geometrically to some extent in this context, would at least be an appropriate means of backing up that therapeutic process repeatedly referred to in this book as "structural gain". Whether or to what extent they find practical application in the implementation of this process cannot, however, be judged on the basis of the findings recorded in this study.

4.2. The /prescribing/ physician and his "relations in public"

In contrast to the pre-Paracelsian period (cf. Chapter 3.2), today's medical students are confronted unanimously in all clinical subjects with the warning that textbook knowledge can never be a substitute for subjective, personal observation. This applies most particularly when dealing with pharmaceutical preparations. The introduction to virtually every pharmacopeia advises the doctor to restrict himself in everyday clinical practice to just a few preparations so that he can first learn the right therapeutic approach with them gradually and within the scope of personal contact with the patient. This advice implies immense concessions to the restriction that both the quality and the quantity of a specific drug effect can be predicted in each individual case only with a marked degree of uncertainty despite all triumphs of standardisation – which are plainly a pipedream from the standpoint of /technology/. So much for the tenor of the textbook recommendation.

Let us take another look at the entire hoard of diagnostically defined and nosologically classified syndromes on the one hand and the stock of all therapeutically effective substances on the other as monoplanar code systems[132] initially independent of one another. Modern pharmacology is then seen to ensure a great deal of what Samuel Hahnemann tried in vain to achieve at the beginning of the nineteenth century (cf. Chapter 3.2): empirically well-founded expertise on dose-dependent structure/effect relationships. Despite persistent gaps, this expertise has meanwhile become so comprehensive that the two systems can hardly be conceived as separate entities even though they are still taught as independent subjects, at least in propedeutics. This correlating expertise enables the physician practising today to segment the complex reality of pathological phenomena for therapeutic purposes. He has – in contrast to Hahnemann's contemporaries – a reliable idea of which substances have a hypotensive, bactericidal, diuretic or antiphlogistic effect. He knows, too, with which pathogen and at what phase of a disease one specific substance is to be given preference over another, although they have a parallel physiological effect. It is pharmacology that furthermore provides him with the expertise needed to recognise his limits, to develop a sceptical eye for the persistent gaps – in other words, not to forget that "liver-protective", "circulation-stimulating", "blood-purifying", "tonicising" substances have yet to be found. In theory, he has at his disposal all means of identification to separate diagnosis and therapy into corresponding segments, using a methodologically exact process.

This process has to deal with the problem of developing clear therapeutic consequences from the diagnosis. Accurate diagnosis is essential to the realisation of an ideal which – within the terms of the textbook recommendation – would have to be called "rationale Therapie" ['rational therapy'] (Kleinsorge 1985). Empirically present everyday prescription practice is far removed from this ideal, and it can be stated without much speculation that this detachment is connected at a very simple pragmatic level with the fact that physicians cannot prescribe substances but almost exclusively //preparations//, in other words industrial products manufactured in large quantities and therefore at economic prices. But the mere fact that each and every therapeutically effective substance on the pharmaceutics market is available in a dozen – and sometimes even in several hundred – different specialised medical preparations would not be a compulsive reason for deviating so far from the ideal of the textbook recommendation. In practical terms, it would not be very difficult to decide on one well-tried active ingredient and one specialised medical preparation for each specific indication and to set out to gain experience gradually. But neither does this strategy comply with empirical findings:

In a regionally based study of the prescribing behaviour of panel doctors with practices in the industrial western German city of Dortmund, Friebel (1988), for example, ascertained

> ... mathematisch gesicherte Beziehungen zwischen der Anzahl der im Quartal von einem Arzt in seiner Praxis mit Arzneimitteln versorgten Patienten und der Anzahl der von ihm im Quartalszeitraum verschriebenen Fertigarzneimittel ... Der durchschnittliche Allgemeinarzt versorgte im ersten Quartal 1985 612 Patienten mit 579 verschiedenen Fertigarzneimitteln. ... Nur wenige Mittel wurden so häufig rezeptiert, daß auf sie ein größerer als zehnprozentiger Anteil indikationsgruppengleicher Fertigarzneimittel entfiel. [... mathematically substantiated correlations between the number of patients provided with drugs by a doctor in his practice in one quarter and the number of different drugs prescribed by him during that quarter. In the first quarter of 1985, the average general practitioner provided 612 patients with 579 different pre-packed drugs. ... Very few preparations were prescribed so frequently as to account for a proportion in excess of ten percent of pre-packed drugs for the same indication group.] (Friebel 1988: 1179–1180)

Even when calculated cumulatively, the number of different syndromes treated in a statistically average practice approached an asymptotic limiting value very rapidly. The cumulative increase in the range of different drugs, however, remained essentially consistent throughout the two-year observation period. The author views his findings somewhat disapprovingly, thoroughly in the sense of the textbook recommendation already referred to in this chapter:

> Die resultierende Aufblähung des Sortiments wird für die arzneitherapeutische Rationalität bedrohlich, wenn mit wachsender Fertigarzneimittelzahl das Informiertsein des Verordnenden über die therapeutisch erwünschten und unerwünschten Wirkungen seiner Arzneimittel abnimmt und auf diese Weise sein Vermögen, den Arzneiverordnungen fundierte Nutzen/Risiko-Abwägungen zu Grunde zu legen leidet. ... Das Sammeln von therapeutischen Erfahrungen an den eigenen Patienten wird von diesem Verfahren nicht begünstigt. [The resulting inflation in the range on offer jeopardises rationality in drug therapy if the level of information attained by the prescriber with respect to the therapeutically desirable and undesirable effects of his drugs decreases with a growing number of pre-packed drugs, and his ability to base his drug prescriptions on benefit/risk considerations is consequently impaired. ... The gleaning of therapeutic experience from his own patients is not assisted by this behaviour.] (Friebel 1988: 1180)

Friebel sums up the nationwide relevance of his data as follows:

> Die in Dortmund angetroffene Situation kann im Großen und Ganzen seit Jahren bestehen. In Berlin hat ein niedergelassener Kollege bereits 1976 ähnliche Daten erhoben. Sie dürfte auch kein auf engeres geographisches Areal begrenzter Sonderfall sein, wie jüngere im südwestdeutschen Raum gesammelte Erfahrungen lehren. Für die Dortmunder Ärzte war sie eine Überraschung, denn Erstaunen war die häufigste Reaktion, wenn ihnen die von den Beratern evaluierten persönlichen Verordnungsdaten vorgelegt wurden. [The situation recorded in Dortmund may, all in all, have existed for years. In Berlin a colleague in private practice collected similar data as early as 1976. Nor is it likely to be a special case confined to a small geographical area, as recent experience gained in southwestern Germany indicates. For the Dortmund doctors it came as a surprise, since astonishment was the most frequent reaction when they were confronted with the personal prescribing data evaluated by the counsellors.] (Friebel 1988: 1180)

The conclusion reached by Friebel, too, is that the question of the causes of this therapeutic "irrationality" – one that is of vast importance to health policy – cannot be answered satisfactorily with the data available to date. It is also of special relevance to the semiotic aspect of drug application developed in the first three chapters of this book, for it is closely related to another question likewise of fundamental significance to the aspect developed in this chapter: What are the motives inducing healthy and sick people, experts and laymen to recommend or to implement the application of a specific preparation?

Following a discussion of this question – a discussion rich in perspectives though less fruitful in findings – in Chapter 1 of this book, Chapter 2 showed that an important part of these motives is derived not from analytical, pharmacologically "specific" expertise on the effects of drugs but from other sources, some of which can be described hypothetically as a semiotic "specificity" and whose empirically most important features are the concrete, sensorily perceptible characteristics of pharmaceutical preparations. Now that these two forms of "specificity" have been shown in Chapter 3 to be related historically and heuristically through their common alignment to one process characterised more closely in that chapter as a "modelling of similarity", the time has come to observe the consequences of this relationship for everyday dealings with pharmaceutical products. The point of departure for this observation is the question: What is the role played by sensorily perceptible qualities of pharmaceutical preparations in the decision to apply them? A concrete example is given in this connection:

Let us first recall the terminological difference between "pseudoplacebos" and so-called "impure placebos", discussed in detail in Chapter 2. Both of them differ from "pure" placebos in that they do contain pharmacologically defined substances. In the case of the "pseudoplacebos", however, these are substances that develop no measurable physiological effects whatsoever in vivo, so that they cannot be termed "active substances" in the narrower sense. "Impure placebos", in contrast, do contain pharmacologically //active substances//, though the effect induced by them has nothing to do with the therapeutically intended change. The application of "impure placebos" was illustrated in Chapter 2 with the /embrocations/ paradigm, i. e. applying //ointments// for local treatment of rheumatic and rheumatoid disease. Whilst producing a subjectively pleasant, pain-alleviating feeling of warmth by stimulating the local cutaneous circulation, the effect induced by these ointments on the phlogistic or degenerative pathological process[133] or on the physiological perception of pain is no greater than that induced by a locally applied hot-water bottle. Yet the ointments are considerably more effective from the therapeutic standpoint, for an annual prescription rate in excess of 6 million packs in the Federal Republic of Germany would be inexplicable unless the effect did indeed satisfy doctors and patients alike.[134]

Now the diseases comprising the rheumatic group form a diagnostically and nosologically highly complex structure. Among these diseases, the diagnostic complex "arthritis, rheumatism" is the leading factor in the prescribing of embrocations. This complex comprises three groups of syndromes:

(1) inflammatory joint disease with the focal diagnosis "arthritis";

(2) degenerative joint disease with the focal diagnosis "arthrosis"; and

(3) rheumatic disease not confined to joints, with the focal diagnosis "non-articular rheumatism syndrome".

In cases of inflammatory joint disease, prescriptions for embrocations – with a relative proportion of 3.2% of all preparations prescribed for this diagnosis – were negligible in the reference year 1983 in the Federal Republic of Germany. For the other two focal diagnoses, this proportion was considerably higher, with 54.7% of all preparations prescribed for arthrosis and 42% of all those prescribed for non-articular rheumatism syndrome. When these two syndromes are broken down according to the frequency with which the leading preparations in this field are prescribed, the result is highly illuminating for the problem being dealt with in this chapter.[135]

Table 6 presents a survey of the diagnosis-specific prescription frequency of the three leading embrocations in the Federal Republic of Germany: /Rheumon/, /Dolo-Arthrosenex/ and /Mobilat/. In addition to substances with no pharmacologically proven internal effect when applied externally, all three preparations contain at least one active substance that stimulates the local cutaneous circulation ("hyperemisation"), giving rise to a subjective sensation

Table 6: Antirheumatic embrocations, their names and 'indications'. Absolute prescription frequency per local diagnosis and relative prescription frequency per preparation of the three leading embrocations for rheumatic diseases in the Federal Republic of Germany (including West Berlin) in 1983 according to Hardenberg (1988). Absolute numbers (in thousand) refer to the diagnosis specified in the column heading, and relative numbers (in %) to the respective preparation listed in the relevant line. Minor deviations from 100% in the line totals are due to prescriptions for inflammatory joint diseases (focal diagnosis: /arthritis/) being ignored. These account for 2 to 3% per preparation.

PREPARATION Total in thousand parts per line in %	Degenerative joint disease /ARTHROSIS/	Non-articular rheumatic disease /NON-ARTICULAR RHEUMATIC SYNDROME/
/RHEUMON/	327 51.9%	273 43.3%
/DOLO-ARTHROSENEX/	824 92.4%	57 6.4%
/MOBILAT/	146 54.7%	116 43.4%

of warmth. It is conspicuous that the preparation /Dolo-Arthrosenex/ is prescribed almost exclusively for the treatment of degenerative joint disease, i. e. arthrosis (in more than 90% of cases of its being prescribed in the diagnostic complex /joint disorders, rheumatism/), whereas the other two preparations are prescribed in roughly equal proportions for "arthrosis" and "non-articular rheumatic disease". Without there being any pharmacological explanation for this manifestation, an analysis of the prescription statistics reveals a clear-cut "differentialindikatorische Zuordnung" ['allocation based on differential indications'] (Hardenberg 1989: 136) of /Dolo-Arthrosenex/ for the focal diagnosis /arthrosis/ despite this indication not being given special emphasis in the applications recommended by the manufacturer, a point emphasised by Hardenberg in his further analysis:

> Grundsätzlich wurde den Salben- und Gelapplikationen ein hoher suggestiver Effekt zugesprochen, der im wesentlichen durch die hyperämisierende Wirkung erklärt wird. Für die Anwendung der zahlreichen verschiedenen sonstigen Wirkstoffe fehlt eine rationale Begründung ebenso, wie der klinisch-pharmakologische Wirksamkeitsnachweis. Fraglos entbehrt die hohe differentialindikatorische Zuordnung der Vielkomponentensalbe Dolo-Arthrosenex^{R} zur Arthrosis deformans einer nachvollziehbaren pharmakologischen oder klinisch-medizinischen Grundlage. Ebensowenig wird von der herstellenden Brenner Arzneimittelfabrik GmbH eine solche spezielle Wirksamkeit des Dolo-Arthrosenex^{R} in den Anwendungsempfehlungen postuliert, sie lauten: "Stumpfe Verletzungen,

Blutergüsse, Schwellungen, Sportverletzungen, oberflächliche Venenerkrankungen, schmerzhafte und entzündliche Erkrankungen an Sehnen, Muskeln, Gelenken und Bändern" (Rote Liste). Dagegen teilen die Troponwerke GmbH und Co. KG zum Rheumon[R] durchaus die Indikation: "Adjuvanstherapie bei degenerativen rheumatischen Erkrankungen", mit (ebenda). Die beschriebene Verordnungsbesonderheit kann nur durch die hohe Suggestivkraft des Namens "Dolo-Arthrosenex" erklärt werden. Er ist mehr als ein Zeichen, durch das das Produkt der Brennerwerke identifizierbar wird. Er suggeriert einen unbestimmten und auf Anspielung beruhenden Zusammenhang zwischen der Salbe und der Entfernung des Schmerzes aus dem arthrotischen Geschehen. Er wird dadurch zum Symbol... Dieses Symbol wird vom Hersteller im typischen – von mehr oder weniger überzeugenden Fachwortkonstruktionen aus antiken Vokabeln oder Silben geprägten medizinischen Kode an die verordnenden Ärzte übermittelt. In dieser durch Symbolik geprägten Kommunikation verwandelt sich die klinisch-pharmakologisch unsichere Vielkomponentenpräparation in ein Arzneimittel mit hochspezifischem Indikationsbereich. Die vorliegenden Daten beweisen die hohe Suggestivkraft des Namens, möglicherweise setzt sie sich in eine gleichfalls starke Suggestionskraft des Arztes gegenüber seinem Rheumapatienten bei der Verordnung des Medikamentes und somit einer im Vergleich hohen Placebowirksamkeit fort. [The ointment and gel applications were fundamentally ascribed a higher suggestive effect, which was explained essentially in terms of hyperemisating action. A rational substantiation for the use of the wide variety of other active substances was lacking, as was any evidence of clinical-pharmacological efficacy. The high differential-diagnostic allocation of the multicomponent ointment Dolo-Arthrosenex[R] to arthritis deformans unquestionably lacks any obvious pharmacological or clinicomedical foundation. The directions given by the manufacturer, Brenner GmbH, attribute no specific efficacy of this kind to Dolo-Arthrosenex[R], stating: "Blunt joint traumatisation, bruising, swelling, sports injuries, superficial venous disorders, painful and inflammatory disorders affecting tendons, muscles, joints and ligaments" (Rote Liste [German pharmacopoeia]). In contrast, the indication "adjuvant therapy of degenerative joint disease" is claimed by the Troponwerke GmbH & Co. KG for Rheumon[R] (ibid.). The special prescribing behaviour detailed can be explained only by the high suggestive force of the name "Dolo-Arthrosenex". It is more than a sign through which the Brenner GmbH product is identifiable. It suggests a non-specific and allusion-based connection between the ointment and the removal of pain from the arthritic process; it becomes a symbol. This symbol is transmitted to the prescribing physicians in a typical medical code composed of more or less convincing technical-term constructions comprising words or syllables deriving from antiquity. In this symbolic communication, the clinicopharmacologically nonspecific multicomponent preparation is transformed into a remedy with a highly specific indication range. The suggestive force of the name, which generates an idea when the preparation is being prescribed, may be continued in a special suggestive force of the physician towards his patient in the prescribing process and thus substantiate a comparatively higher placebo efficacy.] (Hardenberg 1989: 136–137)

The relevance of this finding to the question posed at the end of the preceding section, concerning the semiotic roots of therapeutic "irrationality", could hardly be more fittingly analysed.[136] The finding offers highly distinct empirical evidence that that interpretative activity designated somewhat disparagingly and in a completely different context as "kleinliches Sinnbildeln und Wortdeuteln" ['petty symbolising and subtilizing'] by Boisserée ([1970]: 72) in 1815 can develop an immense therapeutic effect in the search for "structural gain". Both this interpretative activity and the profit obtained from it can be assumed to have been carried out largely unconsciously in the majority of the 824,000 cases (cf. Table 6) in which this "structural gain" was obviously achieved with some measure of success. Such hesitation at the threshold to the sphere of conscious intent appears to be characteristic, in a way that is difficult to divine, of the production of semiotic "specificity". Imaginative exploitation of the resources of sensorily perceptible material permitted by the use of drugs, in the form of their colors, names, aromas and usage rituals, is beneficial to the healing process especially when these resources, though prescribed, are not consciously reflected upon by the partners involved in this process (both of whom benefit from it within their own specific role). This is suggested in all events by the experience gained in a number of double-blind trials that therapeutic placebo effects are exceptionally great when neither of the persons involved is aware that the preparation being applied is a pure placebo.[137] If, then, a doctor searching for that preparation that is /exactly the right one/ for his patient is also directed by the sensory qualities of this preparation, it is nonetheless beneficial to the therapeutic process if he declares this esthetic[138] production of fantasies to himself and the patient as the perception of a pharmacologically "specific" nuance. He does not say: "I am now prescribing you an ointment which, being named "Dolo-Arthrosenex", is ideally suited to your syndrome" or "This tablet will do you good because it comes in your favorite color and tastes of raspberries". He adopts rather the following attitude when prescribing the preparation: "Although there is no drug capable – according to founded pharmacological expertise – of ensuring a rapid and complete cure for your symptoms, there is one preparation with whose composition I have already achieved good results in patients suffering from your syndrome".

The effectiveness of such an attitude need not, of course, remain restricted to the application of "impure" placebos or pseudoplacebos. It can also be beneficial with preparations whose efficacy is pharmacologically assured, either to lend additional support to their efficacy or to keep the development of unpleasant side-effects under control. Gutheil (1977: 82–83) exemplified this with the //phenothiazines//, an important group of substances in the psychiatric treatment of psychoses:

> One area of physician fantasies, linked with the idea of clinical expertise, is the notion of nuances in pharmacology. However often authorities write, for example, that the various phenothiazines are relatively similar in main effects and side effects, most clinicians believe that they have a "feel" for the nuances of a particular drug. "This one is especially good for those left-handed paranoids who are married," say, or "for those patients whose persecutory hallucinations appear in the soprano voice." I do not intend to suggest that nuances do not exist, only that this is an area where fantasy can play a major role. Patients share this kind of individualizing perception of even similar drugs.

Now this attitude conceals a possible explanation – though one admittedly lacking empirical substantiation – for the vast range of specialities to be found in the statistically average prescribing practice. It also explains the persistent preference for multi-component preparations despite the warnings given in textbooks: Doctors may have an almost insuperable aversion to having their "clinical expertise" (Gutheil 1977) capped by pharmacologically founded standard recommendations. From the perspectival standpoint of "commodity esthetics" (Haug 1980), their services to the patient cannot be reduced to the recommendation of one specific chemical substance. When they make a decision in favor of one specific drug preparation in the dialectics between metabolics and metaphysics as exemplified by "Chemie und Chiffre" ['chemistry and cipher'] (Sichrovsky 1984: 28), then they are making a simultaneous preselection concerning the concrete constellation of the sensory treasures provided by it. If this speciality fails to produce the desired results, some doctors will make a second or third attempt with optional drugs. Even if the pharmacological difference between these options and the original therapy are extremely subtle, the obvious difference in their "commodity-esthetic" configurations often provides sufficient motivation to risk this attempt *ut aliquid fiat*[139], as it is termed in clinical jargon. Clinical practice shows that something does indeed happen often enough – the only possible explanation for such attempts being undertaken so frequently.

From the economic standpoint, this practice – with which the physician brings the patient's interest in use value into harmony with the pharmaceutical industry's interest in exchange value – certainly has distinct shortcomings. The price of his service is subjected even less than the price of medical preparations – whose mediation is often the content of this service – to a demand-orientated market mechanism. Neither the physician as an economically uninvolved party nor the patient as a consumer belonging to a health insurance agency will automatically give preference to the cheaper of two products with an identical use value. The price of medical preparations may thus become a semiotically active component of the promise of use value, in the same way as luxury goods whose prices denote /exclusivity/: What costs a lot is worth a lot.

This may well explain the apparently contradictory finding that the frequency with which //Euglucon N// – a successful antidiabetic drug still enjoying a leading position on the German market – was prescribed fell by almost 25% following a repeated reduction in the price of this preparation on intervention by the German Cartel Office. The frequency with which lower-priced but pharmacologically identical optional preparations were precribed in the same period increased by 200 to 350% (Schwabe – Paffrath 1985: 76). With the reduction in price, //Euglucon N// may also have forfeited its special diacritical value as a /luxury preparation/.[140] A similar tendency can be observed in the prescribing of so-called //H2-antagonists// for treating gastric and duodenal ulcers. Newer, higher-priced optional preparations (through which a diacritical status was first introduced) showed distinct gains in 1984 as compared with the former leading product on the German market (Schwabe – Paffrath 1985: 124–125).

Another factor influencing the use of drugs – drug advertising – may also be characterised as a /race for diacritical placings/. This plays an important role in the area of the distributive public, in which producers, mediators and consumers of drugs are involved, a role that might be described in an initial approach with a phrase coined by Negt and Kluge (1972: 22) as a "Produktion der Zirkulations- und Distributionssphäre" ['production of the circulative and distributory sphere'] of medical preparations. The problems of drug advertising were touched upon in Chapter 1 of this book with the concrete example of an advertising campaign for /Aspirin/. One special problem quoted there in dealing with the /advertising/ phenomenon was the tendency to develop either an "integrato" ['integrated'] or an "apocalittico" ['apocalyptic'] relationship to it (Eco 1964).

"Advertising is necessary and beneficial, for it is entertaining and informative and reinforces the supremacy of the consumer, opening up to him the wide range available on the market" on the one hand and "advertising is detrimental and hazardous, for it exudes seductive appeal under the semblance of the informative, creates alienated needs and imposes uncritical acceptance on those to whom it is appealing as 'consumers'" on the other hand are two examples of formulation throwing these relationships into somewhat greater relief. Eco has characterised these two relationship concepts as an important instrument of orientation in his effort towards metacriticism of mass culture. As advertising, for its part, is a particularly disputed phenomenon of mass culture, his orientation framework is clearly applicable in this context too. A comparable perspectival regulation is undertaken by Haug when he writes in his introductory course to the theory of "commodity esthetics":

"Wir werden 'Werbung' und 'Konsum' in diesem Kurs sozialwissenschaftlich analysieren. Wir werden also weder mit den Augen des Werbers oder Unternehmers noch mit denen des privaten Einkäufers (genannt 'Verbraucher') auf die Dinge blicken." ['We shall analyse "advertising" and "consumption" socioscientifically in this course. We shall thus regard the objects neither through the eyes of the advertiser or entrepreneur nor through those of the private buyer (called the "consumer").'] (Haug 1980: 15). This perspectival regulation is applicable in the context of this chapter too.

Closer consideration of the cultural framework conditions of drug consumption makes it difficult to understand at first glance why drugs are advertised at all. Medical preparations traditionally enjoy the reputation of being one of the few enclaves in which the difference between /consumption/ and /indulgence/ – whose elimination "... zu den entscheidenden Voraussetzungen der spezifischen technischen und ökonomischen Entwicklungen der Neuzeit gehört..." ['is one of the decisive preconditions for the specific technical and economic developments of modern times'] (Blumenberg 1951: 465) – is still valid to some degree. The unabated validity of this difference, it might be argued, is illustrated with outstanding clarity in the fact that drugs are not consumed like chewing-gum, quartz watches or convertibles but far more cautiously, critically and rationally. Any vaguely reasonable person would do his best to avoid taking drugs regularly in the long term. Any compulsion for him to take drugs is not the outcome of an inducible or suppressible urge for consumption but is enforced by a chronic illness.[141] At the end of this chain of reasoning, drug advertising really does seem paradoxical. This explains why it is quite feasible from the viewpoint of an "integrated" theoretician to treat this phenomenon as though it were simply nonexistent: "Werbung – man kann das auf einen ganz einfachen Nenner bringen – hat den ausdrücklichen Sinn, den Umsatz einer Ware zu fördern, aber der Krankheitsmarkt läßt sich nun einmal nicht erweitern. Diese beiden Dinge widersprechen sich." ['Advertising ... has the explicit sense of furthering the sales of a commodity, but the illness market is one that cannot be expanded. These two aspects are in contradiction.'] (Schreiber 1974: 1552).

The economic and legislative framework conditions are also designed in certain nuances to retrieve, as it were, the difference between "indulgence" and "consumption" for drug intake. For instance, the law governing the advertising of medical preparations in Germany (Cf. Doepner 1980) specifies in meticulous detail that a large number of those advertising measures that have proved outstandingly successful in general consumer goods advertising from the advertiser's point of view constitute a punishable offence when applied to drugs. Further restrictions are provided for in a "codex", declared as a voluntary self-control instrument and published by the National Association of the German Pharmaceutical Industry (Bundesverband der Pharmazeutischen Industrie 1985).[142]

One factor that should be considerably more effective than any administrative measures in retrieving the "indulgence-consumption differential" is the service assignment of the physician himself. He intervenes in the consumer's decision in a counselling capacity without any direct economic dependence on the concrete implementation of this decision. Since professional segregation of the apothecary in the sixteenth century, this form of consumer counselling has belonged historically to the essential components of his service (for further detail, cf. Zimmermann 1974). If, on the other hand, the everyday situation to which a practising physician is exposed as a participant in the pharmaceutical distributive public is applied to the everyday working life of a consumer counsellor, the following, highly grotesque scenario is revealed:

Let us imagine that a public consumer counselling institution has opened an office in a small town. Now one official is responsible for counselling some 1500 of the citizens living there. Within the framework of his basic and advanced training, he has acquired extensive commodity-specific "Gebrauchswertwissen" ['expertise in use value'] (Haug 1980: 129) even if this has not necessarily the same scope as a degree course specialising in this activity. His level of knowledge is not the same in all spheres of consumer goods, but within a short time a competent colleague to whom he can turn or a publication to which he can refer occurs to him in response to almost any problem with which the citizens confront him. What would be the outcome, though, if manufacturers of consumer goods were to offer to supply him with information material to assist him in his work, or if these manufacturers were to send him unsolicited material totalling some 13,000 letters, 110,000 pages of bound literature and 5 hundredweight of trade journals within the course of one year?[143] Two reactions – which by no means rule out each other – are conceivable: Either the official concerned would suspect attempted manipulation, or he might scrutinise the material offered to him – within the bounds of the time at his disposal – as the somewhat dubious source does not preclude his finding some information of value to his work (since even if he were to conjecture an exceptionally contriving or disreputable advertising strategy, that would be of value to his work and he could give his clients due warning about the product concerned). One particular problem concerning the receipt of this material would probably be that the official would simply not have time to peruse it appropriately. What would be the outcome, then, if he were to be visited in this situation about four times a week[144] by salesmen representing various manufacturers, all of them wishing to have brief talks with him about various products? In the first place, the brief nature of these talks would be an essential prerequisite for such contacts materialising at all. Were they to materialise, the official would certainly be fully aware that the salesman comes to him intending essentially to advertise and that the mediation of useful "Gebrauchswertwissen" ['expertise in use value'] (Haug 1980) must certainly be subordinate to this intent. The salesman, on the other hand, is also aware that he can arouse no interest in his opposite number (and that this may well be his last direct contact with this particular person) if he confines himself to rattling off advertising slogans and handing over glossy brochures. From the salesman's point of view, the success of the discussion in establishing contact will depend in no small measure on how well he manages to make his opposite number forget his or her everyday routine for a while with such strategies as "entertainment" and "flirtation". He can back up these strategies with small advertising handouts or with invitations to publicity events offering a fringe program designed to appeal to the gourmet.[145] He will, however, take great care not to rely too much on these strategies, for he is dealing with an opposite number whose suspicion is always aroused by them, whose professional activity has given him good training in rhetorics and who, having a regular income, can afford to treat himself to a good evening meal.

In addition to the two reactions on the part of the consumer counsellor outlined above as "suspicion" and "sceptical interest", a third reaction is conceivable: He might refuse any contact whatsoever with the manufacturers of consumer goods or with their emissaries, feeling that he owes this to the reputation of his independent counselling institution or because he possibly concludes after some time that the cost in terms of hours spent on these contacts is in an unfavourable ratio to the benefit derived from them for his day-to-day work.

The only grotesque feature in this scenario is the setting. If it is applied to a medical practice or – with certain restrictions – to the workplace of a hospital physician, it is perfectly realistic. It was, in all events, drawn up with marked attention to authenticity and based on a great deal of practical experience, both as a directly involved and as a disinterested party (cf. Schonauer 1986b). The majority of the staff at public counselling centers would probably opt for the third of the possible reactions outlined here. Among doctors, this proportion is presumably much lower, even though it tends in general to be underestimated.[146] Without any empirical data whatsoever, this publicity-created contact between drug manufacturers and doctors as the most competent mediators of consumer decisions can be assumed to assert a marked influence on the implementation of this mediation activity.

This conclusion can be drawn from the mere fact that drug manufacturers, who after all have vast hoards of relevant empirical material at their disposal, would not go to such expense unless it were worth their while.[147] The question most hotly disputed between "integrated" and "apocalyptic" investigators of the drug advertising phenomenon is whether it is only qualitative market shares that are consequently shifted in favor of the manufacturer who is advertising (in comparison with the manufacturer who is advertising less or not at all), or whether the quantitative total volume of drug consumption also undergoes a marked increase.[148] The latter case would imply the end of the "indulgence-consumption differential" handed down within medical culture. In the thematic framework set here, the question of paramount importance is what influence the factor "drug advertising" has on the semiotic aspect of the drug and its role in the doctor-patient relationship.

Langbein, Martin et al. (1983: 54–58) refer to some empirical studies which have shown in the context of research into pharma-marketing that at least half of all doctors rate contact with pharmaceutical representatives as the most important source of information consulted by them when making a decision on prescribing new preparations. The authors conclude that drug manufacturers and their emissaries hold a kind of information monopoly towards the prescribing physician. This finding – one undoubtedly alarming from the health policy standpoint – needs further differentiation for the thematic framework set in this chapter with respect to a decision that is of essential significance to the issue on which attention is focused here:

No one has any monopoly with respect to the pharmacological expertise needed by the physician for reliable assessment and prediction of the effect of pharmaceutical substances. This expertise is socialised, and the physician has acquired it in full in the course of his academic and clinical training. Even if some decades have passed since this period of training, this expertise could be updated perfectly well by taking out a subscription to an industry-independent periodical or by studying the new editions of the relevant pharmacological and clinical therapy manuals. With respect to that expertise required for assessment of the pharmacological "specificity", he cannot derive much benefit from contact with the pharmaceutical representative and the material presented by him.[149] As far as this expertise is concerned, the pharmaceutical representative certainly has no monopoly towards him, though he may well be way ahead in persistence. The situation is, however, completely different with respect to that sphere differentiated in Chapter 2 of this book as semiotic "specificity": To gain a sensory impression of the appearance, smell and name of the drugs that he is considering prescribing, of the "feel" of their application in detail, the physician needs to look at, or preferably to touch, the samples in the salesman's case. And the iconic messages of the pseudo-scientific journals and brochures presented to him by the pharmaceutical representative for his further "information" also tell him most about these aspects, for this literature consists largely of large-scale glossy illustrations in accurate detail. He will find hardly anything about them in pharmacological textbooks; what is more important, he will not even look for them in textbooks, for he has never learnt to regard semiotic "specificity" as a theoretical problem. (Were he to do so, then the possible therapeutic effect of this "specificity" would probably be diminished). In this respect the pharmaceutical representative does have a monopoly towards the physician, though not one concerning information. He will most certainly not say "Do try out the effect of these elegant, bright red tablets" or "We have now developed a fantastic new process that enables us to model similarity". The hoard of sensorily perceptible factors with which the physician is supplied through his contact with the pharmaceutical representative may be an important motive behind his accepting this contact at all and his investing so much of his valuable working time in the – pharmacologically viewed – largely irrational question of what drug speciality he is now to prescribe.[150] His mere contemplation of this question will furthermore enable him to acquire the competency experience of "clinical expertise" (Gutheil 1977: 82). The more often he decides to prescribe fundamentally well-known therapeutic substances in constantly new esthetic forms and constantly new pharmaco-technical forms of preparation, the more his rational "expertise in use value" (Haug 1980) concerning the pharmacological effect of these substances on the patient is jeopardised. It is at this very point that Friebel's (1988) already quoted criticism – that the collecting of therapeutic experiences on one's own patient is not furthered by such erratic prescribing behaviour – was levelled. This risk, however, is the price he pays for the opportunity of prescribing his patient not just any anonymous standard preparations but drugs with a concrete esthetic aura of their very own, selected with only that patient in mind. In the ritual sphere of the doctor-patient relationship, a process is thus realised – generally without those involved being aware of it – that might be described with reference to Haug (1980: 47) as the neglect of pharmacological in favour of esthetical use value.[151]

5. Conclusion: Pharmacomorphism of the doctor–patient relationship and liturgy of the physic

> To write prescriptions is easy, but to come to an understanding with people is hard... Always expecting the impossible from the doctor. They have lost their ancient beliefs; the parson sits at home and unravels his vestments, one after another; but the doctor is supposed to be omnipotent with his merciful surgeons's hand. Well, as it pleases them; I have not thrust my services on them; if they misuse me for sacred ends I let that happen to me too.
>
> Franz Kafka

When Balint (1964) coined the metaphorical "drug-physician" comparison, one of his aims was to direct the scientific study of the doctor-patient relationship towards the hypothesis that the role of the physician in confrontation with illness is in some respect comparable with the effect of drugs. Like these, he suggested, the professional activity of doctors had intended and desirable effects as well as unintended and often undesirable "side-effects". Addictive dependency relationships between patients and doctors might develop in the same way as in the consumption of beneficial and soothing remedies.[152] One of his greatest concerns in this hypothesis was an autocritical reflection of the doctor's understanding of his role.

A study of the scientific literature relating to the role of the drug in the doctor-patient relationship constantly confronts the reader with a term that invites him implicitly – and unfortunately without reflection – to regard the role of the patient within the framework of this relationship on a largely "pharmacomorphic" level: the term /compliance/. What is meant by this is, generally speaking, the degree to which a patient follows the recommendations and instructions given by his doctor in his handling of the prescribed drugs. If he deviates from these in any respect, by changing the intake time, the dose or even the drug, he is – depending on the degree of deviation – "non-compliant". The English-speaking reader may be intrigued to know that this term is generally left untranslated in literature published by German authors. Baier (1988: 1322) therefore refers to an "anglophones Versteckspiel" ['anglophonic game of hide-and-seek'] with the original term "Fügsamkeit" ['docility'], since it ought to be given a lexically correct translation either with that or with far more pedantic lexemes such as /Folgsamkeit/ (obedience), /Verformbarkeit/ (malleability) or /Willfährigkeit/ (compliance). Halhuber (1981: 1130) therefore suggests circumscribing it as a "tragfähiges therapeutisches Arbeitsbündnis" ['stable therapeutic alliance'] or as "therapeutische Kooperation" ['therapeutic cooperation']. This suggestion is undoubtedly meant to be emancipatory; ignoring the history of the term as it does, however, it merely shifts the problem to the question: What kind of cooperation is that to be if the role of one of the cooperators consists by definition in observing the suggestions, instructions and orders of the other? What this question conceals is not so much a problem of emancipation – as would first appear to be the case – as one of communication, a problem that can be traced back to a mechanistic interaction model that transports the construct /compliance/ into the doctor-patient relationship: Very rarely will a patient behave as though under the command of his doctor. If he is dubious about a therapeutic recommendation or confronted with problems in following it, he will not hesitate to modify it or even to ignore it completely on his own initiative. Virtually no provision is made, however, for anticipation of such doubt or problems in the culturally codified form of intercommunication controlling the mediation of pharmacological therapeutic recommendations. This form of intercommunication is referred to traditionally as "prescribing" and it guides the therapeutic processing of the complex symptoms with which the patient has consulted his doctor into a linguistically fixed directive with an enticingly clear structure: the medical /prescription/. To the same extent as the doctor acts as the "drug" in the relationship with his patient, he makes the patient the "receptor". We have to bear in mind at this juncture that a medical prescription can also be referred to as a "recipe". It is not only this terminological[153] conformity that encourages that very "mechanistic interaction model" that transports the concept of compliance into the doctor-patient relationship to be surmised in the /receptor model/. What is far more important in this context is the immense "structural gain" granted by anthropomorphic application of the model in exactly the same way as demonstrated by the protagonists of *Elective Affinities*: it is through this application that the model opens once again a back door to sense imposition. Even the most enlightened, sceptical and emancipated patient finds it quite fascinating to go to his family doctor with a problem and come home with a prescription or a recipe. He has told him what his symptoms are and possibly what marks they have left on his everyday life. The doctor has then examined him, applied his professional diagnostic techniques and finally made a therapeutic proposal that is based at least metaphorically on the assumption that it fits the symptoms like a glove. Once this assumption has proved effective (and just how effective it can be is demonstrated by placebo research), even the most enlightened patient will first guard against jeopardising it by anticipating doubts or difficulties – not because he is afraid of the authoritative power of the doctor but because he has to fear that the promise of "structural gain" will be lost once again. Difficulties arising from this form of contact in the patient's everyday life are referred to in the research field as "non-compliance".

Early in Chapter 1, one important function of the ritual in the doctor-patient relationship was described as being that of staging the distribution of drugs as though they had not yet reached the *age of mechanical reproduction* (Benjamin [1970]). Now this formulation was not coined by Benjamin in the context of drugs; his aim was rather to describe in his essay the influence of the reproducibility of works of art on their cultural function. In a section dedicated to the historical continuity of this function beyond the invention of the technical reproduction, he makes the following statement on this problem:

> Originally the contextual integration of art in tradition found its expression in the cult. We know that the earliest art works originated in the service of a ritual – first the magical, then the religious kind. It is significant that the existence of the work of art with reference to its aura is never entirely separated from its ritual function. In other words, the unique value of the 'authentic' work of art has its basis in ritual, the location of its original use value. (Benjamin 1970: 225–226)

However great the caution and scepticism with which conclusions on analogy are drawn, the semiotically relevant, active aspect of drugs accentuated in this book can be characterised very fittingly with this passage from Benjamin's essay by replacing the term "work of art" with the word "drug". Like the "authentic" – in other words the unique and not mass-produced – work of art, the esthetically unique /medi-cament/, that has acquired its authenticity only within an individual relationship, is also founded in a ritual as an "expressive institutionalisierte ... Handlungssequenz" ['expressive institutionalised ... sequence of action'] (Werlen 1984: 81) in which it – like the work of art – had its first and original use value. Very few service settings in the secular sphere of our culture display so many accessories appropriate to ritual interaction as the doctor's surgery or the hospital. These accessories – from the white overall to the stethoscope, the hypodermic needle and the prescription pad – actually acquire their real liturgical value by being used in an apparently rational way and without much dramatic effect.

In this context it seems plausible that pharmacology somewhat helplessly describes that portion of the drug effect that appears to it to be "non-specific" – and therefore hardly explicable in rational terms – with a word originally coined in late medieval times as a purely liturgical concept: /placebo/. Within the framework of a detailed analysis of this word and its history, an attempt was made in Chapter 2 to classify this alleged "non-specificity" by interpreting this portion of the effect of drugs partly as a function of their sensorily perceptible qualities. This classification eventually flowed into a new semiotic "specificity" developed analogously to the pharmacological specificity concept. Yet neither do these sensory qualities permit much more than an approach to the interpretation of the pharmacologically "non-specific" effect of drugs. They are certainly not the cause of it: "In der Tat, die Realität der Gegenstände liegt nicht in ihren sinnlich wahrnehmbaren Eigenschaften, sondern 'hinter' ihnen. Aber dort liegt keine Welt physischen Seins oder von 'Dingen an sich', sondern eine Welt, die wir in unserer Vorstellung als 'objektive Außenwelt' aus Indizien konstruieren, die unseren täglichen Wahrnehmungen entstammen." ['Indeed, the reality of the objects is not in their sensorily perceptible characteristics but "behind" them. Yet the world out there is not one of physical being or of "things as such" but a world that we construct in our imagination from clues drawn from our daily perceptions as an "objective outside world".'] (Uexküll 1984b: 69).

Applied to the problem being dealt with here, this means that any drug developing a distinct but pharmacologically inexplicable effect has this effect not because it has a specific color or a specific name but because the physician and his patient succeed in attributing an astoundingly contagious meaning to this sensory material below the threshold of what was consciously intended and thus in constituting a beneficial reality for both the physician and the patient. The exploitation of the sensorily perceptible resources of the //drug// as a physic follows for long stretches a program addressed in literary pragmatics under the framework concept of "Rezeptionsästhetik" ['reception esthetics'] (Warning 1975). Within the course of this process, the patient – like the literary reader – becomes, as the consumer of the drug, the author of "geschichtsbildende Energie" ['historioplastic energy'] (Jauss 1975: 127) whose support of additional catalysts permits that very attempt at rescue described by Marquard (1973: 106) as an elementary joint function of esthetics and therapeutics "... unterm Druck einer Übermacht der Natur der Menschlichkeit Präsenz zu bewahren" ['to preserve humanity's presence under Nature's overwhelming force'].

Chapter 3 presented a number of medical, chemical and pharmacological models that were very well suited to catalysing this process, as it were. An obvious point throughout was that these models had not been created for this purpose at all but, on the contrary, rather to prepare the pharmacological specificity concept that is valid today and certainly of outstanding value for "rational" drug therapy. These two apparently contradictory findings may well be interconnected: A pharmacological model for specificity, as described by the relationship between a drug and its receptor, might lend itself to the opening of back doors to "craving for sense" for the very reason that it is empirically so well sustained and heuristically so successful. For it is not least this sustainment that enables both the doctor and the patient to anthropomorphise this model for their relationship and for the production of structural gain without having to transgress the threshold to the consciously intended. The presentation of this structural gain as a semiotic product of "... l'intrecciarsi di gesti, aspettative, credenze e piccole autorità che sembrano coordinati da un potere occulto, ma in realtà si mettono insieme da soli, a livello 'microscopico'" ['the interwoven quality of gestures, expectations, convictions and minor authorities which appear to be coordinated by an occult might but which in reality join up of their own accord at a "microscopic" level'] (Eco in Lilli 1988), has been the objective of this book.

Notes

1. This "red thread" has become a widely used idiom in the German language, referring to what is known in English merely as the "thread" of an argument, discourse etc. The idiomatic use of the color red was coined in early nineteenth century German literature. It was taken from that passage in Goethe's novel *Elective Affinities* which is quoted here, proving that the idiomatic use of "red" originates at least culturally in an English source. Because of its priming function for the mediation between natural and cultural sciences, major parts of Chapter 3.3 in this book are devoted to this novel.
2. Eco also places on the validity of this minimum condition one important restriction that may serve to prevent any axiomatic claim: "... the human adressee is the methodological (and not the empirical) guarantee of the existence of a signification, that is of a sign-function established by a code. But on the other hand the supposed presence of a human sender is not the guarantee of the sign-nature of a supposed sign." (Eco 1976: 16).
3. ['A man named Rotnagel invented a new glue which looked very dependable and smelt of oleander; many women used it to make themselves smell nice. Rotnagel struggled vehemently against this abuse – he wanted his invention to be put to its intended use. But that was the very predicament, for the new glue stuck nothing at all, or at least nothing known to man... So Rotnagel spent three years of his life inventing a new material that could be stuck with this glue, but only with this. After lengthy deliberation, Rotnagel called the new material Nihilit.'] (Kusenberg 1974: 51–52).
4. The English edition seems to omit here one possibly quite important feature of this system. In the Italian edition point (c) is described as follows: "(c) lo studio dei segni in una determinata cultura permette di definire il valore degli interpretanti in termini posizionali e opposizionali all'interno di sistemi semantici." (Eco 1975: 120).
5. I have taken over some examples from a publication by Gipper (1978: 125–129) on the problems of the relationship between propria and appellativa from the linguistics standpoint.
6. The curious reverse path from the measuring unit to the proper name was taken by the American writer Samuel Langhorne Clemens (1835–1910). He chose a literary pseudonym meaning /two fathoms deep/ in the language of the Mississipi boatmen: /Mark Twain/.
7. /Contergan/ was the German proprietary name for //thalidomide//.
8. In the equivalent passage of the English edition (Eco 1976: 87), the phenomen of "homonomy" accompanying the use of proper nouns is not regarded as a "risk" but neutrally referred to as a possible "case".
9. Schuhmacher refers to Meyer-Eppler (1969: 408–434) for concretisation of the concept of "distance".
10. Three- or four-syllable words with an emphasis on the last syllable and with a soft terminal sound (cf. Schuhmacher 1969: 71).
11. For another patent issue with the same result in France cf. Galmiche (1957) and Dillemann (1977), and on the development in the German-speaking world Schlenk (1950).
12. Apart from series products made in small or medium quantities, where each single replica is marked with a consecutive number to make it identifiable, at least potentially, as an individual item. For detailed, trend-setting formulation of this issue, cf. Benjamin (1970).

13. Cf. also Dorfles 1974, Nöth 1975, 1977, Rossi-Landi 1985.
14. A term used by Habermas (1984: 70–71) denoting a form of socio-technological exertion of power whose objectives, rules and principles are kept secret (latin: *arcanus*) from the controlled objects. The concealment of therapeutic principles from the patient as an /arcane/ discipline is indeed a commandment obviously enjoying intercultural respect in almost all medical traditions, and possibly an important factor in their effectiveness. To what extent the application of pharmaceutical therapy can be considered a socio-technological procedure is certainly still a matter of dispute. Since the studies by Stoessel (1973), Illich (1977) and Waitzkin (1984), however, there have been sufficient arguments at least to justify Habermas' term in this sphere. In the English edition of his book (Habermas 1989: 52) the original term "Arkanpraxis" ist translated as "secret practice". For the special status of the term /arcanum/ in Paracelsus, cf. chapter 3.2.
15. For the genetic relationship between division of labour and the rise of notation systems as precedents or analoga of writing cf. Ehlich (1983: 100–102) and Ungeheuer (1980).
16. Taking the Venetian theriac production as an example, Adlung and Urdang (1935: 161) point out that laboratories manufacturing pharmaceutical products for export on a relatively large scale were being set up in some regions as early as the fourteenth century. The proportion of such anonymously produced preparations in the total quantity consumed nevertheless remains negligible until the late nineteenth century.
17. Cf. Sebeok (1979a,b); Bär (1983); Schonauer (1986a); Uexküll and Wesiack (1988); Hucklenbroich (1989); Kahn (1983); Staiano(1986).
18. In the English edition (Eco 1976: 22) this act is very generally referred to as "calling", which would be equivalent to the Italian verb "chiamare". In the Italian edition the verb "denominare" is used and even accentuated by capital letters.
19. Weissbach (1971: 133) refers to August Kekulé, a determining inaugurator of the formular language of organic chemistry in the nineteenth century, as having come to the conclusion that "die Art, wie theoretische Gedanken in Zeichensystemen ausgedrückt werden, sei überhaupt gleichgültig [the way in which theoretical thoughts are expressed in sign systems is of no consequence whatsoever]." Cf. Peirce (1982: 95): "In the first place, it is necessary to show that the hypothesis of atoms, in itself, explains nothing".
20. Martinet's term /moneme/ as a possible *nomen collectivum* for all meaning-bearing units is not used in the further course of this presentation. Within the framework of our comparison, it would /bridge/ two structural levels : the "morphemes" (or "representomorphemes") of the linguistic (or of the representematic) continuum on the one hand and the "functional groups" and "molecules" of the chemical continuum on the other. As a nomen collectivum it would thus de-differentiate precisely that accentuation dealt with below. One important advantage of Koch's terminology used here is its compatibility with Rossi-Landi's (1985: 47–84) comparative analysis of an "omologia fra produzione linguistica e produzione materiale" ['parallelism between linguistic and material production']. With reference to the problem of terminology, cf. in particular Gipper (1978: 112).
21. In further presentation of the history of //salicylic acid//, I keep essentially to the monographs by Schlenk (1947) and Hangarter (1974a), where detailed bibliographical material is provided on the authors referred to below. The richest store of published material relating to the history of aspirin is provided by Alstaedter (1983).
22. On the significance of this mode for Paracelsus and Alexander von Humboldt, cf. Blumenberg (1986: 69, 285–286).
23. Following the initial synthesis in 1859, Kolbe had spent more than 15 years working on technical improvements to his production method. This meant that early patents were

granted at the time of the German Confederation, whereas the comprehensive copyright mentioned here was registered after 1871 and was thus a "German Reich patent" (Deutsches Reichspatent = D. R. P).

24. On the question discussed with considerable momentum in pharmacological history of whether //acetylsalicylic acid// is a German or a French invention, cf. Galmiche (1957), Dillemann (1977) and Schlenk (1947: 11). On 14. 12. 1915, the *Humanité* (Anonymous 1915) published an article entitled "La Fraude de l'Aspirine" that raised the problem from the Socialist aspect but discussed it with such patriotism as if the *Internationale* had never existed.
25. On 9. 11. 1962, the "Medical Tribune" published a tribute to Felix Hoffmann: "The man who 'invented' Aspirin". The author used as a preface a quotation from Thomas.S. Kuhn: "Discovery is seldom a unit event attributable to some particular man, time and place." (Wood 1962)
26. A metaphor that may well link up with Kant's "Verschiebung" ['shifting'] of the *ars naturam imitandi* "auf das fortzeugende Verhältnis von Kunst to Kunst" ['to the generative relation passed on from art to art'] (Blumenberg 1957: 267).
27. This, however, only protected the sale of //acetylsalicylic acid// under the name /Aspirin/. The patents likewise applied for to cover the general production of //acetylsalicylic acid// were refused for the territory of the German Reich on the grounds that the substance had not first been synthetised in the Elberfeld laboratories. The patent was successfully registered, however, in the USA and on some other markets. (For bibliographic references to the patent litigation between 1900 and 1905, cf. Schlenk (1950: 412)).
28. There was a new edition of this campaign, in rapid motion as it were, in Australia during the First World War, when the Australian Lord Chancellor, Hughes, suspended the German patent rights for /Aspirin/ in order to transfer them to the domestic industry. This led to the founding of "Nicholas Ltd.", which began marketing //acetylsalicylic acid// under the name /Aspro/, first in Australia and then in Asia and Africa. The following can be read on this episode of demand production in a leader in the "Medical Journal of Australia" on the occasion of the 60th anniversary of /Aspro/:
Nowhere is this better illustrated than by George Davies, the "extraordinary publicity man" to whom, in 1917, was entrusted the company's entire advertising policy. His campaign began in Queensland and consisted of giving away free samples, and the most incredible, irrelevant, but successful advertising slogans – for example: "Hats off to the great Abe Lincoln because he was a stickler for truth. As such he would recognize a wonderful discovery like Aspro in a minute." As sales grew in Australia, teams were sent to "colonise" Asia and Africa: There even more flamboyant methods of advertising were used. Aspro propaganda vans, complete with loudspeakers extolling the product's virtues, would visit primitive villages bearing free samples and colourful pamphlets. A most ingenious method of spreading information was devised in Egypt, where the local tax collectors were utilised." (Anonymous 1977: 355–356)
29. According to De Ridder (1984: 80), Ortega y Gasset also used the term /Aspirin Age/. The context in which this term was coined is not known to me. Alstaedter (1983: 4) quotes the following passage from Ortega y Gasset's book *The revolt of the masses*, though without specifying the precise page: "Der gewöhnliche Mensch lebt heute leichter, bequemer und sicherer als früher der Mächtigste. Was schert es ihn, daß er nicht reicher ist als andere, wenn die Welt es ist und ihm Straßen, Eisenbahnen, Hotels, Telegraph, körperliche Sicherheit und Aspirin zur Verfügung stellt." ['The common man today has a more relaxed, more comfortable and safer life than the most powerful man used to have. What does he care

that he is no richer than others, when the world is so and places roads, railways, hotels, telegraph, physical safety and aspirin at his disposal.'].

30. The use of this present participle in an ambiguous sense, referring obliquely not only to those years but to an intensity of headaches, has a close parallel in German too.
31. For the history of this threshold in the relationship between nature and technology, cf. Blumenberg (1951: 464–465) and chapter 4.2 below.
32. //Diacytylmorphine//, generally referred to as /Heroin/, can probably still be regarded as such. But because of its prodigious habit-forming potency – a certain dependence may develop even after one single application – it has virtually ceased to be used for therapeutic purposes.
33. Other new interpretations, which can also only be touched upon here, arise from the fact that further pharmacological properties of //acetylsalicylic acid// were discovered in the course of time: their euphorising effect, their growth-inhibiting effect on rapidly proliferating cell populations ("cytostatic effect"), and above all their influence on the thrombocyte-dependent part of blood coagulation (survey in Hangarter 1974b, Lasagna 1983). It is only the last-stated property that has resulted in diffused clinical application, though this has, in contrast to analgesic application, never expanded to the field of self-administration. As //acetylsalicylic acid// lowers the rate of spontaneously agglutinating blood platelets in the circulating blood, it may have a prophylactic effect on thrombosis and a favorable effect on the flow properties of the blood in cases of circulatory disturbances. The main point of interest in the correlations debated here is that the //acetylsalicylic acid// marketed for this range of indications is marketed in Germany by the same manufacturer under another proprietary name: /Colfarit/. Although the //acetylsalicylic acid// contained in /Colfarit/ has a modified formulation, referred to as "micro-encapsulation", making it more suitable for longer-term application, it is chemically absolutely identical with //aspirin// and has the same analgesic properties and also the same single dose. Its advantages could be utilised just as well for the analgesic indication as for its application as a circulation-stimulating agent. The use of a product for a purpose for which it has not yet stood the test obviously puts the stability of the interchange relationship at risk in already established domains. Stabilisation of this interchange relationship is, however – as already shown – probably the most important function of proprietary names.
   There are now indications of a new sphere of application for //acetylsalicylic acid//, also associated with the anticoagulant effect of this substance. The results of an American and a British study carried out in 1988 suggest that regular administration may be of primary prophylactic significance in reducing the risk of cardiac infarction. One outcome of these findings would now be the recommendation – one of momentous significance for the cultural status of //acetylsalicylic acid// – that healthy individuals might consume this substance regularly in order to lower their personal risk of cardiac infarction. There is in all events some pharmacological evidence that such a correlation does indeed exist (cf. relevant survey by Manz – Lüderitz 1988).
34. An introduction to methodological problems of statistical risk surveys in the field of medical preparations is given by Inman (1985).
35. Cf. Blumenberg (1986: 144): "Das Ideal der Lesbarkeit der Welt und ihrer vollendeten Formel schließen sich tendenziell aus." ['The ideal of the legibility of the world and its perfected fomula are mutually exclusive in their tendencies.']
36. The opportunity for large-scale economic utilisation of such macromolecules was provided only very recently by the transition from test tube synthesis to biosynthesis using genetic

engineering. This development has given rise to lively debate with respect to the degree of control over Nature permitted by this method.

37. The admittedly minimisable but hardly completely avoidable use of anthropomorphisms in the description of models taken from the natural sciences may be a rough indicator of their semioticity.
38. If the path taken by a specific substance inside the organism is to be traced in vivo from outside, a computed dose of a radiolabeled fraction of this substance is passed into the organism. The "radiolabeled" substance differs from the reference substance only in that one atom (or one "representeme") is replaced at one, or less frequently at more than one, site with a radioactive "nuclide" with the same atomic number. This change takes place below the first structural level of chemical complexity stages. The reference substance and the "radiolabeled" substance are chemically absolutely identical. They are subject to the same selection restrictions and *attractiones electivae*. Both follow the same metabolic path in spatiotemporal terms. But because the "labeled" substance continues to emit radiation for a multiple of its half-life, its spatial movements can be traced from outside within this period, as long as it is concentrated at specific sites in the organism. In Peirce's terminology, the radiolabeled substance is an "indexical qualisign". Its semiotic efficiency below the lowest complexity stage has an analog in language: the dialectically modified "allophone" that makes a Cockney, a Glaswegian, a Texan or a Bronx taxi driver distinguishable in a circle of speakers of English throughout his life or – in the event of dialectic assimilation – at least for a multiple of its /half-life/.
39. For more detailed presentation of the two studies mentioned here and of other methodologically related studies, cf. Lehrl and Csiske (1980).
40. Cf. Blumenberg (1951: 464–466). This division is dealt with in more detail in Chapter 4.2.
41. For further detail cf.: Sander (1977, vol. II, annex II/51–52) and Doepner (1980).
42. Eco (1972: 271) states within the framework of "Reklamecodes" ['advertising codes'] "daß das verbale Register hauptsächlich die Funktion hat, die Botschaft zu *verankern*, weil die visuelle Botschaft oft als zweideutig und als begrifflich verschieden zu fassen erscheint." ['... the verbal register has primarily the function ... of *anchoring* the message, because the visual message often seems ambiguous and open to different interpretations.']
43. The wording of /T1/ and /T2/ translated into English:
    ['/T1/: In contrast to many other headache remedies, Aspirin contains only one single active substance: acetylsalicylic acid (ASA). This substance acts reliably. It is the most widely used active substance against pain worldwide. Aspirin was developed decades ago by Bayer and is now known throughout the world as an outstanding remedy against...
    /T2/: ...pain and high temperature resulting from colds (influenzal infections). Aspirin is well tolerated. [Change of typeface]
    ASPIRIN against slight to moderate pain, especially headaches, e.g. following stress, overexertion and in cases of exhaustion as well as after alcohol and nicotine abuse, pain and high temperature resulting from colds (influenzal infections); inflammation. ASPIRIN should not be taken in cases of hypersensitivity to salicylates and other non-steroid anti-inflammatory agents and of increased hemorrhagic tendency. In cases of gastric and intestinal ulcers, previously damaged kidneys and during pregnancy, the doctor should be consulted. ASPIRIN should not be taken during the last 4 weeks before the calculated date of confinement. With high-dosage use on a long-term basis, the possibility of a slight increase in the normal discharge of blood from the stomach and bowel should be taken into account (anemia). In rare cases, hypersensitivity reactions (e.g. asthma, skin reactions) and occasionally gastro-intestinal complaints may occur. Like all analgesics, Aspirin should not be

taken on a long-term basis or in high dosages without the doctor being consulted. [Change of typeface]. The economical 50-pack/DM 9.05'].

44. For a commentary on this law ("Heilmittelwerbegesetz"), cf. Sander 1977: vol.II, annex II/5, 2–3.
45. For application of Peirce's trichotomy to advertising messages, cf. Nöth 1975: 29–30.
46. Although the product on offer and the reference to its pain-relieving effect is probably the only substantial connection between the old and the new advertisement, the very structural similarity of the two syntagmas is conspicuous: sequences arranged primarily in reading directing, in each case introduced by a visual embarking focus and terminated by the same company logo.
47. In Larousse (1971:272), the word /aspirine/ is reported to stem from /spiraea ulmaria/ as the natural source product of //salicylic acid//. The prefix is, however, not interpreted as a reference to the //acetic acid residue// (= /acetyl-/; cf. Dreser 1899) but as a privative /a/ intended to indicate that //aspirine// is not a natural but a fully synthetic product.
48. This argument has to be regarded essentially as pure invention. In all events there is no pharmacological evidence for //aspartic acid// having any febrifugal effect. It is a non-essential amino acid that is continuously synthetised in the human body and need not be introduced with food.
49. The biographical connections following are given in somewhat more detail as they are based in part on evaluation of previously unpublished archive material.
50. The chemist concerned was Fritz Hofmann (not to be confused with Felix Hoffmann), whose memoirs have already been quoted in greater detail in this book.
51. This birth was re-enacted, as it were, in Australia 16 years later under thoroughly comparable economic conditions. Cf. note 28.
52. The discussion on this relationship referred to by me as "difficult" as a way out of a dilemma – as I am unable to do justice to its complexity within the confines of this book – has as its main topic the role of the *I. G. Farben* in German Fascism.
53. In substance, this petition was more than well founded, and it was given high-level support by the successor organisation of his former employer, the Leverkusen plant of the *I.G.-Farben.* Briefly, the *UfA – Universum-Film A.-G.*, Germany's then prestigious film company – would have been inconceivable without Eichengrün's //Cellon//. Because of its political explosiveness, however, this last-ditch attempt was virtually hopeless, and the petition was rejected. Eichengrün may even then have been simply too loyal to assess the gravity of his situation realistically.
54. The similarity of the metaphors chosen by Eco and Koch might be evidence of the inductive-synthetic perspective intruding, if the problem dealt with here is to be approached with essentially semiotic interest.
55. In the English edition the term "campione fittizio" (Eco 1975: 288) is translated quite literally as "fictive sample" (Eco 1976: 220), which totally ignores the commodity-esthetic aspect of Eco's terminology.
56. 47 of the 238 Vulgata entries are incidentally preceded by /deo/ or /domino/ as a primary dative object to /placere/.
57. The following entry under the key word /placebo/ in the *Glossarium mediae et infirmiae latinitatis* by du Cange would appear to confirm this:

   "Vesperae pro defunctis ita designantur a prima earundum antiphora, in Testam. Franc. ducis Brit. ann. 1449. ex Bibl. reg.: Un anniversaere solemnel ... à Placebo, vigiles et messes des morts." (du Cange 1845: 275; cf. Steudel 1956).

58. Haas, Fink and Härtfelder (1959); Kissel and Barrucand (1964); Rinkel (1963); Schindel (1967); Rickels (1968); Binz (1977); Jospe (1978); White, Tursky and Schwartz (1985); Hippius, Überla, Laakmann and Hasford (1986).
59. The placebo definition proposed by the two authors at the start of their monograph shows, however, that they, too, obviously maintain the non-specificity of the placebo reaction as a matter of principle – obviously not only from the pharmacological standpoint:
"Mesure thérapeutique, d'efficacité intrinsèque nulle ou faible, sans rapport logique avec la maladie, mais agissant, si le sujet pense recevoir un traitement actif, par un mécanisme psychologique ou psycho-physiologique." ['Therapeutic measure of low or zero intrinsic effectivity, with no logical relation to the illness, but functioning by a psychological or psychophysiological mechanism if the subject believes that he is receiving active treatment.'] (Kissel – Barrucand 1964: 8).
60. Leslie (1954) has dealt with these ethical issues in an overview article, and Brody (1980) in a monograph. For current legal problems of placebo application in the research context, cf. Samson (1986) and Schreiber (1986).
61. From the pharmacological standpoint, the necessity for their terminological differentiation is connected for its part with the specificity problem: Though pharmacologically ineffective, //pseudoplacebos// are not non-specific, as they contain defined components or active substances prepared for therapeutic purposes. Genuine //placebos//, whilst effective in many cases, are in all events non-specific from the pharmacological standpoint, as they contain no defined components or active substances.
62. Attention is focused on this question in Jospe's (1978) monograph on the placebo problem.
63. The contradiction may derive from the fact that all placebo probands were provided with only one out of three possible degrees of information, without any reference to possible side-effects. It is quite feasible that a placebo group with such information would have experienced similar side-effects to those in the adrenalin groups. What speaks against this, however, is the fact that the degree of information had no significant effect on the actual side-effects within the adrenalin groups either. All in all, then, the remarkable finding that remains is that a result contradictory to empirical evidence was observed within the framework of a relatively meticulously planned study that was not carried out within the context of placebo research.
64. This has been described by Cleghorn, for instance (quoted in Beecher 1986) and by Shannon and Isbell (1963) with reference to the injecting of physiological saline solution.
65. This triangle extends between the sternal insertion and the front costal arches. This area is accessible to the examiner's stethoscope even without the patient removing his clothing, an important time-saving factor within the scope of 5-minute medical care. This ritual, sanctioned by German health insurance agencies, enables the physician to perform a clinical examination of all thoracic organs in one maneuver, as it were.
66. The terminological differentiation between "pseudoplacebos" and "impure placebos" is by no means so uniform in the placebo literature, as is shown below. The two terms are used on principle alternately for one of the two contexts differentiated here or as a collective term for both. With reference to the terminology problem, cf. Jospe (1978: XII-XV) and Binz (1977: 51).
67. Hyperemisation = stimulation of the (mostly superficial) blood flow in the tissues of a locally confined region.
68. Empirical counter-arguments for the necessity of this preliminary condition are, for example, Schindel's (1967) good therapeutic results with capsules in the previously ascertained favourite color of the probands, or the "nonblind" test design by Park and Covi

(1965) who achieved good therapeutic success with //placebos// that they had explicitly assured the probands to be pharmacologically ineffective.

69. Nor is this connection explained by the //vitamin C// likewise contained in this preparation. As a defined but (apart from in nutritional deficiency diseases) ineffective pharmacological substance, it is at most the function of a "pseudoplacebo" that is to be attributed to it. It may furthermore have some effect by confirming an attribution in the individual apprehension of many of its users: Vitamin C is good for the health. There are indeed some experimental indications that the localised concentration of //ascorbic acid// (= //vitamin C//) in the adrenal glands is reduced by the effect of //acetylsalicylic acid//. Whether this metabolic fluctuation has any effect at all and, if so, whether it might be compensated by oral administration of //ascorbic acid// is, however, still open to discussion.
70. Who some decades later wrote a book entitled *Die Unfähigkeit zu trauern* ['The inability to grieve'].
71. The relationship of the concept /the detection of similarity/, used here with reference to Meinertz, to the concept of /mimesis/ is, however, slightly clearer and less equivocal. /The detection of similarity/ may be understood as a proto-scientific process that is a preliminary to /mimesis/ when /mimesis/ is taken, according to Feldmann (1988: 17), to be "die Bedeutungs- und Sinnbeziehung menschlicher Sinngebilde zu etwas Wirklichem, das "dargestellt" wird schlechthin" ['the relationship of human symbols in both significance and meaning to something real that is capable of "representation"'].
72. "The articulation of the chaos of sensory impressions, in which definite groups based on similarities are picked out and specific series are formed, is, again, common to both logical and mythical thinking; without it, myth could no more arrive at stable configurations than logical thought at stable concepts." (Cassirer; 1955: 67)
73. For an informative introduction to the history of "Directions for use" leaflets, and for some of the implications of this history with regard to linguistic theory and health policies, see Zacharias; (1985).
74. In Plato's "Phaedo" (Plato 1958: 26–27 [§74a–75c]) /similarity/ is discussed as a precondition of /anamnesis/.
75. "Noch für die Heutigen läßt sich behaupten: Die Fälle, in denen sie im Alltag Ähnlichkeiten bewußt wahrnehmen, sind ein winziger Ausschnitt aus jenen zahllosen, da Ähnlichkeit sie unbewußt bestimmt." ['It is still possible to maintain that the everyday circumstances in which similarities are consciously perceived are only very few, in comparison with the countless number where similarity is unconsciously applied as a shaping force.'] (Benjamin 1984: 125)
76 (Johann Gudrius of Tours: Anatomia et physiognomia simplicium, quoted from Schlegel 1933: 95)
77. An interesting manifestation of diachronous similarity in the context of religious history is the Christian cult of relics during the late Middle Ages, which seems to have been motivated in part, at least, by the battle to regain a lost paradise, and which could be characterised as a cultural codification of collective, rather than individual, transitional objects. More thorough investigation would of course be necessary in order to determine whether this classification is historically appropriate. On the practice of using relics as remedies, see Kroos (1985).
78. In the English edition (Laplanche – Pontalis 1988: 464) this expression is translated as "special value". The literal translation is of special interest here, because the concept of /electivity/ is an important topic of chapter 3.3 below.

79. Virtual repetition of early childhood experience or lack of experience with homeomorphic identification, omnipotence or impotence is, of course, possible. Psychoanalysis groups them together under the heading "narcissistic disorder". Few adults would, however, in fact – like the mythical Narcissus – fall in love with their own mirror image. For the adult, the mirror serves rather as a mechanical aid, enabling him to find out, allowing for distortions, how other adults see him or her in the real world. Eco's comments (1985b: 9–25) are directed at this distinction.
80. Cf. the Old English recipe for a headache remedy, quoted above in Chapter 2, Figure 14. For detailed studies on the use of the //vulture// and parts of its body for medicinal purposes in the late Middle Ages, see Stürmer (1978) and Gerhardt (1981).
81. Maxwell's experimental proposition has caused particular controversy because it assumes that the "sortierende Intellekt" ['sorting intellect'] (Blumenberg 1986) would simply generate energy and not consume it, a proposition running counter to the second law of thermodynamics, according to which differences of temperature existing in a closed system tend to even out. Refutation of Mawell's assumption resulted in the establishment of a connection – of especial interest to a general theory of semiotics – between the thermodynamic concept of entropy, and the concept of entropy deriving from information theory, a "potentially very productive conception, which, however, can occasion incautious comparisons and generalisations" (Monod 1975: 173). The preservation of the second law of thermodynamics coincides temporally at least with its application to the line of enquiry introduced by Shannon and Weaver (1969). This coincidence may be pure chance, and is important and significant for precisely that reason, when related to Monod's argument.
82. "Maxwell consciously developed the use of analogy into a very perspicuous physical method ... The picture is imaginary and based on analogy but nevertheless intuitive: we do not take it as real and we know precisely how it coincides conceptually with the facts to be represented ... Without giving up intuition, Maxwell thus succeeds in preserving his open mind and conceptual purity, combining the advantages of hypothesis and mathematical formulation" (Mach 1976: 168–169)
83. Quecke (1955: 42) discusses the therapeutic recommendation, taken from the old Indian Atharva-Veda tradition, that yellow birds should be tied to the bedside of a person suffering from jaundice, and the Chinese tradition that jaundice should be treated with yellow-flowering plants. Further though rather brief examples of Eastern traditions, also referred to in discussion as "signature remedies", are given by Dann (1975: 11) and Winkler (1926: 946).
84. The dramatic structure of the dialogue's development is especially involved at this point. Immediately after Pausanias has rather abruptly come to the end of his speech on Eros and pederastic practices, the uninvited guest Aristodemos asks Aristophanes, the comic dramatist, if he will speak next. At precisely this moment, however, he has an attack of hiccups and asks his neighbour, the physician Eryximachos, either to cure his hiccups or to speak in his place. Eryximachos replies that he will do both, and then recommends a remedy of the /smelling salts/ variety:
"'I will do both,' replied Eryximachos. 'I will take your turn and you shall take mine when you are better. As for the hiccup, hold your breath for a good time while I am speaking. If that doesn't cure it, gargle with water. If the hiccup is too violent even for that, get something to tickle your nose with, and sneeze. One or two sneezes, and it will stop, however violent.'" (Plato 1951: 53 [§185e])
Eryximachos' contribution represents a kind of intermezzo in the symposium between the theory of a dual love propounded by Pausanias, and Aristophanes' mythological explana-

tion of the two sexes as arising from the violent and punitive dissolution of an original entity. The parable contributed by the fictional Aristophanes will receive more detailed attention in a later section (Chapter 3.3).

85. (Paracelsus 1928b: 145)
86. Heinrich Heine, whose "Almansor" contains the precept so often quoted in debate on Fascism – "Where books are burnt, in the end men too will burn" – wrote as follows on Paracelsus and the Paracelsian dialetic:
"Paracelsus was a great charlatan, and always wore a scarlet coat, breeches, stockings, and hat, and declared that he could make homunculi, or little men; at least he was in confidential relations with occult beings who dwell in different elements, but he was also one of the most profound philosophers, who, with the heart of a true German investigator, understood the pre-Christian popular faith of the German pantheism, and what they did not know they shrewly guessed." (Heine 1982:64)
On the one hand, as an impassioned enemy of authority Paracelsus certainly made an important contribution to the freeing of thought from dogmatism, he even formulated his personal attitude of "anything goes" (Feyerabend) into a kind of creed: "Alterius non sit, qui suus esse potest" ['No one should belong to someone else who could be his own man'] (quoted in Kaiser 1969: 44). On the other hand, he shares with Nietzsche, among others, the posthumous fate of seeing his name on the banner of fanatics intent on burning books. Whether this fate has anything to do with the concept of /free/ science, which the two men possibbly held in common, is a question which must remain open. An article published in 1941 under the title "Über Nietzsche und Paracelsus" ['On Nietzsche and Paracelsus'] contains the following:
"Er [Paracelsus K. S.] ist ein deutsches Schicksal. Sein Bild ist wie ein Symbol für deutsche Wesenheit, deutsche Haltung und deutsche Ritterlichkeit ... Gram, Unruhe, Wanderleben, Armut und Menschenhärte haben ihn nicht zu schwächen vermocht, er blieb zeitlebens der, der er blutgemäß und ererbter seelischer Art war, und sein Erbschicksal rahmt sein Lebensgeschick" ['He [Paracelsus; K..S.] embodies a German destiny. His image is like a symbol for German essence, German attitudes and German chivalry ... Sorrow, unrest, a life of travel, poverty and human hardship could not weaken him, all his life he remained the person which his blood and inherited disposition destined him to be, and the fate which was his inheritance shaped his individual fate'] (Strunz 1941: 243).
87. In connection with development of the "symbolic mode" Eco (1985a: 202) refers explicitly, among other things, to alchemy.
88. The authenticity of this treatise continues to be held in doubt by Paracelsian scholarship, above all because no autograph copies are extant, and because it contains some stylistic peculiarities. For these reasons, Quecke (1955) does not bring it into consideration at all in his article "Paracelsus' doctrine of signatures". Sudhoff (1928: xxxiii) summarises his reservations as follows: "So wie es uns vorliegt ist das Werk nicht aus Hohenheims Feder hervorgegangen ... In den vermutlich überarbeiteten Büchern steckt aber soviel berg- und hüttenmännisches, technisch-chemisches Wissen, daß man Schwierigkeiten haben würde, einen Autor aus dem dritten Viertel des 16. Jahrhnderts und auch noch im vierten Viertel, in dem es überarbeitet wurde (wie es scheint), einen Namen zu finden, dem man dies so ohne weiteres zutrauen könnte als Hohenheim oder Agricola. Es scheint mir doch genug Paracelsischen Wissens in diesen "Büchern" über das Wesen der Naturvorgänge zu stecken, um sie als doch möglicherweise zum Teil Hohenheimsche Ausarbeitungen oder Entwürfe dem Benutzer dieser Paracelsus-Ausgabe nicht vorenthalten zu sollen." ['In its present form, the work does not come from Hohenheim's pen ... However, the presumably revised

work contains so much information on mining and metal-working, as well as on technical and chemical subjects, that it would be difficult to find a writer from the third quarter of the sixteenth century, or from the last quarter, when it appears to have been revised, or to find a name one could more willingly attribute with so much knowledge, as Hohenheim or Agricola. It seems to me that sufficient Paracelsian knowledge is contained in these "books" on the essence of natural processes for them not to be withheld from users of this Paracelsus edition, who may wish to regard them as preliminary plans or drafts in part by Hohenheim himself.']

After a thorough discussion on the question of authenticity, Darmstaedter (1933: 115) draws the following conclusions: "... man kann m.E. doch wohl sagen, daß der Traktat "De Natura Rerum", der neben weniger Wichtigem und Wertvollem auch recht viel Beachtliches enthält, in der Hauptsache doch auf Paracelsus zurückgeht, dessen anderen Schriften dieser Traktat in Form und Inhalt nicht allzu fern steht. Hier und in anderen Fällen sollte m.E. auch der Sprachforscher mehr als bisher mit vergleichendem Studium weiterzukommen suchen." ['In my opinion, it can be said that the treatise "De natura rerum", which contains much that is of real excellence alongside matter of little importance or worth, stems in the main from Paracelsus. His other writings are not too dissimilar in form or content. In this case, as in others, it is my opinion that the question could possibly be resolved by research based on linguistic comparison.']

As far as any contribution to this question by research based on semiotics is concerned, it can be said that the highly differentiated terminology used for semiotic concepts in this treatise is entirely compatible with that used in the authenticated writings. The early work which developed the Paracelsian theory of semiotics furthest during the 1620s even has as its title a German version of the title of the treatise under discussion – "Von den natürlichen Dingen" (Paracelsus 1930).

89. Because the name of Paracelsus' birthplace Einsiedeln could be translated as 'hermitage' an alternative translation of Schipperges' phrase could be 'the magic ass in a forest cell'.
90. On the /chain/ as metaphor, cf. also above, Chapter 1.6.
91. The fact that Paracelsus here takes up an idea first put forward in his *Astronomia magna* and makes it more concrete, may be used as a further argument in evaluation of the authenticity of the treatise and its possible inclusion in his later works. However, the fact that the crucial term from the *Astronomia magna*, /mos et usus/, is not used here tends to argue against the authenticity of the treatise, and in favor of editorial distancing of its contents on the part of a later revision.
92. At this point it must be remembered that the anti-Semitic influence of the German Free Imperial Cities was still very strong, as is indicated by its culmination in the massacre which took place in the Jewish quarter in Cologne on St. Bartholomew's Day 1349. During the years Paracelsus spent travelling, Jewish quarters in many cities were razed to the ground after their inhabitants were charged with /desecrating the sacrament/ or /poisoning wells/ and had their rights to residence withdrawn. From this quotation it is impossible to ascertain whether Paracelsus' "yellow sign" refers to a stigmatising mark of impending pogrom or whether it refers to some badge of status – displayed by its bearer as a means of identification – along the lines of the attributes pertaining to guild-membership, which he also mentions.
93. Reference to Barthes (1985) is again relevant here, but cannot be pursued at this point.
94. Especially in his *De signatura rerum oder von der Geburt und Bezeichnung aller Wesen*, first published in 1622, and available in the Peuckert edition of the collected works (Boehme 1957), and in the Everyman's Library (Boehme 1912).

95. For a more detailed discussion, see Ströker 1982.
96. Schumacher (1944: 249f) tells of an "Angriff von C. H. Schultz auf seinen Zeitgenossen Hahnemann, der durch einen Vergleich der Lehren beider [Hahnemann und Paracelsus; K. S.] feststellen zu können glaubt, daß die "sogenannte neue Methode in all ihren Einzelheiten schon bei einem Schriftsteller der Reformationszeit (nämlich bei Paracelsus; der Verfasser [= Schumacher; K. S.]); von dessen ganzem System diese Methode bloß den verstümmelten praktischen Teil enthält, zu finden" sei; "... daß in der genannten neuen Methode, die physiologisch wohlbegründeten Prinzipien ihres wahren Schöpfers, nachlässig und unrichtig aufgefaßt, entstellt und in eine unbegründete, empirische Form gekleidet sind, von welcher aus sich jedoch alles an ihr auf seinen wirklichen Ursprung so deutlich zurückführen läßt, daß über die eigentlichen Quellen kein Zweifel sein kann." ['attack on Hahnemann made by his contemporary C. H. Schultz, who believed that a comparison of the two men's [i. e. Hahnemann's and Paracelsus'; K. S.] doctrines would prove that "the so-called new method [was present] in every detail in the work of a writer from the time of the Reformation (i. e. Paracelsus; the author [= Schumacher; K. S.]), and that these methods contained merely a garbled version of the practical portion of his complete system," and "that in the so-called new method, the physiologically sound principles of its true creator had been negligently and incorrectly interpreted, distorted, and clothed in an unfounded empirical form, which, however, so clearly betrayed its real origin that there could be no doubt at all of its actual source"."
Carl Heinrich Schultz' quote is taken – according to Schumacher's bibliographical note, which I have not verified – from his work: Die homöobiotische Medizin des Theophrastus Paracelsus, Berlin, 1831.
To judge by what is given here, Schultz' criticism is obviously intended to expose Hahnemann's plagiarism, rather than to call his methodology to task. The reference to Hahnemann's attempt to empiricise the Paracelsian system is, alas, without doubt intended as an accusation. On the accusation of plagiarism and its refutation by later followers and biographers of Hahnemann, see Schadewaldt's summary (1972, 1973).
97. On the nature of his semiotically motivated interest in the concept of symptoms, cf. Fräntzki 1976: 20–21.
98. Here it is by no means suggested that the effect of homeopathic remedies depends exclusively on such symbolisation and subtilisation. The meticulous attention to detail in the rhizomatic structure of homeopathic diagnosis is probably – with regard to its "homage to the unimportant" – far in advance of most current medical systems. One only needs to consider the close-meshed density of cross-references in Kent's (1979) repertoire.
The finding that a certain therapeutic procedure is excellently suited to the production of semiotic specificity does not, however, imply that the therapeutic procedure draws its strength from the semiotic. The observation that //homeotherapeutics// make better //placebos// in clinical practice than many //allotherapeutics// does not lead to the conclusion that they are not pharmacologically effective. The pharmacological basis of homeopathy remains largely unresearched. The placebo question is of vital importance to homeopathy today precisely because it is a topic not covered in homeopathic theory. In this connection, far too few homeopathic double-blind experiments have been conducted.
99. ['For some long years he had almost forgotten what human life was about and that he too had once laughed and grown angry, been foolish and clever, glad and sad. Now he only laughed whenever his chemical substances were the scene of some profusion of comic or unexpected developments.'] Gottfried Keller: A natural scientist discovers a method and travels in order to investigate it.

100. In the following discussion all dates and titles of works are taken from Valentin (1950), unless otherwise acknowledged.
101. Cf. Blumenberg (1986: 408): "Die Theorie bricht die Eselsbrücke der Veranschaulichung, welchen Dienst immer sie bei der Modellbildung geleistet haben mag, hinter sich ab, sobald sie analytisch und funktional vorangekommen ist." ['As it progresses towards analysis and application, theory destroys the fool's path of concrete representation, however valuable it may have been in the construction of hypotheses." And, again on the "fool's path": "The order that our mind imagines is like a net, or like a ladder, built to attain something. But afterward you must throw the ladder away, because you discover that, even if it was useful, it was meaningless. Er muoz gelichesame die leiter abewerfen, so er an ir ufgestigen ... Is that how you say it?" In Eco's novel (1983: 492) William of Baskerville, in conversation with Adson of Melk, attributes this sentence to "a mystic from your land".
The mystic from Adson's land (the monastery at Melk lies in present-day Austria) is, however, none other than Ludwig Wittgenstein, who writes in the Tractatus Logico-Philosophicus: "My propositions serve as elucidations in the following way: anyone who understands me eventually recognises them as nonsensical, when he has used them – as steps – to climb up beyond them. (He must, so to speak, throw away the ladder after he has climbed up it.)" (Wittgenstein 1961: 151)
102. It was not until the twentieth century that such a connection was re-established in processes such as electron microscopy and structural x-ray analysis, which, within certain limited fields, rendered the structure of macromolecules visible in the form of bands of light.
103. Blumenberg (1986: 229) says, for example, that he "hätte weder begriffen noch gebilligt, was Nietzsche schließlich zum Thema machen sollte: den Anthropomorphismus unseres Wirklichkeitsbildes" ['would neither have understood nor agreed with an idea much discussed later by Nietzsche – that our view of reality is conditioned by anthropomorphism'].
104. In German 'affinity' means Verwandtschaft. Adler (1987: 100) discusses the diachronicity of the German adjective /verwandt/, with reference to the dictionaries compiled by Adelung and the Brothers Grimm in the late eighteenth and the nineteenth centuries respectively:
"Tatsächlich wurde das Wort seit dem 16. Jahrhundert vom Verbum "verwenden" losgelöst für Verhältnisse jeder Art benutzt. Die Beschränkung auf Familienverhältnisse war eine Bedeutungsverengung. Spätere Verwendungen im übertragenen Sinne sind derart häufig, daß vielleicht der ältere, eigentliche Sinn fortgelebt hat. Aus diesem Grund dürfte sich das Wort für den chemischen Kontext geeignet haben. Es mußte nicht unbedingt als Anthropomorphismus aufgefaßt werden. Was es aber im chemischen Kontext bedeutete, mußte immer wieder neu erörtert werden." ['In fact, after the sixteenth century the word became detached from its verb "verwenden" (= 'to make use of'), and referred to relationships of every kind. Its limitation to family relationships was a restriction in meaning. Later figurative usage is so frequent that it suggests a survival of the older, literal meaning. This may explain the word's adoption in a chemical context, an adoption that need not necessarily be interpreted as anthropomorphism. Its meaning in this context, however, had to be constantly re-explained.']
Accordingly, the application of the adjective /verwandt/ to relationships other than family relationships was not necessarily metaphorical or anthropomorphic. An interesting hypothesis presents itself in the possible historical connection between development of the concept of affinity (Verwandtschaft) in eighteenth-century theories of chemical combination, and the Paracelsian mos et usus which forms the fourth branch of the doctrine of signatures. The doctrine was developed, of course, before the adjective /verwandt/ became restricted in meaning.

105. On Bergman's importance in the history of chemical terminology, cf. Crosland (1962: 144ff).
106. Adler (1987: 32–39) points out that the term /Wahlverwandtschaft/ cannot have originated in Heinrich Tabor's 1782 translation of Bergman's Disquisitio (the first English translation of this work was published in 1785), as Goethe scholarship had previously assumed. Tabor uses the more neutral formulation "von der Attraction", while /Wahlverwandtschaft/ first appears in the German translation of Bergman's introduction to Henrik Teofilus Scheffer's Chemische Vorlesungen 'chemical lectures' (Adler 1987: 34), a work far less widely known than Bergman's own Disquisitio. Adler also cites several even earlier instances of the concept. Francis Bacon, for example, uses the term /election/ in a context that can be considered chemical in the widest sense (Adler 1987: 47). Some manuscript lecture notes by William Cullen (1710–1790), written in 1748, contain a marginal note in the author's hand where the definitive word-pair /elective attraction/ is used (Adler 1987: 67–68). This reference is of particular interest because Bergman cannot have been familiar with Cullen's unpublished manuscript. Correspondence between their terms is not therefore the result of knowledge gleaned from reading, but of research in a common field. Adler points to a possible route of transmission.
107. In the eighteenth and nineteenth centuries Blutsturz 'hemorrhage' was a nosological term for all diseases whose causes could be attributed to considerable loss of blood (Höfler 1970: 699–700). Signs of external or internal hemorrhage connected, for example, with the expectoration or vomiting of blood, often gave grounds for such an etiological assumption. In many cases, though – as in Goethe's illness in July 1768 – there was no immediate visible evidence of hemorrhage, it was simply assumed to have occurred on the basis of general symptoms such as physical weakness or anemic skin colour. In the late nineteenth century Blutsturz became a specific term for hemorrhage of the lungs in advanced tuberculosis.
108. (Scherer quoted by Kuhn 1972: 268–269)
109. The English edition of the novel (Goethe 1971) translates: "Edward was the name of a wealthy baron in the prime of life", thus obscuring the narratorial act of "naming".
110. Here it is again useful to recall the complicated dramatic structure of the dialogue's development. Immediately after Pausanias has finished his account of the two aspects of love, Aristodemos asks Aristophanes to speak. Aristophanes, however, has an attack of the hiccups, and asks Eryximachos, a doctor, either to heal him or to take his place in the conversation. Eryximachos answers that he will do both at once, and further recommends that Aristophanes should find something to tickle his nose with until he sneezes, a certain cure for hiccups. As a sort of interlude between Pausanias' and Aristophanes' speeches, Eryximachos explains the universal significance which the two aspects of love hold for medicine. (Plato 1951: 53–54 [§185–187]) Aristophanes, fully recovered from the hiccups, then tells his myth, but not before he has marvelled at the nature of his cure: "I can't help wondering whether it is the virtuous love in my body which desires such noises and tickling sensations as a sneeze." (Plato 1951: 58 [§189])
111. "Not a good likeness" would here, in semiotic terminology, have to be translated as /non-iconic/, since it refers, of course, to a picture. There is no doubt, however, that the picture as a sign bears a relationship to something absent which can certainly be described as /similarity/, if not as iconicity.
112. ['In 1932, while I was abroad, I began to realise that I would soon have to leave my native city for a very long time, perhaps for ever. The process of inoculation had often before been salutory in my inner life; I applied it in this situation, too, and deliberately called to

mind those images which in exile can awaken the most powerful sort of homesickness – the memories of childhood. Feelings of longing were to gain as little power over my mind as inoculation does over a healthy body. I tried to contain them through the insight, not that a return to chance biographical past was impossible, but that a return to a past social order had of necessity become impossible.']

113. Cf. Tsouyopoulos 1982: 10–18 for a detailed account.
114. Ehrlich's surname has in the German lexical system the additional meaning of 'honest'. His colleagues used to make fun of his unflagging polychromous enthusiasm by modifying the German proverb "ehrlich währt am längsten" 'honesty is the best policy' into "Ehrlich färbt am längsten" 'Ehrlich's colours are the fastest'.
115. (Marquardt 1951: 82, 84).
116. What is particularly remarkable here is the fact that Ehrlich renounces the expression *Wahlverwandtschaft* although it had been lexicalised in the very context to which he refers in the quoted passage.
117. ['This heart- and nerve-remedy might have been called: lavender-rosmary-goose grass-balm-hop-valerian tonic. But this seemed too long to us. So we called it "Galama" for short. For invigorated nerves, for refreshing sleep and a serene heart: GALAMA!'] (Text of a German television advertisement from the 1970s)
118. Contergan was the German proprietary name for thalidomide.
119. Cf. Jäger (1956), Klickow (1963, 1964), Lemay (1968), Sialm-Bossard (1975), and in the broader sense Praninskas (1968). One exception is to be found in Lötscher's publication; he writes, for example:
"Warennamen sind gewöhnlich «Retortenwörter». Man produziert Wörter in diesem Bereich wie Kunststoffe oder Medikamente: Durch Synthese gewinnt man Stoffe, die so in der Natur nie vorkommen ... Aber sogar diese Kunstsprache teilt das Schicksal jeder Sprache, Gesellschaftsgut einer Gesellschaft zu sein, Traditionen zu bilden und historisch gewachsenen Konventionen zu unterliegen." ['Trade names are customarily «test-tube words». Words are produced in this field like plastics or drugs: substances never occurring in such a form in Nature are gained by synthesis... But even this synthetic language shares the fate of every language: that of being the common property of a society, forming traditions and being subject to conventions rooted in history.'] (Lötscher 1987: 288).
120. During my early internship, I was once in charge of a patient who was being treated with a //cytostatic agent// by the name of /Platinex/ and was suffering from violent nausea. Although the infusion solution of this preparation was colorless, the infusion bottle was always wrapped in metallic foil because the solution had to be kept away from direct sunlight. The patient was keeping his nausea successfully under control by eating regularly, though in small quantities, candies that he had always liked but rarely treated himself to. He was astounded to find that he developed an insuperable repulsion to just one of these candies – chocolate, of which he had once been passionately fond. He himself ascribed this aversion primarily to the fact that the chocolate bars were wrapped in metal foil, just like his infusion bottle of //Platinex//.
121. Surveys on this problem are to be found in Gaus and Kubanek (1984) and in Schultz and Raedler (1986).
122. For criticism of this myth, cf. Gipper (1978: 226–227) and Hörmann (1978: 92–109).
123. In order to accentuate this difference, one should avoid speaking of "semantic differentials" in conjunction with this method. Terms such as /association differential/ or even /connotation differential/ might be more appropriate. But they, too, might suggest the inappropriate

claim of /measurability/, which is – as declared – not to be made here. For this reason it is only /Osgood differentials/ that will be referred to below (except in quotations).

124. This term is used here with reference to Hofstaetter (1955).
125. The consequence of this is that there were fundamentally two different types of questionnaire in circulation: one with partially "forged" names of cytostatic agents and one with partially "forged" names of sedatives. These phonetically minimal (though semiotically quite possibly significant) differences were not taken into account when forming the arithmetical factors from the collected data. With respect to factor formation, this phonetic manipulation was thus taken into the bargain as a confounding, uncontrolled variable.
126. There were two reasons for this assumption: (1) This phonetic combination consists of phonemes classified as exceptionally moving in Ertel's sample (1969: 101) – to which more detailed reference is made below. (2) It contains a preproprial reference to the Latin root sagitta = 'arrow'.
127. Computation was done with the SPSS program installed at the computer center of Cologne University, addressed interactively by a microcomputer in the university's Department of Psychosomatics.
128. For further detail, cf. Überla (1968) and Bortz (1977: 627)
129. Using the "BREAKDOWN" procedure of the SPSS system (cf. Steinhausen – Zörkendörfer 1987: 56).
130. This exception is formed by the pair of names /Galama/ and /Balama/, which records by far the smallest distance among all those investigated. The "genuine" sedative name /Galama/ does, however, play an exceptionally small role in the everyday working situation of doctors and medical students, because the herbal sedative //Galama// is used almost exclusively in the sphere of self-medication, in other words outside hospitals and medical practices.
131. Although no published studies on this aspect are at my disposal, it will even be possible to insinuate that the use of Osgood differentials within the framework of this product design may well play an important methodological role.
132. This observation is inadmissible in so far as the two opposing sides are inseparably interlinked, even interwoven, in the consciousness of the medical profession today. On the other hand, it is justified in that the two systems did indeed arise relatively independently of each other from the heuristic standpoint and that the majority of successful connections established between them in history were chance discoveries.
133. Some of these ointments also contain substances with a proven antiphlogistic effect. But they develop this effect only on reaching the location at which they are to act, e.g. when injected direct into a joint affected with rheumatism or arthritis. The transdermal resorption rate of these //antiphlogistics// is, however, so low that therapeutic concentrations can most likely not be attained even in the skin itself. In addition to the resorption problem, joint diseases present the additional problem of joints – as so-called /bradytrophic/ tissues (= those /slowly absorbing nourishment/) – having virtually no part in the intermediary metabolic process. For this reason it is difficult to attain therapeutic concentrations in the joint even when the substance is injected intravenously to circumvent the resorption problem.
134. This figure refers exclusively to the diagnostic complex "arthritis, rheumatism". The overall prescription rate for these preparations in the Federal Republic of Germany in 1983 was 24.999 million (Hardenberg 1989).
135. The table below is based on a study by Hardenberg (1988) who kindly placed his material, some of it unpublished, at my disposal.

136. The only point possibly worth adding is that the synthetic word /Dolo-Arthrosenex/ generates its semiotic specificity at two different levels of syntagma formation simultaneously, depending on how it is dissected. One of these levels is also accessible to the medically uninformed layman, whereas the other demands a certain pathogenetic concept of the genesis of arthrosis. An appropriate translation, roughly speaking, for the syntagma /dolo-arthrosen-ex/ would be an /agent driving out arthrosis-induced pain/. On dissection into /dolo-arthro-senex/, however, the message imparted by the syntagma would be roughly /agent against painful joint diseases caused by ageing processes, i. e. by biological wear/. This distinction is probably of no significance, however, in realising what is to be designated below, with a term coined by Haug (1980), as "promise of use value".
137. On the other hand, the study by Park and Covi (1965) shows that placebo effects do not vanish completely even when both the doctor and the patient have been informed of the pharmacological ineffectuality of a substance.
138. /Esthetic/ is to be understood here in the sense of Haug's "operational" definition: "Das Ästhetische bestimmen wir hierbei abweichend von der üblichen Begriffsverwendung im Sinne einer vorläufigen operationalen Definition (d. h. einer Definition, mit der wir im Rahmen unserer Untersuchung "arbeiten"/"operieren" können). Und zwar verwenden wir diesen Begriff nicht im Sinne einer Kunsttheorie, sondern näher am ursprünglichen (griechischen) Wortsinn: als die Sinnlichkeit einer Sache, die uns ihren "Sinn" vergegenwärtigt. Unter dem Ästhetischen einer Sache fassen wir aber ihre sinnliche Erscheinung nicht irgendwie, sondern darin, wie sie unsere "Sinnlichkeit" anspricht. Für unseren Zweck brauchen wir also keinen normativen Begriff des Ästhetischen." ['Notwithstanding the conventional use of the term, the esthetic is used here in the sense of a provisional operational definition (i. e. a definition with which we can "work"/"operate" within the framework of our study). We use this term not in the sense of art theory but more closely to the original (Greek) meaning: as the sensuousness of an object that represents its "sense" to us. Under the esthetic of an object, however, we understand its sensory appearance not just in some way but in how it appeals to our "sensuousness". For our purpose, then, we need no normative concept of the esthetic.'] (Haug 1980: 23).
It should be noted that the essential accents of this "operational" definition comply precisely with what is emphasised by a semiotic theory of the esthetic (cf. Mukarovsky 1970).
139. Literally: So that something will happen.
140. In this case too, it is clear that consideration of statistical data of this kind permits no conclusions to be drawn as to the respective motive for prescribing the preparation. The empirical data merely permit or preclude certain interpretations. The trend described here might thus also be due to increasing cost-consciousness among prescribing physicians in general, as propagated by legislation.
141. Among these illnesses – it would have to be admitted within the framework of this debate – special significance is due to addictions, since dependence on consumption is a specific component of their pathological process. This virtually eliminates the role of critical reasoning on the part of the consumer. It is on this weak link within the chain of reasoning set out here that an important part of the "apocalyptic" criticism levelled at drug advertising is also based when it asserts that this generates addiction (cf. Stoessel 1973: 83–88).
142. Cf. the "Dokumentation III (Pharma-Kodex)" published by the A. O. K.-Bundesverband [controlling society of public health insurance agencies] (1986) in which this codex and some examples of its effect on advertising behaviour in general are subjected to critical comment from the standpoint of a consumer association.

143. This was the result reported by a doctor practising in Wiesbaden, Germany, who collected the unsolicited material sent and offered to him in the course of one month, projected the volume to cover one calendar year and reported these data in a reader's letter to the Deutsche Medizinische Wochenschrift (reproduced in: Anonymous: 1985)
144. "Im Durchschnitt wird jeder praktizierende Arzt zwischen 180 und 200 mal im Jahr von Ärztebesuchern besucht." ['On average, each medical practitioner is visited between 180 and 200 times a year by pharmaceutical representatives.'] (Nord 1976: 61; data refer to 1974).
145. "Diese Symposien (die als Gastmähler ihrem Namen Ehre machen) sind nur ein Teil eines dichten PR-Netzes, dem im Wirtschaftszweig "Gesundheit" kaum jemand entgeht." ['These symposia (which, as banquets, do credit to their name) are only part of a dense PR network from which there is virtually no escape in the "health" sector of the economy.'] (Anonymous:1988: 35)
146. I have not succeeded in tracking down any published statistical data relating to this. Personal information provided to me by experienced colleagues – whom I am unable to quote here as a source – suggests, however, that the proportion of medical practitioners refusing contact is between 10 and 20% and that the figure is considerably higher among hospital physicians.
147. "Auf die berufstätigen Ärzte in der Bundesrepublik bezogen wandte die Pharma-Industrie 1969 pro Arzt für Anzeigen in Fachzeitschriften und "die informative Ärztewerbung" DM 5.194,84 auf, 1972 waren es 5.932,97." ['With reference to medical practitioners in the Federal Republic of Germany, the pharmaceutical industry spent DM 5,914.84 on medical journals and "informative medical publicity" for each practitioner in 1969, and DM 5,932.97 in 1972." (Nord 1976: 56)

    Friedrich, Hehn and Rosenbrock (1977: 121) calculated the total cost factor for the reference year 1971 at between DM 0.8 thousand million and DM 1 thousand million per year for "das Werbemedium Ärztebesucher samt den durch sie induzierten Werbeausgaben" ['the advertising medium constituting pharmaceutical representatives together with the expenditure induced by them on advertising.']

    According to a "strictly confidential study" by the pharmaceutical industry, quoted in the economics-orientated periodical "Das Capital" in December 1984 and in the medical journal "Arzneimittelbrief" in May 1988 (Anonymous 1988: 33), the total amount budgeted for advertising purposes by pharmaceutical companies established in the Federal Republic of Germany in the reference year 1983 was DM 1.7 thousand million.
148. A detailed discussion of this question is to be found in Nord (1976: 53–79). From the "integrated" standpoint, repeated reference is made in this context to an empirically interesting constellation: In all reference years for which comparable figures are available, pro capita consumption of analgesics – i. e. on a market sector where a special consumption-raising effect of drug advertising is suspected by some "apocalyptic" critics – was distinctly higher and displayed a distinctly stronger growth trend in the GDR than in the FRG, where expenditure on advertising these preparations was definitely far higher (cf. NORD 1976: 64). This finding is certainly of significance, though hardly a decisive factor, in the question under discussion. Marked appetitive behavior among members of communist societies towards products reputed among the business public in the capitalist world to be guilty of consumer terrorisation is found in many consumer goods areas without permitting conclusions to be drawn on the influence of the advertising factor.
149. Langbein, Martin et al. (1983: 58) also quote in their study a passage from the editorial of the /Pharma-Marketing-Journal/ (vol. 2, 1979, p. 39) which underlines this finding from

the pharmaceutical representative's viewpoint. The question "Würde der Arzt zum (niedergelassenen) Pharmareferenten kommen, um sich seine ... Informationen abzuholen?" ['Would the doctor come to the (practising) pharmaceutical representative ... to obtain his ... information'] is answered there as follows: "Natürlich nicht. Der Arzt würde nicht kommen, weil er kaum Informationen erwartet, weil er die Informationen für (oft) zu banal hält, weil die Informationen zu häufig Informations-Dubletten sind." ['Of course not. The doctor wouldn't come, because he expects hardly any information, because he (often) considers the information too commonplace, because the information is too often duplicated.']

150. The question of the drug speciality is given a certain residue of pharmacological rationality in that the individual specialities are occasionally distinguished not only by their sensory appearance but by the fact that the substances contained in them are processed in different ways or bound to different carriers. This question cannot, though, be clarified by the doctor in contact with the pharmaceutical representative, since the latter will basically have only one standard answer to offer: /Our bio-availability is the best of all/.
151. "Dem ästhetischen Gebrauchswertversprechen zuliebe wird hier der [pharmakologische] Gebrauchswert partiell ... [vernachlässigt]." (Haug 1980: 47)
152. The term /transitional object/ coined by Winnicott (cf. Chapter 3.1) operates with a similar analogisation from the reverse perspective by comparing – inter alia – pharmacological addiction phenomena occurring in adult life with interpersonal dependency relationships in early childhood.
153. In the index to the 11th edition of the Pharmakologie-Lehrbuch by Kuschinsky and Lüllmann (Stuttgart/Thieme 1987, p. VIII), a trace of this terminological proximity has been left in the form of a printing error: The /Rezeptortheorie/ (= receptor theory) section in the /heuristic principles/ subchapter of the general part is listed in this index as /Rezepttheorie/ (= prescription or recipe theory). This printing error does not appear in the earlier editions and is presumably an outcome of the new layout of the type area. For this reason it would hardly be appropriate to regard it as an error in substance by the authors; even so, it must have survived several rounds of attentive proof-reading by experts, in view of its eye-catching position in a high-circulation standard textbook.

References

Ackerknecht, Erwin H.
1973 *Geschichte der Medizin.* Stuttgart: Enke.

Ader, Robert
1981 *Psychoneuroimmunology.* New York: Academic Press.

Adler, Jeremy D.
1987 *Eine fast magische Anziehung – Goethes "Wahlverwandtschaften" und die Chemie seiner Zeit.* Munich: Beck.

Adlung, A. – G. Urdang
1935 *Grundriß der Geschichte der deutschen Pharmazie.* Berlin: Springer.

Adorno, Theodor Wiesengrund – Max Horkheimer
1979 *Dialectic of Enlightenment.* London: Verso.

Ahlheim, Karl-Heinz
1972 *Wie funktioniert das? – Medikamente/Gifte/Drogen.* Mannheim: Bibliographisches Institut.

Alstaedter, Rosemarie
1963 "Unvergleichliche Karriere – Die Aspirin Story", *Euromed* 6. 8. 1963, 714–717.
1983 *Aspirin – Ein Jahrhundertpharmakon.* Leverkusen: Bayer.

Anonymous
(n.d.) *Paul Ehrlich – Forscher für das Leben.* Hoechst: Hoechst. (Catalogue for a rotating exhibition by Hoechst AG, June 1979.)

Anonymous
1915 "La Fraude de l'Aspirine", *Humanité* 14. 12. 1915.

Anonymous
1972 "Drug or Placebo?", *The Lancet* 15. 7. 1972, 122–123.

Anonymous
1977 "Diamond Jubilee of Aspro", *The Medical Journal of Australia 64*, 355–356.

Anonymous
1985 "Altpapier für Ärzte", *Frankfurter Rundschau* 16. 7. 1985.

Anonymous
1988 "Die Abhängigkeit der medizinischen Zeitschriften von der Werbung", *Der Arzneimittelbrief* 22, 33–35.

Anschütz, Felix
1985 "Schmerz und Placebo", *Diagnostik* 18, Nr. 13, 4–4.

AOK Bundesverband
1986 *Dokumentation III – Pharma-Kodex.* Bonn: Bundesverband der Ortskrankenkassen.

Bär, Eugen
1983 "A semiotic history of symptomatology", in: Achim Eschbach – Jürgen Trabant (eds.): *History of semiotics.* Amsterdam: Benjamins, 41–66.

Baier, Horst
1988 "Der Einbruch der Herrschaft in die Medizin", *Deutsches Ärzteblatt* 85, 1321–1322.

Balint, Michael
1960 *Der Arzt, sein Patient und die Krankheit.* Stuttgart: Klett. (2nd edition.)
1964 *The Doctor, his Patient and the Illness.* Edinburgh: Churchill Livingstone. (2nd edition.)

Barthes, Roland
1965 "Eléments de Sémiologie", *Communications* 4, 91–134.
1984 *Writing Degree Zero & Elements of Semiology.* London: Cape.
1985 *The fashion system.* London: Cape.

Bayer AG (section Pharma) (ed.)
(n.d.) *Wer hat hier Aspirin benutzt? – Ein Medikament in der Weltliteratur.* Leverkusen: Bayer.

Bayer-archive
Unpublished archival files (product files "Aspirin", personnel files "Dreser", "Eichengrün", "Hoffmann").

Beecher, Henry K.
1968 "Placebo Effects of Situations, Attitudes, and Drugs – A Quantitative Study of Suggestibility", in: K Rickels (ed.), 27–39.

Benjamin, Walter
1970 "The Work of Art in the Age of Mechanical Reproduction", in: *Walter Benjamin: Illuminations.* London: Cape.
1984 *Allegorien kultureller Erfahrung – Ausgewählte Schriften 1920–1940.* Leipzig: Reclam.
1987 *Berliner Kindheit um neunzehnhundert.* Frankfurt: Suhrkamp.

Bense, Max – Elisabeth Walther
1973 *Wörterbuch der Semiotik.* Cologne: Kiepenheuer & Witsch.

Bentele, Günter – Ivan Bystrina
1978 *Semiotik.* Stuttgart: Kohlhammer.

Bergman, Torbern
1968 *Dissertation on Elective Attractions.* New York: Johnson. (Originally published as *Disquisitio de attractionibus electivis*, Uppsala 1775, translated and edited by J. A. Schufle.)

Binz, Ursula
1977 Das Placebo-Phänomen. (Mannheim: Doctoral thesis submitted to Mannheim Academy of Economics.)

Bliesener, Thomas
1982 *Die Visite – Ein verhinderter Dialog.* Tübingen: Narr.

Bliesener, Thomas – Johannes Siegrist
1981 "Greasing the Wheels – Conflicts on the Round and how they are managed", *Journal of Pragmatics* 5, 181–204.

Bliesener, Thomas – Karl Köhle
1985 *Die Visite – Eine Chance zum Gespräch.* Opladen: Westdeutscher Verlag.

Bloch, Ernst
1919 "Die antike Atomistik in der neueren Geschichte der Chemie", *Isis* 1, 377–415.

Blumenberg, Hans
1951 "Das Verhältnis von Natur und Technik als philosophisches Problem", *Studium Generale* 4, 461–467.
1957 "Nachahmung der Natur – Zur Vorgeschichte der Idee des schöpferischen Menschen", *Studium Generale* 10, 266–283.

1960 "Paradigmen zu einer Metaphorologie", *Archiv für Begriffsgeschichte* 6, 7–142.

1986 *Die Lesbarkeit der Welt.* Frankfurt/M.: Suhrkamp.

Blumenthal, David – Robert Burke – Arthur K. Shapiro

1974 "The Validity of 'Identical Matching Placebos'", *Archives of General Psychiatry* 31, 214–215.

Bock, Henning – Rainald Grosshans

1980 "Das Bildnis – Das autonome Porträt seit der Renaissance", in: Staatliche Museen Preußischer Kulturbesitz (ed.): *Bilder vom Menschen in der Kunst des Abendlandes.* Berlin: Staatliche Museen Preußischer Kulturbesitz, 143–196.

Boehme, Jakob

[1912] *The Signatures of All Things.* London: Dent, New York: Dutton. (Everyman's Library.)

[1957] *De signatura rerum oder von der Geburt und Bezeichnung aller Wesen.* (Will-Erich Peuckert (ed.): Jakob Boehme – Sämtliche Werke, Vol. VI). Stuttgart: Frommann. (Originally published in 1622.)

Boisserée, Sulpiz

[1970] *Briefwechsel / Tagebücher,* Vol. II: "Briefwechsel mit Goethe". Göttingen: Vandenhoeck & Ruprecht. (Facsimile of 1st edition Stuttgart: Cotta 1862.)

Bortz, Jürgen

1977 *Lehrbuch der Statistik für Sozialwissenschaftler.* Berlin: Springer.

Brody, Howard

1980 *Placebos and the philosophy of medicine – Clinical, conceptual and ethical issues.* Chicago: University of Chicago Press.

Brown, Gillian – George Yule

1983 *Discourse Analysis.* Cambridge: Cambridge University Press.

Brüggemann, Rolf

1987 "Pharmakonzerne werben für Drogen", *Psychologie heute* 14, No. 8, 58–65.

Buchholz, Gerhard

1981 *Arzt, Medizin und Heilmittelwerbung im Spiegel einer deutschen Provinzzeitung.* Cologne: Deutscher Ärzte Verlag.

Buchner, Dietrich

1967 Kommunikation zwischen Industrie und Medizin durch Hauszeitschriften für Ärzte. (Cologne: Dissertation submitted to the Faculty of Economics and Social Sciences.)

Bundesverband der pharmazeutischen Industrie (ed.)

1985 *Kodex der Mitglieder des Bundesverbandes der Pharmazeutischen Industrie e. V.* Aulendorf: Cantor.

Bungard, Walter (ed.)

1980 *Die "gute" Versuchsperson denkt nicht – Artefakte in der Sozialpsychologie.* Munich: Urban & Schwarzenberg.

Bynum, William F.

1970 "Chemical Structure and Pharmacological Action – A Chapter in the History of 19th Century Molecular Pharmacology", *Bulletin of the History of Medicine* 44, 519–538.

Campe, Joachim Heinrich

[1970] *Wörterbuch der Deutschen Sprache – Wörterbuch zur Erklärung der unserer Sprache aufgedrungenen fremden Ausdrücke.* Hildesheim: Olms. (Reprint of the 2nd edition Brunswick: Schulbuchhandlung 1813.)

Cange, Charles Dufresne du
1845 *Glossarium mediae et infimiae latinitatis,* Tomus 5. Paris: Didot.
Canguilhem, Georges
1972 *Le normal et le pathologique.* Paris: Presses Universitaires.
1989 *The Normal and the Pathological* (with an introduction by Michel Foucault). New York: Zone Books.
Cassirer, Ernst
1955 *The Philosophy of Symbolic Forms, Volume II.* New Haven, New York: Yale University Press.
1977 *Philosophie der symbolischen Formen, Band 2.* Darmstadt: Wissenschaftliche Buchgesellschaft.
Castelli, Bartolomeo
[1713] *Lexicon medicum Graeco-Latinum.* Leipzig: Fritsch. (Revised and edited by Jacob Pancratius Bruno et al., 1st edition Messina 1598.)
Classen, W. – E. Feingold
1985 "Use of Placebos in Medical Practice", *Pharmacopsychiatry* 18, 131–132.
Cockayne, Thomas Oswald
[1961] *Leechdoms, Wordcunning and Starcraft* (3 Volumes). London: Holland Press. (Reprint of 1st edition 1864–1866.)
Coleman, James – Herbert Menzel – Elihu Katz
1973 "Social Processes in Physicians' Adoption of a New Drug", in: Armitai Etzioni et al. (eds.), *Social Change.* New York: Basic Books, 457–472.
Cornfeld, Betty – Owen Edwards
1985 *Quintessenz – Die schönen Dinge des Lebens.* Munich: Popa.
Coulthard, Malcolm – Margaret Ashby
1975 "Talking with the Doctor", *Journal of Communications* 25, 140–147.
Crosland, Maurice P.
1962 *Historical Studies in the Language of Chemistry.* London: Heinemann.
Dale, Henry H.
1956 "Introduction", in: F. Himmelweit (ed.): *Paul Ehrlich – Gesammelte Arbeiten/ Collected Papers,* Vol I. Berlin/London: Springer/Pergamon.
Danckwardt, Joachim F.
1978 "Zur Interaktion von Psychotherapie und Psychopharmakotherapie", *Psyche* 32, 111–154.
Dann, Georg Edmund
1975 *Einführung in die Pharmaziegeschichte.* Stuttgart: Wissenschaftliche Verlagsgesellschaft.
Darmstaedter, Ernst
1933 "Paracelsus, De Natura Rerum – Eine kritische Studie", *Janus* 37, 1–8, 48–62, 109–115, 323–324.
Debus, Friedhelm
1977 "Aspekte zum Verhältnis Name-Wort", in: Hugo Steger (ed.): *Probleme der Namenforschung im deutschsprachigen Raum.* Darmstadt: Wissenschaftliche Buchgesellschaft, 3–25.
Deleuze, Gilles – Felix Guattari
1977 *Rhizom.* Berlin: Merve.
Deneke, J. F. Volrad
1961 "Arznei- und Heilmittelwerbung in den Zeitungen des 18. Jahrhunderts", *Ärztliche Mitteilungen* 46, 717–720.

Dijk, Teun A. van
1980 *Textwissenschaft.* Munich: dtv.
Dijk, Teun A. van – Walter Kintsch
1983 *Strategies of Discourse Comprehension.* New York: Harcourt.
Dillemann, Georges
1977 "Acide acétylsalicylique et Aspirine", *Revue d'Histoire de la Pharmacie* 24, 99–105.
Doepner, Ulf
1980 *Heilmittelwerbegesetz – Kommentar.* Munich: Vahlen.
Dorfles, Gillo
1974 *Simbolo, communicazione, consumo.* Turin: Einaudi. (3rd edition.)
Dreser, Heinrich
1899 "Pharmakologisches über Aspirin (Acetylsalicylsäure)", *Archiv für die gesamte Physiologie des Menschen und der Thiere* 76, 306–318.
Ebstein, Erich
1923 *Ärzte-Memoiren aus vier Jahrhunderten.* Berlin: Springer.
Eco, Umberto
1964 *Apocalittici e integrati.* Milan: Bompiani.
1972 *Einführung in die Semiotik.* Munich: Fink.
1975 *Trattato di semiotica generale.* Milan: Bompiani.
1976 *A Theory of Semiotics.* Bloomington: Indiana University Press.
1977a *Zeichen – Einführung in einen Begriff und seine Geschichte.* Frankfurt/Main: Suhrkamp.
1977b *Das Offene Kunstwerk.* Frankfurt/Main: Suhrkamp.
1980 *Il nome della rosa.* Milan: Bompiani.
1983 *The Name of the Rose.* London: Secker & Warburg, Picador/Pan Books.
1984a *Semiotica e filosofia del linguaggio.* Turin: Einaudi.
1984b *Semiotics and the Philosophy of Language.* London: Macmillan.
1985a *Semiotik und Philosophie der Sprache.* Munich: Fink.
1985b *Sugli specchi e altri saggi.* Milan: Bompiani.
1987a *Semiotik – Entwurf einer Theorie der Zeichen.* Munich: Fink.
1987b *Lector in fabula.* Munich: Hanser.
Ehlich, Konrad
1983 "Development of writing as social problem solving", in: Konrad Ehlich – Florian Coulmas (eds.): *Writing in Focus.* Berlin: Mouton, 99–129.
1985 "The Language of Pain", *Theoretical Medicine* 6, 177–187.
Ehrlich, Paul
1893 *Constitution, Vertheilung und Wirkung chemischer Körper.* Leipzig: Thieme.
[1956] "Beiträge zur Theorie und Praxis der histologischen Färbung", in: F. Himmelweit (ed.): *Paul Ehrlich – Gesammelte Arbeiten/Collected Papers (vol.I).* Berlin/London: Springer/Pergamon. (1st edition: Leipzig: Medical Dissertation, 1878.)
[1957a] "The Assay of the Activity of Diphtheria-curative Serum", in: F. Himmelweit (ed.): *Paul Ehrlich – Gesammelte Arbeiten/Collected Papers (vol. II).* Berlin/London: Springer/Pergamon. (First published 1897.)
[1957b] "On Immunity with Special Reference to Cell Life – Croonian Lecture", in: F. Himmelweit (ed.): *Paul Ehrlich – Gesammelte Arbeiten/Collected Papers (vol.II).* Berlin/London: Springer/Pergamon. (First published 1900.)

[1957c] "Über moderne Chemotherapie", in: F. Himmelweit (ed.): *Paul Ehrlich – Gesammelte Arbeiten/Collected Papers (vol. III)*. Berlin/London: Springer/Pergamon. (First published 1908.)

Eichengrün, Arthur

1949 "50 Jahre Aspirin", *Die Pharmazie* 4, 582–584.

Eimeren, W. van

1986 "Im Placebo-Konzept implizite Vorstellungen über Wirksamkeit und deren Auswirkungen auf die Pharma-Markt-Gestaltung", in: Hanns Hippius et al. (eds.), 23–28.

Erhard, Hubert

1956 "Paracelsus, die Bienen und die 'Signaturen'", *Gesnerus* 13, 215–218.

Ertel, Suitbert

1969 *Psychophonetik – Untersuchungen über Lautsymbolik und Motivation*. Göttingen: Hogrefe.

Fabrega, Horacio – Stephen Thyma

1976 "Language and Cultural Influences in the Description of Pain", *British Journal of Medical Psychology* 49, 349–371.

Feldmann, Harald

1988 *Mimesis und Wirklichkeit*. Munich: Fink.

Ferreira, Sergio H. – Meire Nakamura

1979 "Prostaglandin Hyperalgesia – A cAMP/Ca2+ Dependant Process", *Prostaglandins* 18, 179–190.

Feyerabend, Paul

1978 *Against Method*. London: Verso.

1986 *Wider den Methodenzwang*. Frankfurt/Main: Suhrkamp.

Fischer, Bonifatius (ed.)

1977 *Novae Concordantia Bibliorum Sacrorum Iuxta Vulgatam Versionem Critice Editam*, Tomus IV. Stuttgart: Frommann-Holzboog.

Fish, Jefferson M.

1973 *Placebo Therapy*. San Francisco: Jossey Bass.

Fleck, Ludwik

1979 *Genesis and Development of a Scientific Fact*. Chicago: University of Chicago Press.

[1982] *Entstehung und Entwicklung einer wissenschaftlichen Tatsache*. Frankfurt/Main: Suhrkamp. (1st edition Basle: Schwabe 1935.)

Folkerts GmbH

1986 TV Spot "Galama", motive No. 34/77. Personal communication.

Foucault, Michel

1970 *The Order of Things*. London: Tavistock Publications.

1974 *Die Ordnung der Dinge*. Frankfurt/Main: Suhrkamp.

1976a *Die Geburt der Klinik*. Frankfurt: Ullstein.

1976b *The Birth of the Clinic*. London. New York: Routledge.

1983a *Dies ist keine Pfeife*. Frankfurt: Ullstein.

1983b *This is Not a Pipe*. Berkeley, Los Angeles, London: University of California Press.

Fräntzki, Ekkehard

1976 *Die Idee der Wissenschaft bei Samuel Hahnemann*. Heidelberg: Haug.

Friebel, Hans

1988 "Kassenärztliche Verordnung – Ist sie rational?", *Deutsches Ärzteblatt* 85, 1179–1180.

Friedrich, Volker – Adam Hehn – Rolf Rosenbrock
1977 *Neunmal teurer als Gold – Die Arzneimittelversorgung in der Bundesrepublik.* Reinbek: Rowohlt.
Gadamer, Hans-Georg
1968 "Antike Atomtheorie", in: H. G. Gadamer (ed.), *Um die Begriffswelt der Vorsokratiker.* Darmstadt: Wissenschaftliche Buchgesellschaft, 512–533.
Gallimore, Ronald G. – Jim L. Turner
1977 "Contemporary Studies of Placebo Phenomena", in: M. E. Jarvik (ed.), *Psychopharmacology in the Practice of Medicine.* New York: Appleton Century Crofts, 47–57.
Galmiche, Paul
1957 "Mais qui a inventé l'Aspirine?" *Presse Médicale* 65, 303–303.
Garfinkel, Harold A.
1972 "Remarks on ethnomethodology", in: John Gumperz – Dell Hymes (eds.), *Directions in Sociolinguistics.* New York: Holt, Rinehart & Winston, 301–324.
Gaus, Eckehard – Bernhard Kubanek
1984 "Psychosoziale Faktoren und Immunkompetenz", *Der Internist* 25, 667–673.
Gerhardt, Christoph
1981 "Arznei und Symbol – Bemerkungen zum altdeutschen Geiertraktat mit einem Ausblick auf das Pelikanexempel", in: Wolfgang Harms – Heimo Reinitzer (eds.): *Natura loquax – Naturkunde und allegorische Naturdeutung vom Mittelalter bis zur frühen Neuzeit.* Frankfurt/M.: Lang, 109–182.
Gerhardt, Dietrich
1950 "Über die Stellung der Namen im lexikalischen System", *Beiträge zur Namenforschung* 1, 1–24.
Giardini, F.
1959 "Gradi di Causalità e di similitudine", *Angelicum* 36, 26–50.
Gipper, Helmut
1978 *Sprachwissenschaftliche Grundbegriffe und Forschungsrichtungen.* Munich: Hueber.
Glauber, Johann Rudolf
1703 *Tractatus De Signatura Salium, Metallorum et Planetarum oder Gründlicher Unterricht, wie oder auf was weise man gar leichtlich nicht allein der Salien, Metallen und Planeten, sondern auch der Wörter, und Nahmen ihre verborgene Kräfften Bedeutung Natur und Eigenschaften nicht aus Büchern oder Schrifften, sondern bloß und allein auß deren signatur, durch ein Circulum und Quadranten, erlernen und außrechnen kann.* (No indication of publisher or place, 1st edition: Amsterdam 1658.)
Göres, Jörn
1981 *Goethes Leben in Bilddokumenten.* Munich: Beck.
Goethe, Johann Wolfgang von
1848–1849 *Goethe's Autobiography.* London: Henry G. Bohn. (Translated by John Oxenford & A. J. W. Morrison.)
1889 *Dichtung und Wahrheit – Zweiter Theil,* in: J. W. Goethe: *Goethes Werke,* Abtheilung I, Band 27. Weimar: Böhlau. (= Sophie edition.)
1954 Vorträge über die ersten drei Kapitel des Entwurfs einer allgemeinen Einleitung in die Vergleichende Anatomie, ausgehend von der Osteologie, in: Rupprecht Mathaei et al. (eds.): *Goethe – Die Schriften zur Naturwissenschaft, Abteilung I, Band 9,* Weimar: Böhlau (= Leopoldina edition.)

1971 *Elective Affinities*, Harmondsworth, Middx.: Penguin Books.
1975 *Die Wahlverwandtschaften.* Stuttgart: Reclam.

Göttling, J. F. A.
1792 *Versuch einer physischen Chemie für Jugendlehrer beim Unterricht, wie auch Gebrauchsanweisung der Sammlung chemischer Präparate zu unterhaltenden und nützlichen Versuchen für Liebhaber der physischen Scheidekunst.* Jena: Mauke.

Goffman, Erving
1971 *Relations in Public. Microstudies of the Public Order.* New York: Basic Books.

Goldammer, Kurt
1966 "Der Beitrag des Paracelsus zur neuen wissenschaftlichen Methodologie und zur Erkenntnislehre", *Medizinhistorisches Journal* 1, 75–95.
1971 "Die Paracelsische Kosmologie und Materietheorie in ihrer wissenschaftsgeschichtlichen Stellung und Eigenart", *Medizinhistorisches Journal* 6, 5–35.

Goltz, Dietlinde
1972 *Studien zur Geschichte der Mineralnamen in Pharmazie, Chemie und Medizin von den Anfängen bis Paracelsus.* Wiesbaden: Steiner.

Gordonoff, T.
1965 "Zur Geschichte der Antipyrese", *Wiener medizinische Wochenschrift* 115, No. 3, 45–46.

Gowdey, C. W. – J. T. Hamilton – R. B. Philp
1967 "A Controlled Clinical Trial Using Placebos in Normal Subjects – A Teaching Exercise", *Canadian Medical Association Journal* 98, 1317–1322.

Grabau, Johann Heinrich Wilhelm
1837, 1838 *Chemisch-physiologisches System der Pharmakodynamik oder vollständiger Parallelismus des chemischen und dynamischen Charakters der anorganischen und organischen Materie.* Kiel: Universitäts-Buchhandlung. (2 Volumes.)

Grassi, Ernesto
1984 *Die Macht der Phantasie.* Frankfurt/Main: Syndikat.

Grattan, J. H. G. – Ch. Singer
1952 *Anglo-Saxon Magic and Medicine.* London: Oxford University Press.

Greimas, Algirdas Julien
1976 *Sémiotique et sciences sociales.* Paris: Du Seuil.

Greimas, Algirdas Julien – Joseph Courtes
1979 *Sémiotique – Dictionnaire Raisonné de la Théorie du Langage.* Paris: Hachette.

Gross, Franz – Henry K. Beecher
1984 *Placebo – Das universelle Medikament?* Mainz: Medizinisch Pharmazeutische Studiengesellschaft.

Grünbaum, Adolf
1985 "Explication and Implications of the Placebo-Concept" in: Leonard White – Bernard Tursky – Gary E. Schwartz, (eds.), 9–36.

Gutheil, Thomas S.
1977 "Psychodynamics in drug prescribing", *Drug Therapy* 7, 82–95.
1978 "Drug Therapy – Alliance and Compliance", Drug Therapy 19, 219–225.

Haas, Hans T. A.
1948 "Theorie und Praxis in der Therapie – Eine medizinhistorische Betrachtung", *Studium Generale* 1, 289–303.
1981 *Ursprung, Geschichte und Idee der Arzneimittelkunde.* Mannheim: Bibliographisches Institut.

Haas, H. – H. Fink – G. Härtfelder
1959 "Das Placeboproblem", *Fortschritte der Arzneimittelforschung* 1, 279–454.
Haberland, H. – J. L. Mey
1981 "Wording and warding – The pragmatics of therapeutical conversation", *Journal of Pragmatics* 5, 103–112.
Habermas, Jürgen
1984 *Strukturwandel der Öffentlichkeit.* Neuwied: Luchterhand. (14th edition.)
1989 *The Structural Transformation of the Public Sphere.* Great Britain: Polity Press.
Hahnemann, Samuel Friedrich Christian
1822–1827 *Reine Arzneimittellehre.* Dresden: Arnoldi. (6 volumes, 2nd edition.)
[1966] *Apothekerlexikon.* Ulm: Haug. (2 volumes, 1st edition: Leipzig: Crusius 1796.)
[1978] *Organon der Heilkunst.* Heidelberg: Haug. (= 6th edition, 1st edition: 1810.)
Halhuber, Carola
1981 "Pharmakotherapie und Arzt-Patient-Verhältnis", *Therapie der Gegenwart* 119, 1129–1147.
Hangarter, W.
1974a *Die Salicylsäure und ihre Abkömmlinge.* Stuttgart: Schattauer.
1974b "Die Evolution eines Jahrhundert-Pharmakons – Acetylsalicylsäure – für die Medizin", *Medizinische Welt* 25, 1968–1974.
Hardenberg, Ralf
1989 Analyse des Diagnose- und Verordnungsverhaltens der niedergelassenen Ärzte in der Bundesrepublik Deutschland einschließlich West Berlin (1983) am Beispiel der Pharmakotherapie rheumatischer Erkrankungen. (Düsseldorf: Medical Dissertation).
Haug, Wolfgang Fritz
1980 *Warenästhetik und kapitalistische Massenkultur.* Berlin: Argument. (1st of 2 volumes.)
Heider, F.
1958 *The psychology of interpersonal relations.* New York: Wiley.
Heine, Heinrich
1982 *History of Religion and Philosophy in Germany.* North Queensland, Australia: James Cook University.
Heischkel, Edith
1958 "Pharmakologie in der Goethezeit", *Sudhoffs Archiv für die Geschichte der Medizin und der Naturwissenschaften* 42, 302–311.
Hemminki, Elina
1975 "Review of Literature on the Factors Affecting Drug Prescribing", *Social Sciences and Medicine* 9, 111–115.
Henne, Heinz
1973 "Hahnemann als Chemiker und Pharmazeut", *Deutsche Apothekerzeitung* 113, 1327–1231.
Herz, Albert
1982 "Endorphine und Schmerz", in: Wolfgang Keeser – Ernst Pöppel – Petra Mitterhusen (eds.): *Schmerz.* Munich: Urban & Schwarzenberg, 69–82.
Hippius, Hanns – Karl Überla – Gregor Laakmann – Jörg Hasford (eds.)
1986 *Das Placebo-Problem.* Stuttgart: G. Fischer.
Höfler, Max
[1970] *Deutsches Krankheitsnamen-Buch.* Hildesheim: Olms. (1st edition: Munich 1899.)

Hörmann, Hans
1978 *Meinen und Verstehen – Grundzüge einer psychologischen Semantik.* Frankfurt/M.: Suhrkamp.
Hoffmann-Richter, Ulrike
1986 *Der Knoten im roten Faden – Eine Untersuchung zur Verständigung von Arzt und Patient in der Visite.* Bern: Lang.
Hofmann, Fritz
1920 "Wie unsere Heilmittel entstehen", *Zeitschrift für angewandte Chemie* 33, 273–277.
Hofstaetter, Peter R.
1955 "Über Ähnlichkeit" *Psyche* 9, No. 1, 54–80.
Hooykaas, Reijer
1939 "Die chemische Verbindung bei Paracelsus". *Sudhoffs Archiv für die Geschichte der Medizin und der Naturwissenschaften* 32, 166–175.
Horkheimer, Max – Theodor W. Adorno
[1971] *Dialektik der Aufklärung.* Frankfurt/M.: Fischer.
Hucklenbroich, Peter
1989 Semiotische Aspekte der Medizin / Medizinsemiotik. (Münster: unpublished manuscript.)
Hunnius, Curt
1962 *Dämonen Ärzte Alchemisten.* Stuttgart: Wissenschaftliche Buchgesellschaft.
Illich, Ivan
1977 *Die Nemesis der Medizin – Von den Grenzen des Gesundheitswesens.* Reinbek: Rowohlt.
Inman, William H. W.
1985 "Risikoüberwachung neu eingeführter Arzneimittel", *pharma dialog,* No. 88, 2–20.
Jäger, Herbert
1956 "Zur Namenkunde der Arzneimittel", *Sprachforum* 2, 55–59.
Janke, W.
1986 "Untersuchungen zur Placeboreaktivität: Vorhersagbarkeit der Reaktion gesunder Personen auf Placebo mit Stimulans-Instruktion", in: Hippius et al. (eds.), 151–170.
Jauß, Hans Robert
1975 "Literaturgeschichte als Provokation der Literaturwissenschaft", in: Warning (ed.), 126–162.
Jenkins, Marianna
1947 *The State Portrait – Its Origin and Evolution.* Cambridge/Mass.: College Art Association of America. (Monographs on Archeology and Fine Arts III.)
Jospe, Michael
1978 *The Placebo Effect in Healing.* Lexington/Mass.: Heath.
Kafka, Franz
1976a *Briefe an Felice.* Frankfurt/Main: Fischer.
1976b *Ein Landarzt,* in: Franz Kafka: *Gesammelte Werke,* Vol.4. Frankfurt/Main: Fischer. (Edited by Max Brod).
1978 *Letters to Felice.* Harmondsworth: Penguin. (With "Kafka's Other Trial" by Elias Canetti.)
1983 "The Penguin Complete Short Stories". Harmondsworth: Penguin.

Kahn, Joan A.
1983 *Modes of Medical Instruction.* Berlin: Mouton de Gruyter.

Kaiser, Ernst
1969 *Paracelsus.* Reinbek: Rowohlt.

Kalverkämper, Hartwig
1978 *Textlinguistik der Eigennamen.* Stuttgart: Klett.

Kampmann, Wanda
1979 *Deutsche und Juden. Die Geschichte der Juden in Deutschland vom Mittelalter bis zum Beginn des Ersten Weltkriegs.* Frankfurt: Fischer.

Kany, Roland
1987 *Mnemosyne als Programm – Geschichte, Erinnerung und die Andacht zum Unbedeutenden im Werk von Usener, Warburg und Benjamin.* Tübingen: Niemeyer.

Katz, Jerrold J. – Jerry A. Fodor
1964 *The Structure of Language.* Englewood Cliffs: Prentice Hall.

Keller, Gottfried
1966 *Das Sinngedicht.* Stuttgart: Reclam.

Kelly, George Alexander
1955 *The Psychology of Personal Constructs.* New York: Norton. (2 volumes.)

Kent, James Tyler
1979 *Repertorium der homoöpathischen Arzneimittellehre.* Stuttgart: Hippokrates. (Edited and translated by Willy Erbe.)

Kissel, P. – D. Barrucand,
1964 *Placebos et effet placebo en médecine.* Paris: Masson.

Kleinsorge, Hellmuth
1985 "Zur Problematik der Rationalen Therapie", in: H. Kleinsorge – H. E. Bock (eds.): *Rationale Therapie – Grundfragen der Arzneiverordnung.* Mainz: Medizinisch Pharmazeutische Studiengesellschaft, 11–19.

Klickow, Reinhard
1963 "Die Sprachphysiognomik und ihre Verwendung bei der Konstruktion von Markennamen", *Der Markenartikel* 25, 960–965.
1964 "Sprachpsychologische Untersuchungs-Methoden bei Markennamen", *Die Anzeige* 40, No. 11, 24–35.

Klinkenberg, Peter
1985 "Der Mensch ein 'beliebig verführbarer, willenloser Konsumidiot'? Argumente und Beweise gegen ein Verbot von Publikumswerbung für Arzneimittel", *Frankfurter Rundschau* 20. 7. 1985, 7.

Kluxen, F.
1971 "Analogie", in: Joachim Ritter (ed.): *Historisches Wörterbuch der Philosophie, Vol.I.* Basle: Schwabe, 214–227.

Koch, Walter Alfred
1971 *Varia Semiotica.* Hildesheim: Olms.

Köhle, Karl – Hans-Heinrich Raspe (eds.)
1982 *Das Gespräch während der ärztlichen Visite.* Munich: Urban & Schwarzenberg.

Kristeva, Julia
1969 *Semeiotiké – Recherches pour une sémanalyse.* Paris: Du Seuil.
1977 "Semiologie – kritische Wissenschaft und/oder Wissenschaftskritik", in: Peter V. Zima (ed.): *Textsemiotik als Ideologiekritik.* Frankfurt/M.: Suhrkamp, 35–53.

Kroos, Renate
1985 "Vom Umgang mit Reliquien", in: Anton Legner (ed.), *Ornamenta Ecclesiae – Kunst und Künstler der Romanik,* Vol.3. Cologne (exhibition catalogue published by Schnütgen Museum), 25–49.
Küpper, Heinz
1982 *Illustriertes Lexikon der deutschen Umgangssprache,* Vol.I. Stuttgart: Klett.
Kuhn, Dorothea
1972 "Goethe und die Chemie", *Medizinhistorisches Journal* 7, 264–278.
Kuhn, Thomas S.
1962 *The Structure of Scientific Revolution.* Chicago: University of Chicago Press.
Kuschinsky, Gustav
1975 "Wirkungen und Indikationen von Placebo", *Deutsches Ärzteblatt* 72, 663–667.
Kuschinsky, Gustav – Heinz Lüllmann
1978 *Kurzes Lehrbuch der Pharmakologie und Toxikologie.* Stuttgart: Thieme. (8th edition.)
Kusenberg, Kurt
1980 *Heiter bis tückisch – 13 Geschichten.* Reinbek: Rowohlt.
Lacan, Jacques
1966 "Le stade du miroir comme formateur de la fonction de Je", in: *Jacques Lacan: Ecrits.* Paris: Du Seuil.
1977 "The mirror stage as formative of the function of the I as revealed in psychoanalytic experience", in: *Jacques Lacan: Ecrits: a selection.* London: Tavistock Publications.
Ladas, Stephen P.
1964 "Die Entwicklung der Marke zur Gattungsbezeichnung", *Gewerblicher Rechtsschutz und Urheberrecht. Auslands- und internationaler Teil* 66, 418–427.
Lämmert, Eberhard
1986 "Die Chemie der Wahlverwandtschaften", *Leviathan* 14, No. 1, 19–36.
Langbein, Kurt – Hans Peter Martin – Hans Weiss – Roland Werner [= Peter Sichrovsky]
1983 *Gesunde Geschäfte – Die Praktiken der Pharma-Industrie.* Cologne: Kiepenheuer & Witsch. (2nd edition.)
Laplanche, J – J. B. Pontalis,
1986 *Das Vokabular der Psychoanalyse.* Frankfurt/M.: Suhrkamp. (7th edition.)
1988 *The Language of Psychoanalysis.* London: Karnac Books.
Grand Larousse de la langue française, Vol.I.
1971 Paris: Larousse.
Lasagna, Louis – Frederick Mosteller – John von Felsinger – Henry K. Beecher
1954 "A Study of the Placebo Response" *American Journal of Medicine* 16, 770–779.
Lasagna, Louis – Victor G. Laties – J. Lawrence Dohan
1958 "Further Studies on the 'Pharmacology' of Placebo Administration", *Journal of Clinical Investigation* 37, 533–537.
Lasagna, Louis
1983 "Introduction: Aspirine's Infinite Variety", *The American Journal of Medicine* 74, Suppl.IV, 1–1.
Lasswitz, Kurd
1889–1890 *Geschichte der Atomistik vom Mittelalter bis zur Neuzeit.* Leipzig: Voss. (2 volumes.)

Lauretis, Teresa de
1981 *Umberto Eco*. Florence: Nuova Italia.
1986 "Das Rätsel der Lösung – Umberto Ecos 'Der Name der Rose' als postmoderner Roman", in: A. Huyssens – K. R. Scherper (eds.): *Postmoderne*. Reinbek: Rowohlt, 251–269.

Lausch, Erwin
1975 "Aspirin, das unbekannte Mittel", *Die Zeit* 14. 11. 1975.

Leibbrand, Werner
1956 *Die spekulative Medizin der Romantik*. Hamburg: Claassen.

Lehrl, Siegfried – Reinhard Csiske
1980 "Messung von Schmerzen durch Adjektiv-Skalen und Untersuchungen zur faktoriellen Stabilität der Schmerzsprache", in: Susanne Davies-Osterkamp – Ernst Pöppel (eds.): *Emotionsforschung*. Göttingen: Vandenhoeck & Ruprecht, 163–181.

Leighton, Isabel (ed.)
1950 *The Aspirin Age 1919–1941*. London: Bodley Head.

Lejeune, F.
1941 "Die Zeit des Paracelsus – Eine politisch-geistesgeschichtliche Studie", *Medizinische Welt* 15, 1004–1008, 1057–1060.

Lemay, René
1968 Dénominations communes et marques des spécialités pharmaceutiques. (Paris: Doctoral thesis of the Academy of Pharmaceutics.)

Leslie, Alan
1954 "Ethics and Practice of Placebo Therapy", *American Journal of Medicine* 16, 854–862.

Levine, John D. – N. C. Gordon – H. L. Fields
1978 "The Mechanism of Placebo Analgesia", *The Lancet* 23. 9. 1978, 654–657.

Lévi-Strauss, Claude
1966 *The Savage Mind*. London: Weidenfield and Nicholson.
1987 *Introduction to the Work of Marcel Mauss*. London: Routledge & Kegan Paul.

Leys, Odo
1977 "Der Eigenname in seinem formalen Verhältnis zum Appellativ", in: H. Steger (ed.): *Probleme der Namenforschung im deutschsprachigen Raum*. Darmstadt: Wissenschaftliche Buchgesellschaft, 26–38.

Lichnowsky, Mechthilde
1925 *Der Kampf mit dem Fachmann*. Vienna: Jahoda & Siegel.

Lienert, Gustav A.
1956 "Die Bedeutung der Suggestion in pharmakopsychologischen Untersuchungen", *Zeitschrift für experimentelle und angewandte Psychologie* 3, 418–438.

Lilli, Laura
1988 "Delirio per delirio", *La Repubblica* 21. 8. 1988 , 24–25. (Interview with Umberto Eco.)

Lillyman, William J.
1983 "Analogies for Love: Goethe's 'Die Wahlverwandtschaften' and Plato's 'Symposium'", in: W. J. Lillyman (ed.): *Goethe's Narrative Fiction – The Irvine Goethe Symposium*. Berlin: De Gruyter, 128–144.

Loewe, Hans
1950 *Paul Ehrlich – Schöpfer der Chemotherapie*. Stuttgart: Wissenschaftliche Verlagsgesellschaft.

Lötscher, Andreas
1987 *Von Ajax bis Xerox*. Zürich: Artemis.
Lomnitz, F.
1925 "Nachruf Heinrich Dreser", *Therapeutische Berichte* 2, No. 3, 78–81.
Lotman, Yuri A. – Boris A. Ouspensky
1976 "Mythe, Nom, Culture", in: Y. A. Lotman – B. Ouspensky (eds.): *Travaux sur les systèmes des signes*. Brüssel: complexe, 18–39.
Mach, Ernst
1925 *Erkenntnis und Irrtum. Skizzen zu einer Psychologie der Forschung*. Leipzig: Voss.
1976 *Knowledge and Error*. Dordrecht, Boston: D. Riedel.
Madaus, Gerhard
1932 "Zur wissenschaftlichen Grundlegung der Signaturenlehre". *Biologische Heilkunst* 13, 649–652.
Magritte, Ren¤
1983 "Brief an Michel Foucault vom 23. 5. 1966", in: *Michel Foucault: Dies ist keine Pfeife*. Berlin: Ullstein.
1983b "Letter to Michel Foucault of May 23, 1966", in: *Michel Foucault: This is Not a Pipe*. Berkeley, Los Angeles, London: University of California Press.
Mahoney, John Thomas
1961 *Vom Heftpflaster bis zum Antihistamin – Bilder aus der Geschichte der pharmazeutischen Industrie*. Düsseldorf: Econ.
Malitz, Sidney
1963 "Variables and Drug Effectiveness", in: Rinkel (ed.), 141–148.
Mann, Thomas
1979 *Tagebücher*, Vol. I. Frankfurt/Main: Fischer. (Edited by Peter de Mendelssohn.)
Manz, Matthias – Bernd Lüderitz
1988 "Aspirin zur Prävention der koronaren Herzkrankheit – Kann die Primärprävention empfohlen werden?", *Deutsches Ärzteblatt* 85, 1134–1138.
Marquard, Odo
1973 "Über einige Beziehungen zwischen Ästhetik und Therapeutik in der Philosophie des neunzehnten Jahrhunderts", in: Odo Marquard: *Schwierigkeiten mit der Geschichtsphilosophie*. Frankfurt/Main: Suhrkamp, 85–106.
Marquardt, Martha
1951 *Paul Ehrlich*. Berlin: Springer.
Martino, Horst Dieter
1986 "Eintragung von Warenzeichen erleichtert – Zur 'Indorektal'-Entscheidung des BGH", *Die Pharmazeutische Industrie* 48, 1396–1399.
Maxwell, James Clerk
1927 *The Scientific Papers*. Paris: Hermann. (Edited by W. D. Niven.)
Mazumdar, Pauline M. H.
1974 "The Antigen-Antibody Reaction and the Physics and Chemistry of Life", *Bulletin of the History of Medicine* 48, 1–21.
McNair, D. M. – R. J. Kahn – L. F. Droppleman – S. Fisher
1968 "Patient Acquiescence and Drug Effects", in: Karl Rickels (ed.), 59–72.
Meinertz, Josef
1949 "Psychosomatische Medizin", *Verhandlungen der deutschen Gesellschaft für Innere Medizin* 55, 58–62.

Melandri, Enzo
1968 *La Linea e il Circulo*. Bologna: Il Mulino.
Melzack, R. – W. S. Torgerson
1971 "On the Language of Pain" *Anesthesiology* 34, 50–59.
Melzack, Ronald – Patrick D. Wall
1982 "Schmerzmechanismen – Eine neue Theorie", in: Wolfgang Keeser – Ernst Pöppel – Petra Mitterhusen (eds.): *Schmerz*. Munich: Urban & Schwarzenberg, 8–29.
Meyer-Eppler, Werner
1969 *Grundlagen und Anwendungen der Informationstheorie*. Berlin: Springer. (2nd edition.)
Moertel, C. G. – D. L. Ahmann – W. F. Taylor – N. Schworton
1972 "A Comparative evaluation of marketed analgesic drugs", *New England Journal of Medicine* 286, 813–815.
Molière [= Poquelin, Jean-Baptiste]
[1959] *The Imaginary Invalid*, in: *The Misanthrope and other Plays*. Harmondsworth: Penguin. (1st edition: Paris 1682.)
Monod, Jacques
1972 *Chance and Necessity*. London: Collins/Fontana.
Morris, Louis A. – Edgar C. O'Neal
1974 "Drug Name Familiarity and Placebo Reaction", *Journal of Clinical Psychology* 30, 280–282.
Morstein, Petra von
1964 "Wittgensteins Untersuchungen des Wortes 'Schmerz'", *Archiv für Philosophie* 13, 131–140.
Müller-Oerlinghausen, Bruno
1986 "Anwendung von Placebos in der ärztlichen Praxis", in: Hippius et al. (eds.), 84–92.
Mukarovsky, Jan
1970 *Kapitel aus der Ästhetik*. Frankfurt/M.: Suhrkamp.
Mumford, Lewis
1971 *The Myth of the Machine*. London: Secker & Warburg. (2 Vols.)
Musil, Robert
1953–1960 *The Man Without Qualities*. London: Secker & Warburg; Picador/Pan Books. (3 Volumes.)
1978 *Der Mann ohne Eigenschaften*. Reinbek: Rowohlt. (2 Volumes.)
Mutschler, Ernst
1982 "Arzneimittelentwicklung – Zufall, Intuition und systematische Suche", *Abhandlungen der Mathematisch-Naturwissenschaftlichen Klasse der Akademie der Wissenschaften und der Literatur Mainz*, No. 2.
Negt, Oskar – Alexander Kluge
1972 *Öffentlichkeit und Erfahrung*. Frankfurt/M.: Suhrkamp.
Netter, Petra
1980 "Suggestibilität und Medikamentenwirkung", in: Susanne Davies-Osterkamp – E. Pöppel (eds.): *Emotionsforschung*. Göttingen: Vandenhoeck & Ruprecht, 195–213.
1986 "Systematik der am Placeboeffekt beteiligten Faktoren und Beispiele für ihre statistischen Wirkungen und Wechselwirkungen", in: Hippius et al. (eds.), 61–73.

Nie, Norman H. – C. Hadlai Hull – Jean Jenkins – Karin Steinbrenner – Dale H. Bend
1975 *Statistical Package for the Social Sciences.* New York: McGraw Hill. (2nd edition.)
Nöth, Winfried
1975 *Semiotik. Eine Einführung mit Beispielen für Reklameanalysen.* Tübingen: Niemeyer.
1977 *Dynamik semiotischer Systeme.* Stuttgart: Metzler.
1985 *Handbuch der Semiotik.* Stuttgart: Metzler.
1990 *Handbook of Semiotics.* Berlin: Mouton De Gruyter.
Nord, Dietrich
1976 *Arzneimittelkonsum in der Bundesrepublik.* Stuttgart: Enke.
Oldenburg, Dieter
1979 *Romantische Naturphilosophie und Arzneimittellehre.* Brunswick: Pharmaziegeschichtliches Seminar.
Ongaro-Basaglia, Franca
1985 *Gesundheit/Krankheit – Das Elend der Medizin.* Frankfurt: Fischer.
Ortega y Gasset, José
1932 *The Revolt of the Masses.* London: Allen & Unwin.
1949 *Betrachtungen über die Technik.* Stuttgart: DVA.
Osgood, Charles Egerton – George J. Suci – Percy H. Tannenbaum
1957 *The measurement of meaning.* Urbana: University of Illinois Press.
Pagel, Walter
1931 "Hahnemann", in: W. Haberling – F. Hübotter – H. Vierordt (eds.): *Biographisches Lexikon der hervorragenden Ärzte aller Zeiten und Völker.* (Vol.III, 2nd edition), Berlin: Urban & Schwarzenberg, 19–21.
Panofsky, Erwin
1979 "Zum Problem der Beschreibung und Inhaltsdeutung von Werken der bildenden Kunst", in: Ekkehard Kaemmerling (ed.): *Ikonographie und Ikonologie.* Cologne: Du Mont, 185–206.
Paracelsus [= Philippus Aureolus Theophrastus Bombastus von Hohenheim]
1650 *A New Light of Alchymie Also Nine Books of the Nature of Things.* London (Publisher not indicated).
[1928a] *De natura rerum.* In: Karl Sudhoff (ed.): *Theophrast von Hohenheim gen. Paracelsus: Sämtliche Werke I. Abteilung: Medizinische und naturwissenschaftliche Schriften, Vol. XI.* Munich: Oldenbourg. (1st edition: 1572.)
[1928b] *Labyrinthus medicorum errantium.* In: Karl Sudhoff (ed.): *Theophrast von Hohenheim gen. Paracelsus: Sämtliche Werke I. Abteilung: Medizinische und naturwissenschaftliche Schriften, Vol.XI.* Munich: Oldenbourg. (1st edition: 1537.)
[1929] *Astronomia magna.* In: Karl Sudhoff (ed.): *Theophrast von Hohenheim gen. Paracelsus: Sämtliche Werke I. Abteilung: Medizinische und naturwissenschaftliche Schriften, Vol. XII.* Munich: Oldenbourg.
[1930] *Von den natürlichen Dingen.* In: Karl Sudhoff (ed.): *Theophrast von Hohenheim gen. Paracelsus: Sämtliche Werke I. Abteilung: Medizinische und naturwissenschaftliche Schriften, Vol.II. Munich:* Oldenbourg.
[1931] "Nachschrift aus der Vorlesung über die Tartarischen Krankheiten", in: Karl Sudhoff (ed.): *Theophrast von Hohenheim gen. Paracelsus: Sämtliche Werke I. Abteilung: Medizinische und naturwissenschaftliche Schriften, Vol.V.* Munich: Oldenbourg.

Parascandola, John – Ronald Jasensky
1974 "Origins of the Receptor Theory of Drug Action", *Bulletin of the History of Medicine* 48, 199–220.

Park, Lee C. – Lico Covi
1965 "Nonblind Placebo Trial", *Archives of General Psychiatry* 12, 336–345.

Peirce, Charles Santiago Sanders
[1982] *Writings, Volume I.* Bloomington: Indiana University Press. (Edited by Max H. Fisch et al..)
[1985] *Die Festigung der Überzeugung und andere Schriften.* Frankfurt: Ullstein. (Edited and translated by Elisabeth Walther.)

Pepper, O. H. P.
1945 "A Note on the Placebo", *American Journal of Pharmacy and the Sciences supporting public health* 117, 409–412.

Peters, Bruce H. – C. J. Fraim – B. E. Masel
1983 "Comparison of 650 mg Aspirin and 1000 mg Acetaminophen with Each Other, and with Placebo in Moderate Severe Headache", *American Journal of Medicine* 74, Suppl. IV, 36–42.

Peters, Georges
1973 *Structure-activity-relationships.* New York: Pergamon.

Petersen, Heiderose
1978 Arzneimitteltheorie und Arzneimittelpraxis im frühen 19. Jahrhundert. Marburg: Doctoral thesis in pharmaceutics.

Peuckert, Will Erich
1935 "Signatur", in: E. Hoffman-Krayer – H. Bächtold-Stäubli (eds.): *Handwörterbuch des deutschen Aberglaubens,* Vol.VII. Berlin: De Gruyter.

Der Physiologus
1960 (edited and translated by Otto Seel), Zürich: Artemis.

Pichot, Pierre – Jacques Perse
1968 "Placebo Effects as Response Set", in: Rickels (ed.), 50–58.

Pilch, Herbert
1965 "Zentrale und periphere Lautsysteme", *Proceedings of the 5th International Congress of Phonetic Sciences,* Münster 1964, 467–473.

Plato
[1951] *The Symposium.* Harmondsworth, Middx.: Penguin Books.
[1957] *Symposion.* In: Plato: *Sämtliche Werke, Vol.II,* Reinbek: Rowohlt. (Edited by W. F. Otto, E. Grassi, G. Plamböck; translated by F. Schleiermacher.)
[1958] *Phaidon.* In: Plato: *Sämtliche Werke, Vol.III,* Reinbek: Rowohlt. (Edited by W. F. Otto, E. Grassi, G. Plamböck; translated by F. Schleiermacher.)

Pörksen, Uwe
1978 "Zur Metaphorik der naturwissenschaftlichen Sprache – Dargestellt am Beispiel Goethes, Darwins und Freuds", *Neue Rundschau 89*, 64–82.

Praninskas, Jean
1968 *Trade Name Creation – Processes and Patterns.* The Hague: Mouton.

Proust, Marcel
1983 *Remenbrance of Things Past.* Harmondsworth: Penguin. (3 volumes, translated by F. Scott Moncrieff.)

Pummerer, Martin
1985 Das Medikamentengespräch – Die medikamentenbezogene Kommunikation von Arzt und Patient während der klinischen Visite. Ulm: Medical Dissertation.

Quecke, Kurt
1955 "Die Signaturenlehre im Schrifttum des Paracelsus", *Beiträge zur Geschichte der Pharmazie und ihrer Nachbargebiete 1*, 41–52.
Quillian, Ross M.
1968 "Semantic Memory", in: Marvin Minsky (ed.): *Semantic Information Processing.* Cambridge/Mass.: MIT-Press, 216–270.
Raspe, Hans-Heinrich
1976 "Institutionalisierte Zumutungen an Krankenhauspatienten", in: Herbert Begemann (ed.): *Patient und Krankenhaus.* Munich: Urban & Schwarzenberg, 1–24.
Rauchfleisch, Udo
1981 *Dissozial.* Göttingen: Vandenhoeck & Ruprecht.
Reichwald-Dietzsch, Ursula
1981 "Soziale Aspekte des ärztlichen Verodnungsverhaltens", *Medizinische Welt* 32, 68–71, 139–142.
Rickels, Karl (ed.)
1968 *Non-Specific Factors in Drug Therapy.* Springfield: Thomas.
Ridder, Michael de
1984 "Das Allerweltpulver", *Der Stern* No. 51, 80–82.
Ridder, Paul
1979 *Die Sprache des Schmerzes.* Konstanz: Universitätsverlag.
Rinkel, Max (ed.)
1963 *Specific and Non-Specific Factors in Psychopharmacology.* New York: Philosophical Library.
Ritzenhoff, Ursula (ed.)
1982 *Erläuterungen und Dokumente: Johann Wolfgang Goethe – Die Wahlverwandtschaften.* Stuttgart: Reclam.
Römer, Ruth
1963 "Schwierigkeiten bei der Benennung von Kunststoffen", *Muttersprache* 73, 108–114.
Röth, F. – S. Lehrl
1973 "Eine mehrdimensionale Beurteilungsskala zur Schmerzerfassung", *Arzneimittelforschung* 23, 997–999.
Rossi-Landi, Ferrucio
1985 *Metodica philosophica e scienza dei segni.* Milan: Bompiani.
Samson, E.
1986 "Rechtliche Aspekte von Placebo-Studien", in: Hippius et al. (eds.), 2–10.
Samuelsson, B.
1965 "Die Prostaglandine", *Angewandte Chemie* 77, 445–452.
Sander, Axel
1977 *Arzneimittelrecht – Kommentar für die juristische und pharmazeutische Praxis zum neuen Gesetz über den Verkehr mit Arzneimitteln 'Arzneimittelgesetz'.* Stuttgart: Kohlhammer. (3 volumes.)
Schachter, Stanley – Jerome E. Singer
1962 "Cognitive, Social, and Physiological Determinants of Emotional States", *Psychological Review 69*, 379–399.
Schadewaldt, Hans
1972, 1973 "Der Ähnlichkeitsgedanke bei Paracelsus", *Allgemeine Homöopathische Zeitung* 217, 265–268; 218, 12–19.

Schindel, Leo
1967 "Placebo und Placebo-Effekte in Klinik und Forschung", *Arzneimittelforschung* 17, 892–917.

Schipperges, Heinrich
1976 "Magia et scientia bei Paracelsus", *Sudhoffs Archiv für die Geschichte der Medizin und der Naturwissenschaften* 60, 76–92.

Schlegel, Emil
1933 *Religion der Arznei – Das ist Herr Gotts Apotheke.* Radebeul: Madaus. (3rd edition.)

Schlenk, Oskar
1947 *Die Salicylsäure.* Berlin: Saenger
1950 "Bemerkungen zu der Arbeit '50 Jahre Aspirin' von Dr. Arthur Eichengrün", *Die Pharmazie* 5, 411–412.

Schneider, Wolfgang
1950 "Über die Signaturenlehre in Pharmazie und Chemie", *Die Pharmazie* 5, 355–358.
1968 *Lexikon zur Arzneimittelgeschichte, Band 2: Pharmakologische Arzneimittelgruppen.* Frankfurt/Main: Govi.

Schöffling, Klaus (ed.)
1983 *Dort wo man Bücher verbrennt.* Frankfurt/Main: Suhrkamp.

Schonauer, Klaus
1986a *Signal Symbol Symptom – Alte und neue Aspekte des medizinischen Symptombegriffs.* Münster: MAkS.
1986b "Marketing im Sprechzimmer oder: Es blinkt das Muco-Regulans – Gespräche zwischen Ärzten und Pharmareferenten", in: Franz Hundsnurscher – Edda Weigand (eds.): *Dialoganalyse.* Tübingen: Niemeyer, 157–169.

Schreiber, G.
1974 "Contribution to Round Table Discussion at the 4th International Advanced Training Course held by the Federal Chamber of Pharmacists", in: Helmut Eberhard: "Arzneimittelwerbung aus der Sicht des Offizinapothekers in Deutschland", *Pharmazeutische Zeitung* 119, 1552–1554.

Schreiber, H. L.
1986 "Rechtliche Grenzen für die Zulässigkeit der Placebo-Anwendung", in: Hippius et al. (eds.), 11–18.

Schuhmacher, W. W.
1969 "Zur Typologie der Markenartikelnamen", *Linguistics* 47, 68–72.

Schultz, K. H. – A. Raedler
1986 "Tumorimmunologie und Psychoimmunologie als Grundlagen für die Psychoonkologie", *Psychotherapie und Medizinische Psychologie* 36, 114–129.

Schultz-Gambard, Jürgen
1983 "Wahrnehmung der eigenen Gefühle: das Experiment von Schachter und Singer", in: Dieter Frey – Siegfried Greif (eds.): *Sozialpsychologie.* Munich: Urban & Schwarzenberg, 465–471.

Schulz, Hans
[1974] *Deutsches Fremdwörterbuch. (Vol.II),* Berlin: De Gruyter (1st edition Strassburg: Trübner 1913.)

Schumacher, Joseph
1944 "Paracelsus und Hahnemann", *Deutsche Medizinische Wochenschrift* 70, 249–251

Schwabe Ulrich – Dieter Paffrath
1985 *Arzneiverordnungs-Report* 85. Stuttgart: G. Fischer.
Sebeok, Thomas Albert
1967 "On Chemical Signs", in: [no editor indicated]: *To Honor Roman Jakobson*. The Hague: Mouton, S. 1775 - 1782.
1976 *Contributions to the Doctrine of Signs*. Bloomington/Lisse: Indiana University/ De Ridder.
1979a *The Sign and its Masters*. Austin: University of Texas Press.
1979b *Theorie und Geschichte der Semiotik*. Reinbek: Rowohlt.
Sebeok, Thomas Albert et al. (eds.)
1986 *Encyclopedic Dictionary of Semiotics*. Berlin: Mouton De Gruyter. (3 volumes.)
Sebeok, Thomas Albert – Jean Umiker-Sebeok
1980 *"You Know My Method" – A Juxtaposition of Charles S. Peirce and Sherlock Holmes*. Bloomington: Gaslight Publications.
1982 *"Du kennst meine Methode" – Charles Sanders Peirce und Sherlock Holmes*. Frankfurt/Main: Suhrkamp.
Shannon, I. L. – G. M. Isbell
1963 "Stress in dental patients", *Dental Digest* 69, 459–461.
Shannon, C. E. – W. Weaver
1969 *The mathematical theory of communication*. Urbana: University of Illinois Press.
Shapiro, Arthur K.
1964 "A Historic and Heuristic Definition of the Placebo", *Psychiatry* 27, 52–58.
Sialm-Bossard, Victor
1975 *Sprachliche Untersuchungen zu den Chemiefaser-Namen*. Bern: Lang.
Sichrovsky, Peter
1984 *Krankheit auf Rezept – Die Praktiken der Praxisärzte*. Cologne: Kiepenheuer & Witsch.
Sieckmann, Hermann E.
1941 "Hahnemann und Goethe" *Hippokrates* 12, 865–868, 891–894.
Siegrist, Johannes
1976 "Der Doppelaspekt der Patientenrolle im Krankenhaus: Empirische Befunde und theoretische Überlegungen", in: Herbert Begemann (ed.): *Patient und Krankenhaus*. Munich: Urban & Schwarzenberg, 25–48.
1982 "Asymmetrische Kommunikation bei klinischen Visiten", in: Karl Köhle – Hans Heinrich Raspe (eds.), 16–22.
Simonton, O. Carl – Stephanie M. Simonton – James L. Creighton
1980 *Getting Well Again*. New York: Bantam Books.
Six, Bernd
1983 "Attribution", in: Dieter Frey – Siegfried Greif (eds.): *Sozialpsychologie*. Munich: Urban & Schwarzenberg, 122–135.
Sowinski, Werner
1979 *Werbeanzeigen und Werbesendungen*. Munich: Oldenbourg.
Sudhoff, Karl
1928 "Vorwort", in: Karl Sudhoff (ed.): *Theophrast von Hohenheim gen. Paracelsus: Sämtliche Werke I. Abteilung: Medizinische und naturwissenschaftliche Schriften*. Vol.XI. Munich: Oldenbourg.
1932 "Paracelsus und Goethe" *Medizinische Welt* 6, 1409–1412.

Stacher, Gerhard
1984 "Analgetika", in: H. P. Kuemmerle – G. Hitzenberger – K. H. Spitzy (eds.): *Klinische Pharmakologie.* (4th edition, Vol.3), [place not indicated]: ecomed, 4. 1. 5/1–4. 1. 5/18.

Stadtlinger, H.
1947 "Dr. Ing. e.h., Dr. phil. Arthur Eichengrün 80 Jahre", *Die Pharmazie* 2, 383–384.

Staiano, Kathryn V.
1986 *Interpreting Signs of Illness. A Case Study in Medical Semiotics.* Berlin: Mouton de Gruyter.

Steinhausen, Delef – Siegfried Zörkendörfer
1987 *Statistische Datenanalyse mit dem Programmsystem SPSSX und SPSS/PC+.* Munich: Oldenbourg.

Stemplinger, Eduard
1925 *Antike und moderne Volksmedizin.* Leipzig: Dieterich.

Steudel, J.
1956 "Woher stammt das Wort Placebo?", *Deutsche Medizinische Wochenschrift* 81, 1482–1482.

Stössel, Jürgen Peter
1973 *Psychopharmaka – Die verordnete Anpassung.* Munich: Piper.

Storz, Eugen:
1984 "Zukunft der Selbstmedikation", *Pharma* 11, No. 10, 31–37.

Ströker, Elisabeth
1982 *Theoriewandel in der Wissenschaftsgeschichte – Chemie im 18. Jahrhundert.* Frankfurt: Klostermann.

Strunz, Franz
1941 "Über Nietzsche und Paracelsus", *Sudhoffs Archiv für die Geschichte der Medizin und der Naturwissenschaften* 34, 243–250.

Stürmer, Joachim
1978 *Von dem gi–re – Untersuchungen zu einer altdeutschen Drogenmonographie des Hochmittelalters.* Hanover: Pattensen.

Toellner, Richard
1971 "Die Umbewertung des Schmerzes im 17. Jahrhundert in ihren Voraussetzungen und Folgen", *Medizinhistorisches Journal* 6, 36–44.

Traut, E. F. – E. W. Passarelli
1959 "Placebos in the Evaluation of treatment in rheumatic diseases", *Illinois Medical Journal* 115, No. 4, 181–183.

Tschirch, August (ed.)
1933 *Handbuch der Pharmakognosie, "III. Abteilung: Allgemeine Pharmakognosie", vol.I.* (2nd edition), Leipzig: Tauchnitz.

Tsouyopoulos, Nelly
1982 *Andreas Röschlaub und die Romantische Medizin – Die philosophischen Grundlagen der modernen Medizin.* Stuttgart: G. Fischer.

Überla, Karl
1968 *Faktorenanalyse.* Berlin: Springer.

Uexküll, Thure von
1984a "Semiotik und Medizin", *Zeitschrift für Semiotik* 6, 3–4.
1984b "Zeichen und Realität als anthroposemiotisches Problem", in: Klaus Oehler (ed.): *Zeichen und Realität.* Tübingen: Stauffenburg, 61–72.

1986 [Personal Communication from 1st of April.]
Uexküll, Thure von – Wesiack, Wolfgang
1988 *Theorie der Humanmedizin.* Munich: Urban & Schwarzenberg.
Ungeheuer, Gerold
1980 "Der Tanzmeister bei den Philosophen: Miszellen aus der Semiotik des 18. Jahrhunderts", *Kodikas* 2, 353–376.
Valentin, Hans
1950 *Geschichte der Pharmazie und Chemie in Form von Zeittafeln unter besonderer Berücksichtigung der Verhältnisse in Deutschland.* Stuttgart: Wissenschaftliche Verlagsgesellschaft.
Valéry, Paul
1957–1975 *The Collected Works.* London: Routledge & Kegan Paul. (15 Volumes.)
1960 "Pièces sur l'art", in: Paul Valéry: *Oeuvres.* (Vol.II), Paris: Gallimard.
Vane, J. R.
1971 "Inhibition of prostaglandin synthesis as a mechanism of action for aspirin-like drugs", *Nature/New Biology* 231, 232–235.
Vinar, Oldrych
1969 "Dependance on a placebo – A case report", *British Journal of Psychiatry* 115, 1189–1190.
Waitzkin, Howard
1984 "The Micropolitics of Medicine: A Contextual Analysis", *International Journal of Health Services* 14, 339–378.
Warning, Rainer (ed.)
1975 *Rezeptionsästhetik.* Munich: Fink/UTB.
Weiss, Georg
1984 "Beziehungs-Pharma-Marketing", *Pharma* 11, No. 10, 22–30.
Weissbach, Helmut
1971 *Strukturdenken in der organischen Chemie.* Berlin: VEB Deutscher Verlag der Wissenschaften.
Werlen, Iwar
1984 *Ritual und Sprache.* Tübingen: Niemeyer.
Westermann, Claus
1977 *Lob und Klage in den Psalmen.* Göttingen: Vandenhoeck & Ruprecht.
1984 *Ausgewählte Psalmen.* Göttingen: Vandenhoeck & Ruprecht.
Wheatley, David
1968 "Effects of Doctors' and Patients' Attitudes and Other Factors on Response to Drugs", in: Rickels (ed.), 73–79.
White, Leonard – Bernard Tursky – Gary E. Schwartz (eds.)
1985 *Placebo – Theory, Research, and Mechanisms.* New York: Guilford.
Whitehorn, J. C.
1958 "Psychiatric Implications of the Placebo effect", *American Journal of Psychiatry* 111, 662–664.
Wiegleb, Johann Christian
1792 *Geschichte des Wachstums und der Erfindungen in der Chemie.* Berlin: Nicolai. (= Annotated translation of two Latin manuscripts by Torbern Bergman: "De primordiis Chemiae", Uppsala 1779 and: "Historiae Chemiae medium seu obscurum aevum, a medio seculi VII ad medium seculi XVII", Uppsala 1782).

Wildenstein, Georges
1956 *The Paintings of J. A. D. Ingres.* London: Phaidon.
Winkler, Leo
1926 "Signaturtherapie", in: Hermann Thoms (ed.): *Handbuch der praktischen und wissenschaftlichen Pharmazie.* (Vol.IV), Berlin: Saenger, 946–957.
Winnicott, David Wark
1969 "Übergangsobjekte und Übergangsphänomene", *Psyche* 23, 666–682.
1974 *Playing and Reality.* Harmondsworth, Middx.: Penguin Books.
Wissenschaftliche Zentralstelle des Schweizerischen Apothekervereins
1984 *Index Nominum 1984 – Arzneistoffsynonymverzeichnis.* Zürich: Schweizerischer Apothekerverein.
Wittgenstein, Ludwig
1967 *Philosophical Investigations.* Oxford: Blackwell.
1961 *Tractatus Logico-Philosophicus.* London: Routledge & Kegan Paul, New York: The Humanities Press. (With a translation by D. F. Pears & B. F. McGuinness.)
1973 Tractatus logico-philosophicus. (9th edition), Frankfurt/M. Suhrkamp.
Witthauer, Kurt
1899 "Aspirin, ein neues Salicylpräparat", *Die Heilkunde* 3, 396–397.
Wood, Philip
1962 "The man who 'invented' Aspirin", *Medical News* 9. 11. 1972.
Wurster, Carl
n.d. "Justus von Liebig", in: H. Heimpel – Th. Heuss – B. Reifenberg (eds.): *Genius der Deutschen. Die großen Forscher, Erfinder, Ärzte.* Berlin: Propyläen.
Zacharias, Sylvia
1985 *Arzneimittelzulassung und Verbraucherschutz.* Frankfurt: P. Lang.
Zimmermann, H.
1974 *Arzneimittelwerbung in Deutschland von Beginn des 16. bis Ende des 18. Jahrhunderts.* Würzburg: jal.
Zimmermann, Manfred
1982 "Neurophysiologische Mechanismen von Schmerz und Schmerztherapie", in: Wolfgang Keeser – Ernst Pöppel – Petra Mitterhusen (eds.): *Schmerz.* Munich: Urban & Schwarzenberg, 46–68.

Index

FSC
www.fsc.org
MIX
Papier | Fördert gute Waldnutzung
FSC® C083411

Kolibri 360 GmbH
Ferdinand-Jühlke-Straße 7
99095 Erfurt, Deutschland
produktsicherheit@kolibri360.de